THE AMAZING HEALING BENEFITS OF CHINESE HERBAL MEDICINE ARE RIGHT AT YOUR FINGERTIPS.

Don't Miss . . .

- A common seed to restore normal hair coloring in premature graying

- The recipe for "the food of the gods," the safest and most healing food the world has ever known

- A wonderful high-protein food that can be substituted for animal products

- The best known remedy for nausea and motion sickness

- A coffee-like beverage to lower blood pressure and cholesterol

- A favorite remedy for infertility and impotence

- A detoxifying tea that helps clear the skin of acne, eczema, and other conditions

- "White Tiger" decoction for an effective treatment for flu and high fevers

- Night Sight Pills for improving vision and early stages of cataract

- The secret of an oat-based complex for both male and female libido

- "Four Noble Gentlemen" tonic to combat chronic fatigue

- And more!

Books by Michael Tierra

The Natural Remedy Bible (*with John Lust*)
The Way of Herbs
The Way of Chinese Herbs

Published by POCKET BOOKS

THE WAY OF
CHINESE
HERBS

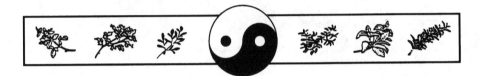

MICHAEL TIERRA
L.Ac., O.M.D.

POCKET BOOKS
New York   London   Toronto   Sydney   Tokyo   Singapore

The author of this book is not a physician and the ideas, procedures, and suggestions in this book are not intended as a substitute for the medical advice of a trained health professional. All matters regarding your health require medical supervision. Consult your physician before adopting the suggestions in this book, as well as about any condition that may require diagnosis or medical attention. In addition, the statements made by the author regarding certain products and services represent the views of the author alone, and do not constitute a recommendation or endorsement of any product or service by the publisher. The author and publisher disclaim any liability arising directly or indirectly from the use of the book, or of any products mentioned herein.

An *Original* Publication of POCKET BOOKS

POCKET BOOKS, a division of Simon & Schuster Inc.
1230 Avenue of the Americas, New York, NY 10020

Copyright © 1998 by Dr. Michael Tierra

All rights reserved, including the right to reproduce
this book or portions thereof in any form whatsoever.
For information address Pocket Books, 1230 Avenue
of the Americas, New York, NY 10020

Library of Congress Cataloging-in-Publication Data

Tierra, Michael, 1939–
    The way of Chinese herbs / Michael Tierra.
        p.   cm.
    Includes bibliographical references and index.
    ISBN: 0-671-89869-8
    1. Herbs—Therapeutic use. 2. Medicine, Chinese. I. Title.
RM666.H33.T527   1998
615'.321'0951—dc21   98-15715
                                                    CIP

First Pocket Books trade paperback printing August 1998

10   9   8   7   6   5   4   3   2   1

POCKET and colophon are registered trademarks of
Simon & Schuster Inc.

Cover design by Joseph Perez
Front cover illustration by Amy Panzer

Text design by Stanley S. Drate/Folio Graphics Co. Inc.

Printed in the U.S.A.

Dedicated to the Chinese people
in gratitude for preserving the wisdom of the ancient world
for all humanity

CONTENTS

INTRODUCTION

Just as North Americans and Europeans are accustomed to using a multitude of over-the-counter drugs as well as vitamins and other supplements for various conditions, the Chinese people know the use of a wide variety of herbs and other natural substances that are available in their local pharmacies. Because of the growing popularity of acupuncture and traditional Chinese medicine in the West and the increasing popularity of many Chinese herbs and products, this book is intended to serve as an introduction and practical guide.

Unlike most Western drugs, traditional Chinese herbs and products not only help relieve symptoms of disease but also work to alleviate the underlying causes. Supplements, such as vitamins and minerals, may overload and imbalance the body with nutrients and substances that it does not need. Chinese herbs can help the body regain strength and balance. One can purchase these in various forms, such as Chinese tonic, including *dang gui* (*Angelica sinensis*), which nourishes the blood and strengthens and regulates the female reproductive cycle; astragalus root (*Astragalus membranaceus*), which powerfully strengthens the body's immune system to prevent sickness; ginseng (*Panax ginseng*) or codonopsis (*Codonopsis pilosula*), which builds energy and vitality; and delicious Chinese lycii berries (*Lycium chinensis*), which the Chinese call "red raisins" and are high in easily assimilable betacarotene and act as a powerful blood tonic. Any of these can be simply cooked with rice or in soup according to one's personal needs or the needs of members of one's immediate family, or they may be purchased in the form of pills, syrups, or alcoholic wines.

My first impression of Chinese herbal medicine came from visits to Chinese pharmacies in San Francisco's Chinatown. Instead of seeming a part of a North American metropolis, San Francisco's Chinatown could be a transplant of similar shopping centers throughout Southeast Asia such as in Hong Kong, Shanghai, or Taiwan, where a variety of businesses are situated below close-quartered residential apartments. In an incongruous juxtaposition, Chinatown offers clothing boutiques, small mom-and-pop Chinese corner grocery stores, and shops featuring such exotic foods as sea slugs and winter melon. There are stores selling gaudy tourist souvenirs and others featuring a range of semiprecious Chinese jade jewelry or other valuable Chinese art and antiques. Among this mundane yet exotic din of market activity, there are a remarkable number of traditional Chinese pharmacies, indicative of the importance of health and well being in Chinese culture.

I vividly remember one such pharmacy located on Washington Street, which I was told later happens to be one of the oldest Chinese pharmacies in San Francisco's Chinatown. In the early 1970s, for a hippie *may gwo ren* (North American) like me, it evoked a shadowy world of mystery, a medieval time warp where abacus and hand-balanced scales prevailed. Representative of a unique cultural phenomenon, the pharmacy serves a dual function as a business and a neighborhood hangout for a group of older Chinese men, always smoking and gambling or playing cards or Chinese dominos (Mah Jong) in the back of the shop. To my naive mindset, it conjured flashbacks of suspenseful scenes from TV reruns of 1940s Charlie Chan mysteries I had seen as a child. It was an attraction to herbal medicine that guided my efforts to overcome my uneasiness and inhibitions and explore such arcane haunts that seemed to represent the widest cultural gap between East and West.

The average Western visitor is fascinated by and curious about the lively interest the Chinese have had in indigenous medicine for over 3,000 years. Typically, one may find a storefront exhibit of various grades of ginseng (*Panax ginseng*), *dang gui* (*Angelica sinensis*), *huang qi* or astragalus (*Astragalus membranaceus*), and innumerable other herbs, roots and barks. Besides these, placed on red satin displays, there are such oddities as Sitka red deer antlers, used to treat low metabolism, coldness, and sexual frigidity and impotence; antelope horns, whose shavings are used in teas and pills to reduce fevers; and strange bundles of wormlike fungi (*Cordyceps sinensis*), harvested from the high Tibetan plateaus and recently discovered by Western athletes as a cutting-edge treatment to increase stamina and endurance. Another curiosity is the hardened multiformed red or black reishi mushroom (*Ganoderma lucidum*), the type that one frequently sees at the bottom of countless antique Chinese scroll paintings. As if all this were not enough, imagine a window display of pickled snakes suspended in clear alcohol or dried gecko lizards skewered on slices of bamboo, hanging on the display backboard.

It is only in retrospect that I have come to appreciate how pharmacies and medicine are reflections of the integrated philosophy and cultural lifestyle of the Chinese people. To them, a pharmacy is not simply a dispensary for chemically based pharmaceuticals, but a symbol of a culture with its roots deep in nature and antiquity, a place where the sacred traditions and healing wisdom are common topics of conversation as they are passed down and preserved. To the Chinese people, a traditional herbal pharmacy is a lifeline affirming their connection with primal nature.

While highly skilled herb doctors write and fill compound herbal prescriptions with expert efficiency, practically all herbs and drugs are available to everyone regardless of their professional standing and expertise. A Chinese herbal pharmacy is foremost a people's pharmacy, serving the needs of the majority of Chinese people, who appreciate and understand the use of herbs for self-treatment for a wide variety of conditions as well as for ongoing health maintenance.

From approximately the 1920s through the 1950s, with the rise of medical technology, synthetic drugs, and powerful multibillion-dollar pharmaceutical companies, American herbalism became obsolete. The strong counterculture movement in the late 1960s and early 1970s, however, with its alternative lifestyle that sought a return to nature and communal interdependence, began the twentieth-century herbal renaissance. For me, as for many of my then-unknown colleagues who were similarly but independently exploring the North American continent, nature, through her plant kingdom, cast a spell of inexorable attraction. As a result, some of us found ourselves living in small wilderness communities, relearning the medicinal and food uses for a variety of wild plants.

Naive as we may have been then about the political repression of Maoist China, during the early 1970s many of us identified with mainland Chinese who lived communally in the countryside. To us, this meant growing our own food, composting, building simple structures out of recycled material, home birthing, and rediscovering herbal and other natural forms of healing.

At the same time, around 1971, when it was announced that *New York Times* journalist James Reston, who was on assignment in China, was successfully treated with acupuncture for pain after an appendectomy, front-page stories carried his story: "I've seen the past, and it works!" The Western world began to learn about acupuncture. Some of our group, who were living in a community in the Klamath National Forest in the Northern California mountains, found their way to study in England to learn acupuncture. We did not fully appreciate then that acupuncture is in fact regarded as only a relatively minor part of a powerful ancient healing system. As a result, the thousands of acupuncturists who practice traditional Chinese medicine through the United States and Europe, integrating therapeutic diet and herbal medicine, are primarily known even today only as acupuncturists rather than traditional Chinese medical doctors, which is how their Chinese counterparts are known.

I vividly remember that after exhausting the few books on Western herbal medicine, such as *Back to Eden* by Jethro Kloss and *The Herbalist* by Joseph Meyer, I felt a desperate thirst for more practical knowledge from someone who was actually practicing herbal medicine. Shortly thereafter, I initiated a part-time apprenticeship with John Christopher, N.D, M.H., who was then the "lone herbal voice in the wilderness." I also studied with Norma Meyers, an herbalist living in Vancouver, British Columbia, who was very knowledgeable about Native American herbalism. Despite all I learned from these beloved mentors, I felt I had gone as far as the existing knowledge of Western herbal medicine could take me. I gradually found myself gravitating toward traditional Chinese medicine, which included both acupuncture and Chinese herbalism. This was facilitated by a mutual exchange of newly acquired knowledge and teachings with my fellow commune members, Efrem and Harriet Korngold. Since then, I have been a clinical practitioner and devoted lifetime student of traditional Chinese medicine.

Many of my Western herbalist colleagues, knowing that I had learned a great deal about Western herbs and Native American plants in my early studies, have asked me why I have focused so much of my attention on an ethnic healing system that is so culturally distant from my own and relies on plants and other materials from animals and minerals from distant shores.

The answer is that unlike traditions of herbal medicine in the West that have historically been fractured several times over the last 2,000 years, traditional Chinese herbal medicine represents a vast body of knowledge of practical health and healing that extends back at least 3,000 years. I believe, like Chinese people and others around the world, that traditional Chinese medicine, especially acupuncture and Chinese herbalism, is a treasured gift from the ancient world that comes to us at a time when such practical wisdom is so desperately needed. Beyond obvious cultural differences, traditional Chinese herbal medicine is not so unlike the ancient traditional medicine of the West represented by the Greco-Roman teachings of Hippocrites and Galen. We chuckle at the famous "eye of newt" scene in *Macbeth*, while realizing that Shakespeare's son-in-law, John Hall, was a famous doctor of the time whose materia medica, a mere 400 years ago, regularly included a wide assortment of medicinal plants, minerals, and what seems to us today to include some bizarre insect and animal parts. All of this is remarkably like traditional Chinese herbal medicine. While we offhandedly dismiss such sixteenth-century prescriptions as "superstitious" and "worthless" without ever considering the possibility of their efficacy, the Chinese maintain respect for traditional medicine. In recent years, they have subjected its theories, along with the various plants, minerals, and animal parts used in traditional Chinese medicine, to scientific scrutiny and research. As a result, the world is coming to acknowledge that there is a genuine pharmacological scientific basis to the efficacy long claimed for most of these traditional herbs, as well as for the other substances traditionally used. Further, these approaches and treatments, in most cases, offer a safer and more inexpensive alternative to what is currently the trend in contemporary medicine.

Even today, a number of pharmaceutical drugs are still derived from mineral and animal sources. These include vaccines derived from the blood and urine of various domestic and wild animals, such as horses and monkeys; drugs manufactured from insects, such as cantharides from the Spanish fly; and drugs made from venomous snakes and frogs. It is a purely cultural preference that causes many people to reject as "superstitious" and "disgusting" the use of insect- and animal-derived drugs from traditional cultures while accepting chemotherapy, the injection of cellular poisons, as a valid treatment for cancer.

Ultimately, traditional Chinese medicine is a gift from which all countries throughout the world can benefit. As its use spreads throughout the world, its practitioners will continue to classify and incorporate non-Chinese medicinal plants and substances as part of its treatment protocol. This is what I call planetary herbology, described in my book of the same title (Lotus Light Press, 1992). One of the most famous non-Chinese herbs, used for over 300 years by the Chinese, is American ginseng (*Panax quinquefolium*). Others, such as epimedium (*yin yang huo*), ophiopogon (*mai men dong*), Japanese privet (*Ligustrum japonicum*), and asparagus root (*tian men dong*), are found as ornamental cultivars in Western nurseries. Still others include many of the wild plants and escaped weeds that abound in various countries, such as Solomon's seal (*Polygonatum* species), wild peony root (*Paeonia* species), burdock (*Arctium lappa*), and dandelion (*Taraxacum officinalis*). We are also discovering similar or closely related species of Chinese medicinal herbs that grow both in North and South America, such as reishi mushroom (*Ganoderma lucidum*) and uncaria (gambir, or *gou teng*, as it is called in Chinese medicine), which seems to be related to the famous cat's-claw of the South American rain forest. The difference is that the Chinese use only the "claws" or grasping thorns for their antispasmodic properties, while the entire vine of the South American species is used as a potent antiviral and antibacterial. The list of traditional herbs used in Chinese herbalism continues to expand as we experiment with growing certain Chinese herbs in the West, such as the valuable immune tonics: astragalus root (*huang qi*), schizandra (*wu wei zi*), and Chinese dioscorea (*shan yao*).

Beyond the medicinal plants used in traditional Chinese herbalism, it is the profound holistic theory and philosophy that is of even greater value. Traditional Chinese medicine is, like most ancient medical systems, truly holistic because it understands and addresses all aspects of the mind–body connection, something that contemporary Western medicine has only recently come to recognize. It also sees a close relationship between health and all external factors such as climate, season, diet, work, lifestyle, and relationships. The depth of its holism extends to a profound nonmechanical understanding of complex mind–body physiological processes that simultaneously involve, to varying degrees, all systems of the body, including the digestive, excretory, urinary, circulatory, respiratory, neurological, and endocrinological functions. It further integrates its theoretical understanding with the classification of disease imbalances and the classification of medicinal herbs and formulas on the same related continuum. For instance, if one describes a cold disease in traditional Chinese medicine, there are specific foods, herbs, and herbal formulas, whose energetic classification is warm, that can be used to treat the condition. Conversely, hot (or inflammatory) diseases are treated with cool or cold medicinal herbs and substances that probably have antibiotic and/or antiviral properties.

Besides the concept of supplementing or freeing the circulation of qi and blood, this latter approach of integrating diagnosis and treatment is the unique and most valuable contribution of traditional Chinese medicine. One of the problems of Western medicine is that it tends to name specific diseases based on the presumed offending pathogen. Unfortunately, without an overriding theory of medicine, there is little connection between the named disease and its treatment. As a result, Western scientific medicine is too often limited in the effective treatment of many "unbalanced" conditions, which include a varying complex of symptoms and are then managed only symptomatically, rather than assisting the body to reinstate balance or homeostasis through diet, herbs, and lifestyle.

Currently, the issue of how much we should attempt to redefine the great theories and tenets of traditional Chinese medicine in light of contemporary understanding of anatomy, physiology, pathology, and biochemistry is controversial among practitioners of traditional Chinese medicine. Truth is truth, regardless of the language or jargon in which it is expressed. It does neither the traditional Chinese medical viewpoint nor the ancient world that brought it to life any homage to avoid actively seeking to understand its profound tenets in terms of modern science. Even rudimentary attempts to do so have led many to a deeper appreciation of the profound understanding of the processes of health and healing that the ancient Chinese possessed. This is probably true of many other traditional cultures as well, including the East Indian Ayurvedic medicine tradition and even our own traditional Western medical tradition, epitomized in the teachings of Hippocrites, Dioscorides, Avicenna, and Galen. This book is therefore offered as a practical overview of the essential theoretical principles of traditional Chinese medicine. Beyond this, it should serve as a useful guide to the appropriate treatment and use of Chinese herbs and formulas for many common diseases and conditions and as a reference for the increasing numbers of Westerners who are undergoing treatment by traditional Chinese medicine doctors and practitioners.

THE WAY OF
CHINESE
HERBS

· ONE ·

A PHILOSOPHY
OF BEING

YIN AND YANG:
QI, BLOOD, AND ESSENCE

Legend describes how Emperor Shen Nung (3494 B.C.), the "divine farmer" revered as the founder of agriculture, out of his compassion for the sick set forth to discover the healing properties of plants. It is said that each day he would taste various plants to determine their medicinal properties, poisoning himself 100 times, each time necessitating his finding the corresponding antidote. The trial-and-error method exemplified by Shen Nung may be viewed as a synthesis of the discovery of healing plants by people throughout the world. Whether his story is mythology or fact, we can appreciate that over 3,000 to 5,000 years, a unique system of holistic healing evolved that today is highly respected not only by the Chinese but by many peoples of most countries of Asia, Africa, and more recently, of the West.

One major difference between the traditional medicine of China and other countries is that the Chinese were able to pass their knowledge down in relative continuity over millennia. This is represented by the fact that the attributed discoveries of Emperor Shen Nung were originally recorded in the first Chinese herbal handbook, lost for some time, called the *Shen Nung Pen T'sao*, or *Shen Nung's Herbal*. Since that time, all Chinese herbal handbooks have been respectfully called *pen t'sao* in honor of Shen Nung.

Historically, the greatest strides in medicine have tended to occur during periods of strife and war. The codification of the knowledge and wisdom of traditional Chinese medicine (TCM) evolved from the socialist and naturalist philosophies of Confucianism and Taoism as a tempering reaction to a prolonged period of feudal strife called the Warring States (481–221 B.C.).

There are several philosophies that are central to the practice of TCM. The philosophy of yin–yang dates back to somewhere between 1000 and 700 B.C. and represents opposite but complementary forces that exist throughout the universe. The Five Elements of wood, fire, earth, metal, and water embrace all aspects of being and transformation in nature, as embodied by the cycles of day into night and the passing of seasons. To this day, regardless of the centuries of overlays of various religious, social, and political influences—including Communist and socialist philosophies in recent times, Confucian and Taoist philosophies imbue the Chinese outlook with a relativistic attitude based on the ancient perspectives of yin–yang and Five Elements that are at the heart of TCM. Since both of these philosophical systems had a profound effect on the theoretical evolution of Chinese medicine, it is worth understanding the basic tenets of each. Confucianism, based on the teachings of Confucius (551–479 B.C.), holds that a well-ordered society is the result of everyone's assuming and properly executing their respective social duties and obligations. This belief extended through all strata of society, from the emperor down to the lowliest subject. Similarly, the TCM understanding of physiology assigns a complex pattern of interdependencies between the 12 primary organ systems of the body, based on the Five Element theory, to achieve order or health. The Five Elements offer a better depiction of an orderly functional relationship between the various aspects of each of the five elements in nature. When in harmony with each other, they reflect health; when in disharmony, they are the cause of disease. Taoism, represented by the teachings of Lao-tzu and the *Tao-te Ching,* is more interested in our spontaneous relationship with inner and outer nature, while Confucian philosophy focused more on the orderly relationship with natural cycles and society. The yin–yang theory is better able to include spontaneous irregularities of experiences and so it is more reflective of early Taoist thought. TCM looks for the balance in the separate natures, and that balance reflects health.

Qi: The Supreme Energy

Chinese medicine is founded on the principle of *qi* as the absolute energy of all phenomena. The characteristics of *qi* are ephemerality, activity, constant change, and warmth. It forms the basis for all organic life, meaning people, animals, and plants, as well as for all inorganic substances, such as minerals. In life, *qi* is expressed both specifically and generally. Generally, one who is youthful and energetic exudes abundant *qi*, but *qi* wanes with age, exposing one to accompanying infirmities, weaknesses, and degenerative symptoms. It is in this area of health maintenance and longevity that Chinese herbalism, with its highly evolved concept of tonics, can prove a very positive asset. Specifically, *qi* is expressed in the strength of the individual organs, including respiration, nerve force, reproductive power, and digestion. The *qi* of plants is perceived in their growth, odor, flavor, texture, and color. Minerals have a slower *qi* that undergoes transformation and change almost imperceptibly over great periods of time.

From the Chinese perspective, the fundamental principle of health and healing is dependent on *qi* flow and removing its blockage. This is accomplished with all of the Chinese healing modalities, including the science of herbalism and dietetics (which use the various textures and flavors to stimulate organic processes), acupuncture, Chinese massage (*tui'na*) and exercise, such as *qi gong* and *tai chi*. In contrast, Western herbalism and dietetics are primarily based on micronutrients and biochemical constituents. Chinese herbalism and dietetics more obviously use both energetic responses, classifying herbs and foods "organoleptically," according to their flavors, energies, textures, and colors. Today, these are considered along with the various quantifiable components, such as protein, carbohydrate, fats, vitamins, and minerals, according to individual indications. The immune system is also seen as a form of *qi* that it can be negatively influenced by pollution, bad diet, physical and emotional stress, and other factors. This eventually becomes the underlying cause for disease.

Yin and Yang

Under heaven all can see beauty as beauty only because there is ugliness,
All can know good as good only because there is evil.

Therefore having and not having arise together.
Difficult and easy complement each other.

Long and short contrast each other;
High and low rest upon each other;
Voice and sound harmonize each other;
Front and back follow one another.

Therefore the sage goes about doing nothing, teaching no-talking.
The ten thousand things rise and fall without cease,
Creating, yet not possessing,
Working, yet not taking credit.
Work is done, then forgotten.
*Therefore it lasts forever.**

First mentioned in the *I Ching*, or *Book of Changes*, attributed to Lao-tzu (around 1250 B.C.), yin and yang represent the bipolar manifestation of all phenomena. Whatever has a front has a back; if there is above, there is below; heat and cold are relative to each other; great strength is accompanied by great weakness and vice versa; night is followed by day; where there is male, there is also female. Through all of creation, *qi* appears to subdivide and manifest in the duality called yin and yang. Yin–yang is aptly represented in the ancient symbol as two parts of a whole, a dance, as it were, depicting at once both complement and opposition. Literally, *yin* means the "shady side of the mountain" and *yang* means the "sunny side of the mountain." These terms are also used to describe the opposite and complementary energies of male and female, hot and cold, day and night, summer and winter, and so forth. This also becomes the foundation of TCM, including dietetics, herbalism, acupuncture, and all other physiotherapies.

Yang is hot, moving, energetic, external, dry, masculine, aggressive, bold, light, day, sky or heaven. Yin is cold, slow, without energy, internal, moist, feminine, receptive, timid, dark, night, and earth. While yang rises upward, yin descends; yang expresses itself externally, while yin is internal. Yang is hot and inflammatory; yin is cold; yang is dry, yin is moist; yang is acute, yin is chronic. Health is represented as a balance of yin and yang.

Qualities of Yin and Yang

The qualities of yin and yang are summarized in the following table and then explained in more detail in the text following it.

---

*From *Tao-Te Ching*, by Lao-tzu, translated by Gia-Fu Feng and Jane English, Vintage Books (New York), 1972, with permission.

QUALITIES OF YIN AND YANG

ASPECT	YANG	YIN
	Heaven	Earth
	Sun	Moon
	Immaterial	Material
	Generation	Growth
	Energy	Form
	Creation	Materialization
	Activity	Rest
TENDENCIES	Develop, expand	Condense, contract
POSITION	Outward	Inward
STRUCTURE	Time	Space
DIRECTION	Ascending—left	Descending—right
COLOR	Bright	Dark
TEMPERATURE	Hot	Cold
WEIGHT	Light	Heavy
CATALYST	Fire	Water
LIGHT	Light	Dark
CONSTRUCTION	Exterior	Interior
WORK	Psychological	Physiological
ATTITUDE	Extrovert	Introvert
BIOLOGY	Animal	Vegetable
ENERGY	Aggressive	Receptive
NERVOUS SYSTEM	Sympathetic	Parasympathetic
TASTES	Spicy/sweet	Sour/bitter/salty
SEASON	Summer	Winter
PHYSIOLOGICAL ORGANS	Small intestine, triple warmer (an organ function; that is, the relation of all parts of the body with each other), large intestine, bladder, gallbladder	Heart, pericardium, spleen–pancreas, lungs, kidneys–adrenal glands, liver

Tendencies: The power of yin is grounding, while Yang develops outwardly. The positive manifestation of yin is patience, tolerance, sensitivity, and receptivity, while its negative manifestation is dullness and lack of motivation and will. The positive manifestation of yang is action, drive, and motivation, while its negative manifestation is aggressiveness, rigidity, and insensitivity. In humans, yin manifests as greater sensitivity, compassion, and stillness, while yang is active, outgoing, and may lack compassion and sensitivity. Excess yang activity can lead to "yin deficiency," which we recognize in the West as burnout. An excess of yin can lower one's immunity and make one more vulnerable to disease. It also makes one overly sensitive to emotional stresses and pain.

Structure: Space is emptiness or hollowness out of which the motivating force of yang occurs. Whereas space is unlimited, time is limited; therefore, what occurs in time belongs to yang, while that which ceases to occur and returns to space is yin.

Color and light: Yin is expressed in the darker colors, such as black or dark blue. Herbs that are black, such as the Chinese herb *Rehmannia glutinosa,* are used to tonify yin energy in the body. Yang is expressed as lighter and brighter colors. Herbs that are bright red, such as cayenne pepper, are yang because they have a warm circulating energy. Physiologically, individuals—irrespective of race—who exhibit a dark pallor and a sullen, introspective attitude have a stagnant yin condition, while yang manifests as bright or red complexion and more aggressive, outgoing disposition.

Temperature: Coldness, in terms of seasons, body temperature and metabolism, and even emotional disposition, expresses a yin state, while heat, in terms of the warmer seasons, body temperature and metabolism, and emotional disposition, expresses yang.

Weight: Heaviness is yin because it is slower and more inert, while lightness is yang because it has a greater potential for agility and speed. Generally speaking, those body types in both animals and plants that are heavier and more expanded are more yin. Lighter bodies and lifeforms of more compact shape and form have the potential for increased functional activity, which makes them more yang.

Work: Individuals who are more philosophically and psychologically oriented are more yin than those who are more physical. Of course, in this area, balance is the ideal. Nevertheless, an individual who is more mental, receptive, and introspective in nature expresses yin more than one who is more physical, aggressive, and extroverted.

Biology: The vegetable kingdom, having little or no potential for expressing movement and warmth, is yin in relationship to the animal kingdom. This is why vegetable food as a whole, irrespective of the relative yin–yang relationships between specific items, represents a more yin diet than does one that includes more animal food.

Nervous system: The essential yin physiological energy is expressed through the complex functions of the parasympathetic nervous system. These involve bodily repair and maintenance, reproductive capacity, digestion, cooling, and anti-inflammatory aspects, such as the secretion of cortical hormones and other complex physiological mechanisms that tend to control heat and inflammation. Yang physiological energy is embodied in the sympathetic nervous system that allows us to react to danger and stress, manifest ambition and motivation, and act on our impulses.

Flavors: A flavor can be misleading if one does not understand the underlying types of biochemical components and physiological activity they generate. Generally, the sour taste naturally found in some foods indicates the presence of the anti-inflammatory vitamin C. Sour can also be an acid that, ingested in excess, can cause heat and irritation. In small amounts, it will stimulate a cooling alkaline reaction in the body. Similarly, salty and bitter generally indicate an innate alkaline biochemistry that, taken in excess, especially in the case of salt, can cause acidity and heat. In general, the reason these flavors are broadly classified as yin is because sour is astringent, condensing, and cooling; salty causes us to retain fluids; and bitter-tasting herbs are cooling and generally possess anti-inflammatory, antibiotic, and antiviral properties.

From this, we see that it is not so easy to simply say that acid, for instance, is heating and alkaline is cooling. This is because the relative degree of acidity or alkalinity of a food or herb determines the type of reaction the body will have. Spicy flavors tend to be mildly irritating and dispersing; therefore, they activate an internal sympathetic response that in some individuals causes sweating and flushing of the face. Sweet flavors include not only sugar and honey but also the majority of nutritious high-carbohydrate and proteinaceous foods, such as dairy, meat, whole grains, and beans. When these are digested and me-tabolized, they produce heat and vital energy, which is what makes them yang.

In traditional Chinese herbalism, great emphasis is placed on the classification of herbs and foods first according to their energies—expressed as heating, neutral, or cooling—and second, but of no lesser importance, on their flavors.

Organs: Yin conditions are reflected as more chronic and internal diseases. Usually these involve organic disorders with the solid yin organs of transformation: liver, heart, spleen–pancreas, lungs, and kidneys–endocrine system. Yang conditions are more functional imbalances and manifest as external, acute diseases, such as skin diseases, muscular aches and pains, and colds and flus. These tend to involve functional problems that involve the hollow yang organs of transportation: gallbladder, small intestine, stomach, large intestine, and bladder.

Theorems of Yin and Yang

Yin and yang are two dynamically interdependent parts of a whole, expressed by the following theorems:

- Infinity divides itself into yin and yang.
- Yin and yang result from the infinite movement of the universe.
- Although they are opposite ends of a continuum, yin and yang are complementary and form a unity.
- Yang contains the seed of yin and yin contains the seed of yang.
- Yin is centripetal and yang is centrifugal; together, they produce all energy and phenomena.
- Yin attracts yang and yang attracts yin.
- Yin repels yin and yang repels yang.
- The force of attraction and repulsion between any two phenomena is proportional to the difference between their yin–yang constitution.
- All things are ephemeral and constantly changing their yin–yang constitution.
- Nothing is neutral; either yin or yang is dominant.
- Nothing is solely yin or yang; everything involves polarity.
- Yin and yang are relative: large yin attracts small yin and large yang attracts small yang.

- At the extreme of manifestation, yin produces yang and yang produces yin.
- All physical forms are yin at the center and yang on the surface.

Infinity divides itself into Yin and Yang: Everything exists in polarity. This is the essential way that energy manifests itself to our normal perception. Integration and health always represents a balance of positive and negative aspects of being. Disease, disintegration, and death are therefore an expression of the imbalance and separation of yin and yang.

Yin and Yang result from the infinite movement of the universe: The basis of all transformation and change is the cyclical evolution of yin and yang. This is most obviously expressed in the cycles of night and day and the seasons but also in our own body–mind process, in which we are continually transforming yin-earth into heavenly yang and vice versa. Chinese physiology describes the yang of heaven as descending through the top of the head to a point below the navel (called Conception Vessel 6, "the sea of *qi*") where it combines and mixes with the yin energy of earth. It is here that they mutually transform each other.

Although they are opposite ends of a continuum, yin and yang are complementary and form a unity: Yin and yang are two parts of a dynamic whole. Throughout all of nature, we see that balance is achieved through a process of checks and balances. Nature needs the cold wet of winter to produce the harvest of summer. Male requires female for most species to survive. Practically speaking, every organ in the body has a yin and a yang function. Those that are classified as yin are only predominantly so, as are those that are classified as yang. For instance, this is most embodied in the adrenals, which are part of Chinese kidney *qi*. These small pealike glands attached to the kidneys are distinguished by their outer cortex that produces primarily yin, or cortical hormones that regulate the parasympathetic nervous system, which is involved with maintenance and repair. The inner medulla of the adrenals secretes adrenergenic hormones that are more stimulatory (yang) and regulate the sympathetic nervous system, which is involved with the "flight or fight" response. The sympathetic nervous system is what the Chinese call kidney yang, while the parasympathetic nervous system is kidney yin.

Yang contains the seed of yin and yin contains the seed of yang: Within yin, there is yang, and within yang, there is yin. Most seeds have a strong outer coating to preserve their precious nucleus for sprouting and growth. The yangness of the outer coat of some seeds is so protective and strong that certain seeds found in the burial chambers of ancient Egyptians have been able to sprout after thousands of years. Yet when this strong outer yang seed coat is subjected to yin moisture, its inner yin contents begin to germinate and display such strength as to literally break open the outer yang seed coat. Thus, what was once yin becomes yang, as expressed by its growth, and what was once yang becomes yin by being broken open.

Yin is centripetal and yang is centrifugal; together, they produce all energy and phenomena: Yin arises from the earth. It mixes with and is transformed by yang, which descends from above. This is the expression of the direction of yin and yang: yin is below and yang is above.

Yin attracts yang and yang attracts yin: The very nature of yin and yang is one of relationship and change; therefore, this energy of transformation and change is the basis of magnetic attraction between all things. Yin female and yang male are mutually attractive based on individual biochemical hormonal reactions, which in turn leads to procreation.

Yin repels yin and yang repels yang: By definition, yin and yang can be attracted only to what is opposite and repelled only by what is similar. For example, the two magnetic north and south poles attract each other, while north repels north and south repels south.

The force of attraction and repulsion between any two phenomena is proportional to the difference between their yin-yang constitution: Yin and yang represent a continual process of transformation. The degree to which two things are yin-negative or yang-positive determines the energy or force of attraction between them.

All things are ephemeral and constantly changing their yin–yang constitution: We should not be deceived into believing that anything stays the same forever. The principle of change implied in the concept of yin and yang is the basis of all that can be known about any future outcome. In healing, we need to understand disease as a dynamic expression of the body attempting to compensate for and/or correct a physiological imbalance. Eventually, any extreme yin or yang condition will change to its opposite.

Nothing is neutral; either yin or yang is dominant: Because all phenomena have a yin-negative or yang-positive relationship to each other, everything must therefore have an effect and purpose. Physiologically, anything we do or eat has, to some degree, a positive or negative effect.

Nothing is solely yin or yang: Just as the Chinese character describes yin–yang as the shady and sunny side of a hill respectively, the two are always present in all phenomena. In life, as in recovery from illness, knowing that the opposite is true forms the basis of faith.

Yin and yang are relative: large yin attracts small yin and large yang attracts small yang: To the degree that a thing can be either more yin or yang, it is possible to transform it into its opposite yin–yang polarity. This principle is occasionally employed in Chinese herbalism by using a yin tonic herb to produce a yang reaction and a yang tonic herb to produce a yin reaction. For instance, cayenne pepper is yang and in excess can make one weak through excessive perspiration and stimulation of the nervous system. Cold water is the essence of yin, yet in small amounts, as in a brief cold plunge after a hot sweat bath, can stimulate greater yang warmth.

At the extreme of manifestation, yin produces yang and yang produces yin: An extreme of any strong yin or yang energy will stimulate its opposite. Often, through stress and poor nutrition, an individual can become critically run down and weakened and yet manifest apparent high (though ungrounded) energy. We would say that such an individual is running on empty, or nervous energy. Nervous energy is excess yang arising out of deficiency of yin. This condition is called "yin deficiency" and is a pivotal concept in understanding traditional Chinese medical theory. In all wasting diseases, with symptoms of autoconsumption and heat, yin deficiency is a manifestation of extreme yin weakness and deficiency producing symptoms of yang heat and inflammation. Conversely, individuals who manifest extreme yang congestion and heaviness from overindulgence in heavy, rich foods, can experience yin exhaustion and fatigue.

All physical forms are yin at the center and yang on the surface: Since nothing is purely yin or yang, as one manifests the quality of yin or yang on the surface, its opposite is contained at one's center. This has many therapeutic implications. Children appear weaker and more yin on the surface but have a tendency to have more internal heat. As a result, they generally have a faster pulse rate and their diseases are usually caused by heat rather than coldness. With maturity and age, we achieve our maximum strength and size (a yang phenomenon), but our internal metabolic process slows and becomes colder and more yin.

Laws Governing Yin and Yang

Yin and yang are governed by several laws:

- All things are the differentiated apparatus of one infinity.
- Everything changes.
- All antagonisms are complementary.
- No two things are identical.
- All things have their opposite.
- Extremes always produce their opposite.
- Whatever begins has an end.

All things are the differentiated apparatus of one infinity: Everything emanates from one essential source. That source is invisible and nonapparent and can be perceived only through its expression in duality.

Everything changes: Since yin and yang represent a complement or opposing expression of a given phenomenon, everything is subject to the law of infinite change. Because there is a positive-yang and a negative-yin aspect to everything, wisdom upholds the view that behind all adversity and suffering, there is the possibility of great joy and fulfillment. An overindulgence in pleasure in any form contains the lurking threat of pain and suffering. We see this in everything from our overindulgence in food and sexual promiscuity, which too often leads to disease and sickness, to emotional and physical struggles, which ultimately lead to some positive changes or realization that could not be foreseen.

All antagonisms are complementary: Too often, conflicts we have with others, especially those to whom we are closest, reflect the deep inner frustrations and conflicts within ourselves. It is therefore misplaced anger at and frustration with ourselves that in turn causes us to lash out uncontrollably against another. It is strange to consider the possibility that for reasons that ultimately foster greater personal growth and change in ourselves, we attract and often are attracted to seemingly negative experiences and individuals. From this perspective, we are often compelled to acknowledge that a particular affliction or disease we may have can actually be the source of deeper psychological and spiritual growth.

No two things are identical: Anything that is perceived is seen through the eyes of yin–yang duality. One is never two. Again, this reminds us to appreciate whatever differences that we perceive, at the same time remaining cautious of any possible negative consequences.

All things have their opposite: Yin–yang reminds us that there are always two sides to everything. We should thus be cautious of any excesses and indulgences in food, drink, sex, anger, sadness, fear, joy, and so on, knowing that behind each of these, whether positive or negative, is its opposite.

Extremes always produce their opposite: Yin and yang are not static. One is always in a constant state of transforming into the other. An excess of any experience, whether positive or negative, including food, herbs, and physical therapies, can produce a paradoxical opposite reaction. Vitamin C, for instance, is essentially anti-inflammatory and cooling, but used in excess, it can cause heat and inflammatory reactions. Coffee helps some to sleep. Ritalin, a form of speed, is occasionally given to hyperactive children to help them become more focused and settled. These are just a few examples of how an extreme can indeed produce an opposite reaction.

Whatever begins has an end: Many see the idea of an end as an occasion for sadness and regret. For the wise, however, this law is the essential definition of grace. No matter how wonderful we may see life as being, because it exists in duality, we must always struggle and suffer on some level. How can anyone be completely happy knowing that somewhere, someone is suffering? It is this law that embodies the promise of relief and peace. This law is particularly relevant to individuals who are experiencing physical and emotional pain and in need of hope and reassurance.

The Four Primary Aspects of Yin and Yang

There are four primary aspects of yin and yang.

Yin and yang represent opposing aspects of energy: Everything in the natural world is in yin–yang relationship to all other things. This relationship is in a state of constant change and transformation, however. In healing, one uses yin cooling energy, for instance, to counteract a yang inflammatory imbalance. If there is an excess of coldness, one would use yang herbs and foods to assist in restoring balance.

Yin and yang are interdependent: While yin and yang are in opposition or complementary relationship with each other, they are nevertheless always interdependent. Day contrasts with night, heat with cold, activity with rest, expansion with contraction. One cannot exist without the other.

Yin and yang mutually consume each other: Yin and yang are in a constant state of adjustment to each other. If one is greater, the other is always attempting to compensate and readjust. It is this propensity for the body to energetically adjust itself that makes it possible to use mild experiences, foods, and herbs to restore balance. When yin is in excess, it tends to consume yang. When yang is in excess, it consumes yin. When yin is deficient, it can cause deficiency of yang. When yang is deficient, it can cause deficiency of yin. At the same time, a deficiency of yin will manifest as an apparent excess of yang, and the apparent yang excess is therefore termed "empty heat" or "deficiency heat." If yang is deficient, it will manifest as an apparent excess of yin. This is also only apparent, and the condition is called "empty cold" or "deficiency cold."

Ying and yang mutually transform into each other: Yin and yang represent the very essence of change, so that one is always in the process of transforming into the other. This is what creates movement and life. In health, the transformation of yin and yang is orderly and cyclic. In disease, it is blocked or irregular. If food does not transform in the stomach, it putrefies and causes gas and possibly inflammation. Herbs that have carminative properties and are high in digestive enzymes help regulate the transformation of food. If desires and ambitions are not transformed, they can lead to despair and depression. This in turn will cause emotionally charged hormones and neurotransmitter secretions to produce symptoms of chronic depression and negativity. Whenever the vital energy of the body is not flowing smoothly, it is classified as irregular liver *Qi*. Herbs that regulate liver *qi*, such as cyperus (*xiang fu*), vitex, and bupleurum (*Chai hu*) can be used to relieve stagnant liver *Qi* and depression.

Therapeutic Applications of Yin and Yang

The basis of traditional Chinese herbalism is either to reduce, tonify, or regulate yin or yang. All diseases represent an imbalance of either or both of these qualities. Herbs and other therapeutic substances used for treatment of yin–yang imbalances must embody to a greater or lesser extent the energy of both. In general, herbs that are heating, tending to stimulate and raise metabolism, are yang, while those that are cooling, tending to sedate or lower metabolism, are yin. Medicinal plants and foods are classified by their heating or cooling energy according to their flavors and bodily effects. Because in nature yin and yang embody aspects of each other, every plant or food has both a yin or yang aspect. The exceptions, in many cases, are seeds that represent a balance of yin and yang energy. It is the most predominant quality that determines the classification of medicinal herbs and therapeutic foods. Generally speaking, herbs that have spicy or sweet flavors and somehow stimulate or raise body metabolism have a warm energy. Cinnamon, cayenne pepper, and ginger would be classified as yang, for instance. The exceptions are plants like mint that have a spicy flavor and a cool energy and tend to be surface relaxants.

Sugar has a strong yang effect, but extremes of either yin or yang tend to produce their opposite, and the secondary reaction to sugar is yin. Sweet substances are warming, providing metabolic fuel for the production yang Qi. In excess, however, sweet taste overloads the body's Fire mechanisms and causes an excess of yin. Many fruits that have more of an empty-sweet energy (lacking in protein) are cooling and therefore have a yin energy. Herbs and foods that are cool eliminate excess yang. Again, we can speak only in generalities because nature represents a complex embodiment and interaction of yin and yang qualities. From this perspective, substances with a cool yin energy generally have bitter, salty, or sour flavors. They tend to lower metabolism, relieve inflammation, and calm the mind.

In the kingdom of herbs, plants with a bitter flavor are cooling, antipathogenic, reducing, and eliminative. These include strongly bitter substances such as rhubarb, cascara, and goldenseal, for instance, that are very cooling and detoxifying. A substance's effect on the body, besides the intrinsic energy of the therapeutic substance, ultimately depends, however, on the amount used and the condition of the individual to whom it is administered. In Chinese medicine, gentian, a strong bitter anti-inflammatory herb, is used in small amounts before meals as a digestive tonic. Small doses of gentian will stimulate the secretion of hydrochloric acid, a yang secretion of the stomach that is necessary for the breakdown of food. It is the presence of hydrochloric acid in the stomach that produces the sensation of hunger.

Salty herbs are mostly seaweeds that can be used both as an herb and a part of one's diet. In contrast, sodium chloride is a concentrated essence of salt, and following the principle that an excess of anything will produce its opposite, salt sprinkled on food brings out its yang flavor and ultimately produces a strong yang physiological reaction. Again, going beyond this level, long-term excessive salt intake causes fluid retention, which is a yin physiological reaction.

A sour flavor is found in many fruits that are high in vitamin C, such as citrus fruits. These are extremely cool and damp and therefore extremely yin. Following the principle that what is strongly yin on the inside is strongly Yang on the outside, we can observe that the peel of many citrus fruits contains a lot of yang-warming volatile oils useful for drying mucus and stimulating digestion. Fermented foods also have a sour flavor. Because they embody a denser nutritional package of virtually predigested proteins, carbohydrates, and other nutrients, fermented foods can generate a deeper yang effect through improved digestion, assimilation, and elimination. Fermented foods include vegetables, such as sauerkraut, and dairy products, such as yogurt and acidophillus, for instance.

Therapeutically, the principle of balancing yin and yang is to use heating herbs and foods to eliminate cold pathological symptoms (asthenic), such as general hypofunctioning of various organs and metabolic processes, and to use cooling herbs and foods to counteract hyperfunctioning and inflammation or hot pathological symptoms (sthenic). The appropriate level of yin and yang for any individual varies, so that there can be either an excess or deficiency of either quality. This commonly results in diseases that have a combined imbalance of both yin and yang. This is the reason that for serious diseases, herbalists tend to use a balance of yin and yang herbs according to the particular organ or areas of the body that are affected. Herbs and foods are then also classified according to their affinity for the specific organ meridians they affect. We will discuss the individual organs in more detail later, but for now it is enough to understand that by combining substances that affect specific organ territories of the body, such as heat in the liver treated with dandelion root or cold in the lung treated with ginger, an herbalist is able to combine both heating and cooling herbs together in complex formulation. When used in combination, herbs of both a heating and cooling energy can be combined to regulate the transformation of yin and yang.

Qi, Blood, and Essence: The Three Humors

Yin–yang is further subdivided into *qi*, Blood, and Essence. The essential aspects of yang are ephemerality, *qi*, warmth, and movement, and the essential aspects of yin are substantiality, fluidity (including blood), coolness, and inertia. *Qi* represents a part of yang, while blood represents a part of yin. Men are predisposed to *qi* problems, while women tend to have problems with blood. Since *qi* is considered "the commander of blood and blood is the mother of *qi*," there is a reciprocal relationship between the two that is similar to that of yin and yang. If there is a deficiency of *qi*, a *qi* tonic, such as ginseng, is indicated. For a deficiency of blood, on the other hand, a blood tonic, such as *dang gui* (*Angelica sinensis*) is used. The physiological qualities of yang and yin are as follows:

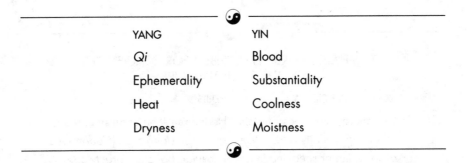

YANG	YIN
Qi	Blood
Ephemerality	Substantiality
Heat	Coolness
Dryness	Moistness

From the above table, we understand that it is possible to have *qi* deficiency with coolness, for instance, or blood deficiency with heat. The symptoms of *qi* deficiency imply lack of energy and weakness, while the symptoms of yang deficiency are coldness, frigidity, and impotence. Symptoms of blood deficiency are pale complexion and scanty menstruation in women, while symptoms of yin deficiency are emaciation and lack of fluid, dryness, and heat caused by deficiency. For this reason, such herbs as ginseng, astragalus, and codonopsis are used to tonify *qi*, while herbs such as cinnamon, which have a warm and spicy energy, are used to tonify yang. Similarly, herbs such as rehmannia and *dang gui* can be used to nourish Blood while asparagus and ophiopogon root nourish yin.

Essence or *jing* represents a further refinement from a grosser material. This is subdivided into preheaven essence, which represents one's inherited potential, and postheaven essence, which is that which is refined after birth from food and fluids. Kidney essence represents a combination of both preheaven essence, one's innate constitutional strength, and postheaven essence, from food and fluids that are stored as the body's reserves in the kidneys. Here, the kidneys refer to the adrenals and the endocrine glands that regulate growth, reproduction, and constitutional strength.

The Four Treasures

The Four Treasures are *qi*, yang, blood and yin. This is an important classification because certain herbs and formulas are specifically designated as *qi*, yang, blood, or yin tonics and can be used when there are signs of deficiency in any one or a combination of these. The table below gives examples of each:

SAMPLE OF HERBS PRESCRIBED FOR DEFICIENCIES OF THE FOUR TREASURES

	SIGNS OF DEFICIENCY	HERBS
Qi	Low energy, weakness, feeble breathing, timidity and dislike of speaking or speaking in a low voice, aversion to wind, spontaneous sweating, pale tongue, and weak pulse	Herbs: *ren shen* or ginseng (*Panax ginseng*), *dang shen* (*Codonopsis pilosula*), *bai zhu* (*Atractylodes macrocephala*), *huang qi* (*Astragalus membranaceus*), *shan yao* (*Dioscorea batatas*), *gan cao* or licorice root (*Glycyrrhiza uralensis*). Representative formula: Four Gentlemen Combination (*Si jun zi tang*)
YANG	Coldness, lack of motivation, poor circulation, weak digestion and low libido,	Herbs: *rou gui* or cinnamon bark (*Cinnamomum cassia*), *fu zi* or prepared aconite (*Aconitum carmichaeli*), *xu*

SIGNS OF DEFICIENCY	HERBS
white tongue coat, and a deep or submerged pulse	*duan* or teasel root (*Dipsacus asperi*), *yin yang huo* (*Epimedium grandiflorum*) Representative herbal formula: *You Gui Wan*
BLOOD Paleness, poor circulation, dizziness, restlessness, insomnia with dream-disturbed sleep, thin, thready pulse, pale tongue, and (in women) insufficient menstruation	Herbs: *dang gui* (*Angelica sinensis*), *he shou wou* (*Polygonum multiflorum*), *shu di huang* (*Rehmannia glutinosa*) Representative herbal formula: Dang Gui Four (*Si Wu Tang*)
YIN Sensation of heat in the palms and/or soles, insomnia, restlessness, malar flush, night sweats, red tongue with little or no coat, and thin, thready, rapid pulse	Herbs: *xi yang shen* or American ginseng (*Panax quinquefolium*), *yu zhu* (*Polygonati odoratum*), *bai he* or tiger lily bulb (*Lilium brownii*), *mai men dong* or Japanese turf lily (*Ophiopogonis japonicus*), *tian men dong* (*Asparagus cochinchinensis*) Representative formula: Rehmannia Six Combination (*Liu Wei Di Huang Tang*)

In other chapters, we will discuss each herb and formula in detail, including their appropriate indications and uses.

Yin and Yang in the Body

All living beings contain aspects of both yin and yang because life, with all its psychophysiological functions, is the result of the interplay of yin and yang. The lung's inward breath is a result of yang (grasping), while its outward breath is a manifestation of yin (releasing); the contraction and expansion of the heart is also a manifestation of yang and yin. The front and right sides of the body are governed by yin blood, while the back and left side are governed by yang *qi*. If during conception the sperm is more active than the egg, a boy will result; if the egg is stronger, a girl will result. The nervous system is more yang, so that a predominance of the father is seen more on the left side. The father contributes to a strong nervous system in the offspring. The internal organs are substantive and more yin, so a predominance of the mother will show on the right side more and contribute to a stronger digestive system. The father's influence during conception is also responsible for the mental ability of the offspring, while the mother's will tend to dominate its physical, sensory, and emotional development.

How can we determine our basic yin–yang constitution? There are four kinds of Chinese medical diagnosis: observation, listening/smelling, interrogation, and palpation. These are described in further detail in later chapters. Remember, in traditional Chinese differential diagnosis, the practitioner does not attempt to make a diagnosis based on one indication alone. Rather, the practitioner seeks to determine the most predominant characteristics until they emerge into a pattern. Even then, a diagnosis is not complete until some remedial measures are tried, such as a change of diet or an herbal prescription. Barring the manifestation of a temporary cleansing or healing reaction from the change, the patient should feel a fundamental core improvement overall.

Conclusion

Yin–yang theory is a profound doctrine that is in many ways contrary to contemporary Western thought processes. While Western thought tends to exemplify a rational, linear process, where A leads to B to C and so on, in an infinite progression of phenomena and events, yin–yang philosophy allows B and C, for instance, to embody and return to A, forming a circular thought process. While linear thought leads to hierarchy and intolerance, circular thought leads to a greater accommodation of seemingly opposing viewpoints and differences. Of more poignant concern for our time is that linear thought processes, represented by Judeo-Christian and Western rationalistic philosophies, lead us away from the planet, ultimately toward a denial of natural law in favor of divine redemption and intercession, with the reward of a good life in "heaven." In contrast, Taoist yin–yang philosophy centers us within nature and the self: the life force is around us and inside us. In medicine, this embodies the very essence of mind-body-spirit holistic healing.

· TWO ·

THE FIVE ELEMENTS

The Chinese Five Elements, also called *Wu Xing* or Five Phases, are wood, fire, earth, metal, and water. The first recorded reference to the Five Elements was between 476 and 221 B.C. It was mentioned in the *Yellow Emperor's Classic of Internal Medicine (Huangdi Nei Jing)*: "Heaven has four seasons and five elements to allow cultivation, growth, harvesting, and storing. It produces cold, heat, drought, humidity, and wind. Man has five vital organs that transform the five influences to engender happiness, anger, vexation, sadness, and fear."

The Chinese Five Elements represent interactive phases or processes that are fundamental to the natural cycles of existence. Originally, they were probably a further division of yin–yang relationships into four parts, with earth in the center. Eventually, the concept of *earth* evolved to form its distinct interrelationships and it became one of the five.

The term *xing* in Chinese suggests a process of one thing acting upon another. For example, wood feeds fire; fire produces ashes, which become earth; within earth is metal; metal, when heated, liquefies and produces steam (water); and water in turn produces trees (wood). Thus, each element in turn feeds or nurtures the one that follows. This is called the *shen* or engendering cycle. It is also called the "mother-child law" because it is like a mother nurturing her child.

There is also a controlling or *ko* cycle in which the elements exert a restraining or controlling action on each other. In this cycle, earth is broken by wood, water is restrained by earth, fire is extinguished by water, metal is melted by fire, and wood is chopped by metal. This is called the "grandparent-grandchild law" because it resembles the controlling influence of the elders and grandparents in traditional Chinese society.

Another cycle of interdependency is called the "husband-wife" law, and it reflects the relationship of specific yin and yang organs within each element and between each other. These are as follows: the stomach is the yang "husband" of the yin spleen, which is the "wife"; the large intestine is the yang "husband" of the yin lungs; the bladder is the yang "husband" of the yin kidneys; the gallbladder is the yang "husband" of the yin liver; the small intestine is the yang "husband" of the yin heart; and the triple warmer is the yang "husband" of the yin pericardium.

The Five Element concept evolved from an ancient people who lived closely with the earth and its natural cycles. Today, with an overcrowded urban lifestyle and such amenities as central heating, electrical lighting, automobile and airplane travel, and imported foods, many of us forget the powerful influence the seasons exert over our lives. Ancient sages, however, respected the cycles of night and day and the seasons, as well as the various stages of human life. As a result, the Five Elements are a reflection of various relationships and natural cycles. In human existence, they include body–mind relationships, the relationship of diet, physical activities, internal organ relationships, and all aspects of health and disease with each other. The following table outlines the primary correspondences of the Five Elements:

THE FIVE ELEMENTS AND THEIR PRIMARY CORRESPONDENCES

	WOOD	FIRE	EARTH	METAL	WATER
PLANET	Jupiter	Mars	Saturn	Venus	Mercury
DIRECTION	East	South	Center	West	North
COLORS	Green	Red	Yellow	White	Black
SEASON	Spring	Summer	Indian summer	Autumn	Winter
INJURIOUS CLIMATE	Wind	Heat	Dampness	Dryness	Cold
YIN ORGAN	Liver	Heart	Spleen–pancreas	Lungs	Kidneys–endocrine

	WOOD	FIRE	EARTH	METAL	WATER
YANG ORGAN	Gall-bladder	Small intestine	Stomach	Large intestine	Bladder
POWER	Birth	Growth	Transformation	Harvest	Storage
SENSE	Sight	Speech	Taste	Smell	Hearing
BODY PART	Tendons–ligaments	Blood vessels	Flesh	Skin	Bones
EXTERNAL MANIFESTATION	Nails	Complexion	Lips	Body hair	Head hair
BODY ORIFICE	Eyes	Tongue	Mouth	Nose	Ears, anus, urinary organs
BODILY SECRETION	Tears	Sweat	Lymph	Mucus	Saliva
BODILY SOUND	Shouting	Laughter	Singing	Sobbing	Groaning
SPIRITUAL QUALITY	Ethereal soul: *hun*	Spirit: *shen*	Thought: *yi*	Corporal soul: *po*	Will: *zhi*
EMOTION	Anger	Joy/levity	Worry	Grief	Paranoia
DYNAMIC	Spirituality	Visionary	Intellect	Vitality	Will
CONTROLS	Spleen	Lungs	Kidneys	Liver	Heart
ACTIVITY	Seeing	Walking	Sitting	Reclining	Standing
FOODS					
GRAINS	Wheat	Beans	Rice	Hemp	Millet
VEGETABLE	Leek	Shallot	Hollyhock	Scallions	Leaf of bean plant
ANIMAL	Sheep	Fowl	Ox	Dog	Pig
FRUITS	Plum	Apricot	Date	Peach	Chestnut
FLAVORS THAT ARE BENEFICIAL WHEN EATEN	Sweet	Sour	Salty	Bitter	Spicy
FLAVORS THAT INJURE WHEN OVEREATEN	Spicy	Salty	Sweet	Sour	Bitter

In the following, we can see the Confucian organizing influence that assigns specific duties for each organ as an "official" in charge of specific bodily functions.

Fire

The heart (yin) and small intestine (yang) are under the fire element. Consider how fire is hot, flaring upward, light, and energy, all of which are embodied in the traditional Chinese medicine (TCM) functions of the heart and small intestine. The heart is responsible for heat and the circulation of blood and nourishment throughout the body. Psychologically, the heart houses the spirit and represents the clear light of consciousness. Warmth from the heart gives it control over the process of sweat. Recognized as the "supreme controller" over the entire body, the heart governs the blood and its vessels and finds expression in the complexion of the face. It opens to the tongue and influences speech. The small intestine is the official responsible for "the separation of the pure from the impure" because it governs the metabolic breakdown and absorption of food and the initial discharge of waste.

There are two complementary organ processes: the pericardium (yin), as the sac that encases the heart in TCM, serves as an extension of the heart, while the triple warmer (yang) represents the coordination of the upper, middle, and lower parts of the body and the circulation of fluids through the various pathways.

Joy is the emotion associated with fire. In this sense, *joy* refers to exuberant celebrating and all that generally accompanies such activities, such as overeating and overindulging all the senses. Conversely, since the heart governs the mind, individuals who have imbalanced heart *qi* may manifest manic tendencies accompanied with inappropriate giggling or laughter.

Earth

The earth element includes the stomach, which is yang, and the spleen, which is yin. The stomach is the "official" in charge of "ripening and rotting" because it initially receives ingested food for digestion. The stomach is also the origin of fluids and moves *qi* downward. The spleen is the official governing "transformation and transportation." While the

stomach begins the process of digestive breakdown, the spleen transforms and transports the energy from food and drink throughout the
body down to the cellular level. Poor appetite and digestion or malnutrition are therefore considered primarily an imbalance of the spleen
and secondarily of the stomach. The spleen is regarded as the source of
"acquired *qi*," which is the energy one derives and uses daily from food,
air, and water. It also controls blood and the ability to support or up-
hold the energy and vital organs of the body. Menstrual irregularities
involving blood, therefore, often imply spleen imbalance, as does any
prolapsed internal organ. Because the spleen is deeply responsible for
nourishment, it also governs the muscles and limbs. The spleen also
opens to the mouth and manifests on the lips. Finally, the spleen governs the process of contemplation and thought. This implies that excessive thought or being spaced out or off center (associated with
hypoglycemia, a spleen–pancreas imbalance) are both symptoms of
earth imbalance. In addition, activities such as worry or excessive study
can injure earth-element energy. This will commonly manifest as digestive weakness, edema, and obesity (sitting is also the position or movement of the earth element).

Metal

The metal element includes the lungs, metal yin, and the large intestine, metal yang. The lungs are the officials in charge of controlling
the vital energy of the whole body. They extract *qi* from the air during
respiration and transfer it through the respiratory passages to the blood.
It is then circulated throughout the body. The lungs also have direct
contact with the outer environment through breathing and are considered to be directly related to the skin. Because of this, they are the
most prone to external pernicious influences and thus are often called a
delicate organ, or the "princess" of the organs. The lungs are also the
uppermost organ in the body and consequently are often seen as a "lid"
on the other organs.

The official of the large intestine is in charge of receiving and discharging waste. Its dysfunctions have to do with disturbances in bowel
movements, including the substance and amount of feces and the frequency of defecation. The emotion associated with metal is sadness or
grieving. The energy of metal is "letting go," so that an appropriate

amount of sadness and grief is necessary for balance. Excessive tendency toward sadness can be either a sign or a cause of metal imbalance.

Water

Water includes the urinary bladder (water yang) and the kidney (water yin). The function of the bladder is to be the official in charge of receiving, storing, and excreting urine. Through water metabolism, fluids are dissipated all over the body to moisten and then accumulate in the kidneys. Urine is produced from the final portions of turbid fluids sent from the lungs, small intestines, and large intestines. It is then sent down to the bladder, where it is stored until excreted.

The kidneys are the officials that store the *jing* essence (reproductive secretions) and the refined aspect of the body that represents the essential "inherited" constitution of the individual. They are divided into kidney yang (sympathetic nervous system) and kidney yin (parasympathetic nervous system), which serve as the root of yin and yang for the entire body. The kidneys are therefore regarded as the basis of life, governing birth, growth, development, and reproduction. They control the brain, generate marrow, and govern the bones. They also rule the ears and hearing and manifest in head hair. Finally, kidney *qi* is responsible for willpower.

Fear and paranoia are the emotions of water. Again, either an excess of these emotions or a tendency toward inappropriate paranoia are signs of water imbalance.

Wood

Wood includes the liver as wood yin and the gallbladder as wood yang. In all cases, the yin organs are considered the deeper organs with more profound effects; they store blood and regulate the smooth flow of *qi*. In this, the liver is comparable to an army general who is responsible for the overall planning (or strategy) of the body's functions. The liver manifests itself in the nails and ligaments of the body. It opens into the eyes and houses the ethereal soul.

The gallbladder is the officer in charge of making decisions. It is responsible for storing and excreting bile, which is regarded as a pure substance. This capacity of the gallbladder to make decisions links well to the liver's capacity to plan one's life. The gallbladder also provides initiative to make the decisions and the bravery or courage to carry them out. Thus, timidity, indecisiveness, lack of drive or initiative to make decisions, and being easily discouraged reflect a gallbladder disharmony. As with the liver, the gallbladder also rules the sinews and ligaments of the body.

Anger and frustration are the emotions associated with the liver, while indecisiveness or lack of courage are associated with the gallbladder. Again these emotions can either be a symptom or cause of the corresponding physiological processes. Walking, the activity of the liver, is useful because it helps spread or harmonize liver *qi*. *Spread,* as the term is used in TCM, refers to what we in the West experience as a kind of equalizing of our thoughts and feelings. Whenever we feel extreme anger and frustration, one of the best and most immediate remedies is to take a walk.

The Five Elements and Herbalism

In Chinese herbalism, the heating or cooling energies, flavors, textures, and colors are of utmost importance. The bitter flavor is used to clear and detoxify excess heat and therefore help clear the fire heart and small intestine; the sweet flavor is used to tonify and nourish the earth spleen and stomach; the spicy flavor is used to stimulate, warm, and dry dampness and therefore help a condition of excess dampness or mucus affecting metal lungs; the salty flavor helps retain bodily fluids, moistens the tissues, and assists the water kidneys; the sour flavor is associated with fermented foods and lemons and complements the process of wood-liver enzyme formation.

Some herbs have a rough, dry texture and are good for excessively damp conditions, such as edema or mucous discharge, while others have a slippery, smooth, moist texture that is good for promoting the granulation and healing of injuries and ameliorating dryness.

In Chinese herbalism, a disease that appears in one element may actually be caused by a weakness or excess in another. By treating the "mother" element, therefore, it is possible to calm or subdue symptoms associated with the corresponding "child." Another approach might be to subdue the "child" to strengthen the "mother." In the controlling cycle, the bitter flavor associated with fire can be used to help dry or otherwise control mucus associated with the lungs and metal.

Practically speaking, while the Five Elements represent a powerful tool for healing and transformation on the body–mind level, this level may not be the most efficient one at which to expeditiously treat most diseases. It offers a deeper understanding, however, of the influences of seasons, diet, relationships, occupation, and other factors that are the underlying cause of disease or that hamper the recovery process.

· THREE ·

THE CAUSES OF DISEASE

In traditional Chinese medicine (TCM), there are six external causes of disease (Six External Evils) and seven emotions that cause internal disease. This may seem like an oversimplification, but it is in fact quite comprehensive. Again, the principles of diagnostic classification, unlike contemporary Western scientific medicine, which can produce the name of a disease with no apparent treatment, is strictly a guide for arriving at corresponding treatment modalities. There is no traditional understanding of specific micropathogenic organisms, such as bacteria and viruses, as the causes of disease. On the external level, disease is caused by the body's reserves being lowered or compromised by overexposure to one of the Six External Causes, which leaves us vulnerable to pathogenic invasion. On the internal level, it is the stress and dysfunction of the internal organs, with their emotional correspondences, that are considered the Seven Internal Causes.

As with other diagnostic indications, the Six External and Seven Internal Causes are not necessarily exclusive of each other. External conditions can be precipitated by internal weakness and deficiencies, and internal chronic conditions can be exacerbated by external diseases. As with all traditional diagnostic indications, the purpose is to arrive at an appropriate treatment.

The Six External Causes of Disease

Wind

Wind, the most pervasive of the Six Evils, is a yang evil that tends to rise and disperse outward. Pathogenic wind usually attacks the upper and outer yang areas of the body first, with symptoms such as headache, skin diseases, dizziness, spasms, muscle rigidity, deviation of the mouth and eyes (Bell's palsy), and arthritic and rheumatic conditions. It is also closely associated with sudden colds, fevers, influenzas, allergies, headaches, nasal congestion, chills, fever, and stiff neck and shoulders. These are called external wind. Here, *wind* refers to the ability of a disease pathogen to spread and proliferate. Internal wind comes from an imbalance of the liver and other vital organs. Symptoms of internal wind involve an imbalance of the nervous system and include hypertension, strokes, vertigo, dizziness, twitches, blurred vision, and so forth. Parkinson's disease, an epilepsy, is characteristically an internal wind condition. See the following tables for diagnostic indications for wind diseases.

EXTERNAL WIND

TYPE OF WIND	SYMPTOMS
EXTERNAL WIND	Fever, cold phobia, perspiration, shivers, headache, nasal congestion, cough, thin white coat on tongue (practically normal appearance), floating pulse
WIND ATTACK	Fainting, convulsions, coma, twitching, wry mouth and eyes, tongue possibly curved to one side, floating and leisurely pulse
WIND COLD	Fever, cold phobia, absence of perspiration, headache, joint pains, thin white coat on tongue (practically normal appearance), and floating, tight, and slower pulse
WIND HEAT	Headache, sore throat, pink eyes, yellow pus discharges, thirst, darker colored

TYPE OF WIND	SYMPTOMS
	urine, red-bodied and yellow-coated tongue, fast and perhaps more forceful pulse
WIND DAMPNESS	Feeling of heaviness, joint pains that move around, headache, moderate swelling, perspiration, fear of wind, fever that worsens in the afternoon, scanty urination, moist and scalloped tongue, gliding or slippery pulse
WIND DRYNESS	Dryness of the throat and respiratory passages, thirst, dry cough, dry and withered skin, dry nails, dry tongue, short and rough pulse

INTERNAL WIND

TYPE OF WIND	SYMPTOMS
INTERNAL WIND	Diseases involving cerebral damage, such as strokes, coma, Parkinson's, chorea, epilepsy
WIND CAUSED BY BLOOD DEFICIENCY	Same as wind attack but with accompanying symptoms of blood deficiency with internal dryness, pale-bodied tongue, thin or thready pulse
WIND CAUSED BY HEAT	Same as wind attack but with symptoms of excess heat

Cold

Cold imbalances represent conditions that are cold, slow, and typically aggravated by cold weather and cold outdoor temperatures. These include chronic or subacute internal conditions such as anemia, poor circulation, weak digestion, and all low metabolic hypofunctioning of the various glands and organs, such as hypothyroid, hypoadrenalism, and hypoglycemia. Cold can also include sexual debility, such as impotence and frigidity, and rheumatic conditions. The emotion associated with coldness is shyness or timidity. External cold represents the penetration of cold climatic influences from the outside, taxing the body's immune reserves and manifesting ailments such as the common cold, cough, and upper-respiratory allergies and diseases. Symptoms of coldness include pale complexion, pale-colored tongue, loose stool, clear urine, clear or whitish mucous discharges, and a slow pulse of less than 60 beats per minute. Cold diseases, therefore, are aggravated by cold weather and ameliorated by warmth. By their nature, all cold diseases are yin.

☯

COLD DISEASES

TYPE OF COLD	SYMPTOMS
EXTERNAL COLD	Fever, cold phobia, absence of perspiration, headache, joint pains, thin white coat on tongue, and floating, tight, slow pulse
COLD ATTACK	Sudden and extreme cold, shivering, blue complexion, coma with body stiffness, abdominal pains relieved with warmth, lying down with feet and legs curled inward, vomiting and diarrhea, pale- or blue-bodied tongue with a white coat, slow pulse
INTERNAL COLD	Pale complexion, fear of cold, diarrhea, cold extremities, pale tongue with a white coat, slow pulse

☯

Heat

Heat imbalances are diseases and conditions that are hot and inflammatory, aggravated by hot weather and heat exposure. They tend to be acute, excessive, and quickly evolving. Diseases that are inflammatory or feverish in nature are described as hot and represent excessive metabolic processes, causing a variety of hyperfunctions, such as hypertension and hyperthyroid, ulcers, or colitis. Individuals with excessive heat tend to be aggressive, loud, and overbearing. Also, external heat includes acute skin rashes that are red or dry, feverish diseases such as influenza, acute traumas and injuries, and inflamed arthritic joints. When confirming symptoms of heat, the TCM practitioner looks for a red, swollen appearance of the affected part, ruddy complexion, red tongue, yellow coating, yellow or blood-streaked discharges, dark-colored urine, constipation or dry stool, and a pulse of more than 80 beats per minute. Heat diseases are aggravated by external hot weather and ameliorated by coolness. By nature, all hot diseases and conditions are yang.

HEAT CONDITIONS

TYPE OF HEAT	SYMPTOMS
EXCESS HEAT	High fever, thirst, sore throat, ruddy complexion, constipation, dark and even blood-tinged urine, mental irritability, fast and forceful pulse, red-bodied tongue with yellow coat
DEFICIENT HEAT	Feeling of heat in the Five Spaces (hands, feet, and/or chest) sore throat, light and intermittent fever, coughing up of blood, dryness of the mouth and throat, mental irritability, fast and thin pulse, red-bodied or mirrorlike tongue with little or no coat

Dampness

Dampness represents a class of symptoms that are aggravated by damp weather and the intake of oily and fluidic foods. Symptoms of dampness include swelling and impaired fluid metabolism, such as edema, abdominal swelling, obesity, and the formation of cysts, tumors, and lumps. Dampness is also manifested with oozing sores and with damp or fluid discharges, described as damp heat. When dampness congeals, it causes phlegm, which affects the sinuses and upper-respiratory passages, including the lungs and bronchioles. Dampness is differentiated as external or internal and hot or cold. Swelling with characteristic oozing and weeping sores is described as external damp heat. Allergies with abundant mucous, vaginal, or other discharges are also a sign of external dampness, and they may represent either cold, if the discharge is clear or whitish, or hot, if it is thick and yellowish or blood tinged. Abdominal swelling, obesity, tumors, and cysts are described as internal dampness. Signs of dampness are a swollen appearance, edema with excessively moist and swollen tongue with scalloped edges, and a gliding or slippery-feeling pulse.

DAMPNESS

TYPE OF DAMPNESS	SYMPTOMS
WIND DAMPNESS	See External Wind above
COLD DAMPNESS	Joint stiffness and pains, no perspiration, edema of the extremities, scanty and clear urine, sticky and muddy stool
SUMMER HEAT DAMPNESS	Nausea, vomiting, diarrhea, dysentery, fever, perspiration
DAMP HEAT	Inflammation, fever, yellowish discharges and appearance, pain and swelling of the extremities, thirst, depression, chest congestion, reddish and scanty urine, greasy tongue with a yellow coat, full and slippery pulse
INTERNAL DAMPNESS	Feeling of congestion and fullness, abdominal swelling, craving for hot drinks but little thirst (internal damp cold), tasteless but greasy sensation in the mouth, scanty and cloudy urination, scalloped and swollen tongue, gliding and slippery pulse, sticky, muddy, and loose stool

Dryness

Dryness corresponds with autumn and represents symptoms that are aggravated by dry climates. As with each of the other evils, dryness is commonly found combined with other evils, such as dry cold, dry heat, or wind dryness. As such, it adversely affects the lungs, sinuses, large intestine, skin, digestion, and reproductive organs. Inordinate thirst is an important symptom for dryness. Typically, herbalists prescribe oily, mucilaginous substances, such as oils, demulcent and mucilaginous herbs, and yin tonics.

DRYNESS

TYPE OF DRYNESS	SYMPTOMS
COLD DRYNESS	Sensitivity to cold and drafts, dry and stuffy nasal passages and throat, headache, dry lips, lack of perspiration, panting, dry and pale tongue, slow pulse
WARM DRYNESS	Feeling of heat in the body with perspiration, thirst, sore throat, lack of mucus and/or chest pain with red-tainted sputum, dry nasal passages, cough, red-bodied and dry tongue, faster pulse
INTERNAL DRYNESS	Dry skin, dry and lusterless hair that breaks easily, constipation and dry stool, dry tongue with little or no coat, deep and thin pulse

---

Summer Heat

Summer heat occurs as heat stroke from an extreme exposure to heat. With overexposure to sunlight and hot weather, the body experiences high fever, dizziness, nausea, heavy sweating, diarrhea, and extreme thirst that can ultimately lead to exhaustion, delirium, and coma. Such diseases as summer colds may also be treated as summer heat. For

Western-trained practitioners, this is an unusual classification. One of the most common formulas is a patented formula called Agastache Formula (*Huo Xiang Zheng Qi San*).

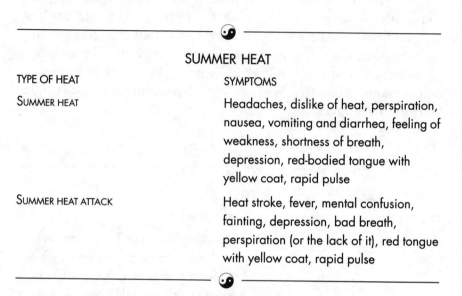

SUMMER HEAT

TYPE OF HEAT	SYMPTOMS
SUMMER HEAT	Headaches, dislike of heat, perspiration, nausea, vomiting and diarrhea, feeling of weakness, shortness of breath, depression, red-bodied tongue with yellow coat, rapid pulse
SUMMER HEAT ATTACK	Heat stroke, fever, mental confusion, fainting, depression, bad breath, perspiration (or the lack of it), red tongue with yellow coat, rapid pulse

The Seven Emotions as Causes of Internal Disease

Internal disease refers to chronic conditions that exemplify the mind–body relationship through emotions and the effects they have on the body. The Seven Emotions or Seven Internal Causes are joy, anger, sadness, pensiveness, grief, fear, and fright.

Joy

Here, *joy* refers to diseases caused by too much celebrating. TCM practitioners believe that an excess of joy can damage the heart and is associated with such symptoms as insomnia, muddled thought, inappropriate tears or laughter, fits, hysteria, and insanity.

Anger

Anger, which includes resentment, frustration, irritability, rage, indignation, bitterness, and animosity, both disturbs and indicates liver imbalance. Anger causes the *qi* to inappropriately rise, causing hypertension, headaches, tinnitus, dizziness, blurred vision, mental confusion, red face, and vomiting of blood.

Sadness

Sadness depletes the *qi* of the lungs and heart and results in diseases associated with breathlessness, depression, crying, tiredness, amenorrhea, shortness of breath, asthma, emphysema, allergies, and frequent colds and bouts of influenza.

Pensiveness

Pensiveness, or excessive worry, thinking, studying, and/or mental work, weakens spleen *qi* and can lead to symptoms of edema (obesity), low appetite, digestive disorders, and fatigue.

Grief

Grief, like sadness, injures the lungs and can weaken one's resistance to colds and influenza and cause chronic upper-respiratory diseases, such as asthma, emphysema, and allergies.

Fear (Paranoia)

Fear depletes and injures the kidneys. Because it causes the *qi* to descend, fear can be an underlying cause of many chronic urinary complaints such as bed-wetting and urinary incontinence, as well as lower back and joint pains and libido imbalance.

Fright (Shock)

Shock is different from fear in that it is more sudden and causes the *qi* to scatter. First, it injures the heart, causing such symptoms as palpitations, breathlessness, and insomnia. Next, it will adversely effect the kidneys, causing urinary incontinence, night sweats, dizziness, or tinnitus.

· F O U R ·

THE WAY OF
DIAGNOSIS

THE FOUR DIAGNOSES

In 1982, I was fortunate to be part of the first group of Americans to travel to China specifically to study herbal medicine. Previous groups had gone and returned, but their focus was on Chinese acupuncture. I suppose we were part of the first wave of licensed North American acupuncturists whose interest extended to traditional Chinese herbalism.

Our destination was Kunming, a city located on the frontier bordering the Himalayas. We were told that Kunming was called the "spring city" because the weather was always warm and temperate. It wasn't long after we were settled in our adequate but stark hotel accommodations, freezing in our rooms, that we reinterpreted the happy Chinese image of "spring city" as a kind of Chinese mental exercise to help save on central heating expenses. In fact, despite the exceptional availability of health care characteristic of Communist countries, where medical practitioners are considered only slightly higher in status than any other respectable worker, we found that the compact city abounded in fully equipped worker's hospitals that were also unheated. Patients had to remain under heavy covers to keep warm. At first, we admired the picturesque sight of the entire hospital staff, all dressed in their white uniforms and caps, gathering in the front of the hospital each morning for calisthenics. After a few days, our admiration for Chinese health care, apart from any health considerations, became recognition that the staff were attempting to warm themselves for the day's work in the cold hospital.

Notwithstanding this situation, which existed only because of economic shortcomings, the doctors and hospital staff seemed professional and highly qualified and provided excellent person-to-person care. In America today, the training of a traditional Chinese medicine (TCM) doctor in most schools lasts 3 or 4 years. Presumably, that will increase in years to come. In China, however, the training is in both Western and traditional medicine and takes at least 8 years. So what makes up the extensive training of a TCM doctor in China? A good part of it involves the study of materia medica and classical formulas, but most important are the infinite subtleties of traditional diagnosis. Without a sound diagnosis, treatment will be hit-or-miss.

The most outstanding doctor there, who was our teacher at the time, was Dr. Zhen Wen Tao, M.D. He was a young, innovative herb doctor at the time specializing in cardiovascular disease in a ward in the hospital where we made our daily rounds. The most remarkable thing I still remember and appreciate was watching him diagnose and treat a patient who had suffered a heart attack. Among the symptoms he was treating in this patient were heart palpitations and angina pains. For these, he prescribed a tea made of anywhere from nine to a dozen herbs to be taken two or three times daily. When we went back in a week, Dr. Zhen noted how after the patient had taken the tea for a week, the palpitations and heart pains were gone, but the patient still seemed to have a considerable amount of mucus in his lungs, which was related to his heart condition. Dr. Zhen, feeling his pulse, said to us that there were indeed some conditions he had not treated with the previous prescription. He added another couple of herbs to the prescription for the week to come. Sure enough, 1 week later, like an arrow hitting its mark, Dr. Zhen's revised formula encompassed all the imbalances in this particular patient and he was completely symptom free. The happy but well-bundled patient would be allowed to stay on in the hospital another couple of weeks for observation and to regain his strength.

It is said that in North America today, the average M.D. spends about 7 minutes with each patient. This is not the way medicine was always practiced in the West. I remember how as recently as the 1950s, most medical doctors would still make house calls. They used a full range of diagnostic skills similar to those of TCM: palpating the abdomen, observing the tongue, identifying several different pulse qualities, and so forth. Unfortunately, in today's litigious climate, the human element is lacking and the art of medicine has been largely replaced by technology and machines.

Certain aspects of diagnosis presented here are obvious and can be prudently learned by the layperson. These include the differentiation of the Eight Principles—external/internal, hot/cold, excess/deficient, yin/yang—and some of the basic organ symptom diagnoses. Anyone with a watch with a second hand can determine whether a pulse is fast or slow, whether it is regular or irregular. With a little more practice, one can learn to recognize a full or strong pulse from a weak one. Similarly, anyone can recognize a pale, swollen tongue or a cardinal red tongue, or a tongue with a yellow or white coat. Even with this simple knowledge, it is possible to have a basic understanding of hot or cold and excess or deficient conditions, which is very valuable. Mastering the interpretation of these signs, in respect to other seemingly conflicting symptoms and signs, can take years of practice under the guidance of a qualified practitioner.

Traditional Chinese diagnosis is a useful guide to identifying some of the more obvious diagnostic signs and symptoms. It can also serve as a warning by aiding in the recognition of possibly life-threatening conditions for which one is better advised to seek experienced help and guidance.

Chinese herbal medicine is based on the Four Diagnoses: observation, palpation, interrogation, and listening. The practitioner first begins by listening and evaluating the patient's primary and secondary complaints, noting at the same time complexion, level of vitality, physical appearance, openness, and emotional demeanor. All of these are evaluated according to yin–yang principles. Ten basic questions encompassing symptoms that are not obvious through assessment by any other method are asked:

1. Ask about chills and fever and sensitivity to heat and cold.
2. Ask about perspiration: spontaneous perspiration with no unusual physical exertion or night sweats are important diagnostic considerations.
3. Ask about pains, such as headaches, chest or abdominal pains, or pains anywhere else on the body.

4. Ask about urination and defecation and their frequency, urgency, color, consistency, and so on.

5. Ask about appetite—its lack or excess—and cravings for particular kinds of food.

6. Ask about mental and emotional state, including tendency to depression, anger, fear, melancholy, and so on. All have relevance in terms of the Five Elements.

7. Ask about hearing or unusual ear sounds.

8. Ask about thirst, discerning whether there is a depletion of fluid as a result of heat and dryness.

9. Ask about the history of past diseases, including those of immediate family members. At the same time, inquire as to whether the patient has any ideas about the cause of his or her present condition.

10. If the patient is female, inquire concerning menstruation, leukorrhea, number of children, childbirth, miscarriages, and abortions.

Whenever possible, determine the underlying cause of the complaint. This usually involves such aspects as exposure to inclement weather, lifestyle, diet, work, appetite, elimination, sleep, exercise, and so forth. The final stages of diagnosis may involve observing and palpating affected areas of the body. Finally, the tongue is observed and the pulse is studied to help confirm the diagnosis. The object of traditional diagnosis is to allow the practitioner to become more informed about the condition and underlying cause of the disease. This involves the study of symptoms and signs and their integration into one or a number of functional patterns of imbalance of which the disease is composed. Various approaches and theories are used, including the Eight Principles, the Five Elements, the Three Humors (qi, Blood, and fluid), or the corroboration of symptoms and patterns based on functional organ imbalances, called zang-fu diagnosis.

Given the complex psychophysiological response capabilities of the body, healing will always be at best as much an art as it is a science. One can spend a lifetime studying, only to find that any attempt to oversimplify diagnostic processes or classification of diseases is often complicated by paradoxical irregularities. In TCM, understanding symptoms in terms of the Eight Principles is pivotal for successfully treating any disease. In practice, however, it is not always so easy to discern between patterns of hot and cold, external and internal, or excess and deficiency.

On rare occasions, a practitioner may prescribe a test herb or formula with a particular set of strong characteristics, such as being extremely spicy, bitter, hot, or cold, in an attempt to further clarify the patient's condition. In any case, the practitioner should not permaturely reckon a single indication to be definitive before evaluating various parameters, following the principles of differential diagnosis. The beginning approach to treatment should be considered as tentative, based on the patient's response in a week or so. In addition, there should be periodic reevaluation and adjustment of the treatment protocol as the condition changes and improves.

Because TCM diagnosis is not based on named diseases as is Western medicine (at least in theory), with the treatment of a relatively unique pattern of signs and symptoms, no condition is considered untreatable. This includes both acute infectious diseases, such as colds and influenza, and a variety of chronic conditions, such as arthritis, cancer, and certain types of cardiovascular diseases.

The practitioner begins by evaluating signs and symptoms based on yin and yang, using the Eight Principles. Other diagnostic theories, such as the Five Element theory or the Three Humors, are used, based on their relevance and appearance. Symptom–sign diagnosis is, along with Eight Principles, another approach most commonly employed.

Treatment then consists in providing guidance regarding lifestyle, diet, herbs, exercises, and appropriate physiotherapies, such as Chinese massage (tui'na) and acupuncture to alter the course of disease. From this perspective, disease represents an adjustment by the body to an underlying condition of imbalance.

Branch and Root

We cannot eradicate a tree by simply trimming the outer leaves and branches; instead, we must eradicate the root. Like we peel back the layers of an onion, we attend to the outer manifestation of chronic disease symptoms as they present themselves, with the understanding that eventually the root must be eradicated. This can occur either simultaneously or after the acute symptoms have subsided.

Examples of branch and root treatment are myriad. A most obvious one is someone who frequently catches a cold or develops a fever. Here, the cold and fever are the branch, while a weak immune system is the root. Another example is lower back pain, the branch, for which the root is often the kidneys. In acute conditions, treatment gives priority to the branch before the root. In more chronic conditions, such as lower back pain, both branch and root must be treated simultaneously. Symptoms of arthritis or lower back pain may be regarded as the outer acute branch symptoms, and the underlying weakness and deficiency of the kidneys–adrenals is the root cause. In this case, it may be necessary to simultaneously treat the "branch"—joint pains—with herbs and a formula that also tonifies the kidney–adrenal deficiency as the underlying root.

A patient who visits a Western medical doctor complaining of a recurring headache, for instance, might either be given simple analgesic medication or be subjected to an expensive battery of tests to rule out the possibility of a brain tumor. In the end, the patient may feel consoled to learn that there is no brain tumor, but there is also no satisfactory treatment for the headache. The same patient, evaluated with traditional Chinese low-tech diagnostic approaches based on direct observation, achieves complete relief with minor lifestyle adjustments along with therapeutic diet and herbs.

While TCM is not capable of discovering the presence of a brain tumor through a holistic differential diagnosis of the symptoms, it is likely to find the most effective treatment approach for most other types of headaches. For this reason, a diagnostic approach that combines both Western medicine and TCM can provide the best strategy for treatment.

Diet, herbs, noninvasive physiotherapies, and lifestyle adjustments are the primary methods of effecting change in Chinese herbalism. Such comparatively mild approaches to treatment can be effective only if they begin with the premise of mobilizing the body's innate healing capacities.

Once again, the beginner is cautioned against making too hasty a judgment based on a single indication. Treatment will result in either a positive or negative reaction. It is easy to evaluate a positive reaction, but an adverse reaction may signify either a deepening of the imbalance or a healing crisis.

Healing Crisis

As the body begins recovery from a debilitated state, it takes on new levels of energy. This new energy can increase its ability to push out or complete latent disease processes, which may show up in the form of minor acute symptoms. At first, this may seem confusing because the attempt to eradicate one set of symptoms brings on either a temporary aggravation or the manifestation of seemingly unrelated symptoms, such as a cold, fever, or skin eruptions. To distinguish between a healing crisis and a worsening of the disease, consider the following points:

- A healing crisis often involves a retracing of an older disease process. For this reason, it is important to take a good preliminary case history.
- A healing crisis is always of short duration—a few days to a week at most.
- Although during a healing crisis there are seemingly new symptoms, the primary complaint is lessened, and often the patient feels better in some other way, such as having more energy, sleeping more deeply, and so on.

From the perspective of the body, disease represents an adaptation to an underlying condition of imbalance. We can view these imbalances as an accumulation of toxins or, from another perspective, an imbalance of yin and yang. The objective of natural healing, therefore, is to stimulate or supply the necessary ingredients for the body to eliminate its stored toxins and regain yin–yang homeostasis. It may seem ironic that the very methods and herbs that are most likely to aggravate a condition can, in many instances, have just the opposite effect. It is always important to first recognize the direction the energy of the body is attempting to take, regardless of the pathology involved. Many times, the best treatment, rather than opposing or suppressing a symptomatic physical reaction, is to assist the seemingly negative condition to completion. Examples of this includes the use of warming diaphoretic herbs for the treatment of fevers and skin eruptions, the use of herbal diuretics for urinary frequency, the use of laxatives for dysentery and diarrhea, and the application of warming and stimulating herbs to relieve arthritic and rheumatic pains.

Inflammatory diseases of various kinds can occur as a result of heat congestion caused by excess or coldness caused by weakness. The latter occurs when the body lacks the energy to adequately eliminate its own metabolic waste. The use of strong cooling herbs or antibiotic drugs for inflammatory conditions caused by weakness, coldness, and deficiency is regarded as suppression and ultimately deepens the imbalance. This may occur whether or not the primary viral or bacterial inflammation is alleviated, with the result being a more chronic cold and deficient state.

It is becoming more recognized and understood that the abuse of antibiotics, cortisone, or other suppressive drugs can ultimately weaken the immune system, leaving one with somewhat vague symptoms of chronic fatigue, weak digestion, allergies of various forms, and possible candidiasis. Adding insult to injury, there is a good possibility that the primary inflammatory symptoms will return at the same or some different physical site after the antibiotics are stopped. In general, when herbs are used, because they are milder and more foodlike, there is less chance of such long-term adverse reactions occurring. The overall result of taking antibiotic drugs is exhaustion of the body's internal reserves. This can also be caused by stress. When this is the case, it is better to rest and rehabilitate while supplementing the underlying deficiency with appropriate foods and taking tonic herbs to strengthen the body's innate potential to overcome pathological conditions.

In life-threatening cases or conditions that show no favorable response to natural therapies, the inexperienced person should refer patients, whenever possible, to a qualified traditional Chinese medicine practitioner or a Western medical doctor for further guidance. In all appropriate cases, treatment should first involve the simplest, most noninvasive natural approach, dealing with diet, herbs, lifestyle and so forth.

Making a Diagnosis

In TCM, the diagnostic process involves assessing the patient on several levels.

Observation

Observing several aspects can provide a great deal of useful information.

1. **Expression, energy level, and emotional state:** Much of the initial observation is based on the assessment of the eyes, complexion, posture, and body movement. Bright eyes and an exuberant manner indicate a high state of healthful energy and vitality. Such an individual is likely to respond well to treatment. Listless expression and eyes may indicate serious illness and a

protracted period of recovery. An abnormal or strange expression may indicate mental depression and other problems.

2. **Body structure:** A yin individual has a thinner, more frail appearance.

3. **Complexion:** A white or pale complexion represents a weakened, cold, or hypotonic condition. It is often associated with yang deficiency. A bright yellow or jaundiced condition with possible yellowing of the whites of the eyes indicates damp Heat. A slight yellowish cast all over the entire body may indicate damp Cold. A red or ruddy complexion indicates heat. If the red color is deeper, it represents excess heat; if it is more on the surface, around the nose and eyes, it represents yin deficiency or superficial heat. A blue or cyanotic complexion indicates coldness or pain. A bluish black complexion indicates severe internal cold with possible gastrointestinal symptoms.

4. **Head size:** The size and shape of the head is an indication of intelligence and innate vitality. Those with a yin constitution have more elongated heads, with broad foreheads tapering down to their chins. Those with a yang constitution have more square-shaped heads. In children, a head that is either too large or too small indicates impaired mental development and essence deficiency. Bulging of the fontanel in infants is normal when they are upset and crying. In sickness, it indicates the upward attack of fire. Head shaking or facial twitches are considered a wind imbalance possibly caused by a deficiency of *qi* and blood.

5. **Facial features:** A yin individual will have more expanded facial features, as in a greater distance between the nose and the mouth. The eyes are horizontally placed further apart and large. The eyebrows of a yang person tend to be more bushy and thick and tilt downward toward the nose, while those for a yin individual slant downward toward the temples. The nose of a yin individual is longer and larger. A yang individual presents a generally more contracted and compact appearance, with a shorter distance between the eyes and mouth and eyes that are smaller and more closely set together. The nose is more flattened. Famous individuals with a more yin-type face are D. H. Lawrence, Frédéric Chopin, and the actress Julia Roberts. Famous individuals with more yang facial features include George Washington,

Winston Churchill, Franklin Roosevelt, Margaret Thatcher, and Ronald Reagan.

6. **Hair:** Those who have a strong inherited constitution with an abundance of blood and essence will have thick, sleek, and glossy hair. Those with dry, sparse, withered hair with split ends have a deficiency of blood and essence. Alopecia, or hair loss, when it is not inherited pattern baldness, is the result of wind arising because of blood deficiency. It occurs in some women after childbirth. It is treated with blood tonics, such as Dang Gui Four (Si Wu Tang), and local shallow tapping over the affected area with a disinfected needle. This procedure is repeated daily. The kidneys also govern head hair, while the lungs govern body hair. A lack of body hair can be an indication of lung weakness. Prematurely gray hair is a sign of kidney–adrenal deficiency. The kidneys–adrenals in TCM are the source qi for yin and yang of the entire body. It houses the constitutional reserves. Many times, when an individual experiences extreme stress, more than their reserves can buffer, they experience their hair suddenly turning gray or falling out. This proves TCM wisdom relating to profound and deep physiological processes. Thin hair with split ends is a yin-deficient condition, while thick hair is an indication of rich yin energy. In TCM, blood and yin tonics such as *Rehmannia glutinosa (di huang)* and *Polygonum multiflorum (he shou wou)* are used to promote hair growth and color.

7. **Neck and nape:** A swelling or lump at the frontal base of the neck is indicative of a goiter. This is especially true if the individual also has bulging eyes. It is considered a stagnation of qi with an accumulation of phlegm. Such seaweeds as kelp are usually used to treat goiters. Swollen glands, also called scrofula, are indicative of inflammation, for which heat clearing or alterative herbs are used. Stiff neck, or opisthotonos, can be a sign of influenza or fever or an ongoing condition of wind caused by an accumulation of stress and tension. The herb pueraria (ge gen) is specifically useful for neck and shoulder conditions. It is usually taken in a formula called Pueraria Combination (Ge Gen Tang).

8. **Posture, configuration, and body movement:** Generally, individuals who are obese have excessive dampness and phlegm and are deficient in yang qi. They are likely to suffer from cardiovascular diseases. Thin individuals, on the other hand, are deficient

in essence and yin and may have symptoms of deficient heat or fire. Restlessness and outer agitation indicates yang heat, while listlessness and susceptibility to chills indicates a yin cold condition. Individuals who appear droopy and slow in their responses and movement are lacking in *qi*. Twitching of any part of the body is indicative of internal liver wind, while twitching of the lips, cheeks, eyelids, or fingers is indicative of internal wind caused by deficient blood. Arthritic or rheumatic conditions are usually classified as wind, cold, and dampness.

9. **Eyes:** Different parts of the eyes correspond to different internal organs.

RELATIONSHIP OF EYES TO THE REST OF THE BODY

EYE PART	CORRESPONDENCE	RELATED ORGAN
Canthus	Blood	Heart
Black rim of the pupil	Wind	Liver
The sclera or white part of the eye	Vital energy	Lungs
Pupil	Water	Kidneys
Eyelid	Flesh	Spleen

Vitality: The general liveliness and alertness of the eyes indicates vitality. For weakness and low vitality, such formulas as Major Four Herbs (*Si Jun Zi Tang*) or Six Major Herbs (*Liu Jun Zi Tang*) are used if there is digestive weakness; Ginseng and Astragalus Combination (*Bu Zhong Yi Qi Tang*) or Eight Precious Herbs (*Ba Zhen Tang*) are indicated if there is both *qi* and blood deficiency.

Color: Redness of the conjunctiva or whites of the eyes is an indication of heat. If it is general, it indicates lung heat; if it is more at the inner canthus near the nose, it indicates heart fire. A general redness over the entire pupil and white area is indicative of liver heat. A sty is an indication of damp heat, usually caused by too much digestive fire. In all cases, heat-clearing herbs are indicated, such Coptis and Scutellaria Combination (*Huang Lian Jie Du Tang*) and Lonicera and Forsythia Combination (*Yin Qiao San*); for damp heat, Gentiana Combination (*Long Dan Xie Gan Tang*) is used.

Puffiness or swollen eyelids: If the lower eyelids are puffy or there are swollen areas under the eyes, it indicates deficient kidney *qi* and yang, for which Rehmannia Eight Combination (*Ba Wei Di Huang Wan*) is used. Swollen upper eyelids indicate spleen dampness, for which Poria Five Herb Combination (*Wu Ling San*) can be used.

Sunken eye orbits: Sunken orbits indicate a depletion of body fluids with a deficiency of both yin and yang. Rehmannia Six Combination (*Liu Wei Di Huang Tang*) can be used for yin deficiency or Rehmannia Eight Combination (*Ba Wei Di Huang Tang*) can be used for both yin and yang deficiency.

Pterygium or fatty tissue on the eye: Pterygium may have several causes, including wind heat affecting the heart and lung or damp heat of the spleen and stomach. In either case, heat-clearing herbs are indicated, such as Coptis and Scutellaria Combination (*Huang Lian Jie Du Tang*) and Lonicera and Forsythia Combination (*Yin Qiao San*); for damp heat, Gentiana Combination (*Long Dan Xie Gan Tang*) is indicated. Another cause can be liver and kidney yin deficiency, for which Rehmannia Six Combination (*Liu Wei Di Huang Tang*) can be used.

Pupils: A markedly dilated pupil (mydriasis), when the pupil hardly contracts under exposure to light, can be determined by shining a small flashlight into the eye. This generally indicates weakness of the nervous system, opiate addiction with weakness, or injury of kidney *qi,* for which Ginseng and Dang Gui Ten Combination (*Shi Quan Da Bu Tang*) is used. Markedly contracted pupils can indicate hypertension and extreme nervousness, for which Zizyphus Combination (*Suan Zao Ren Tang*) is useful.

Eyeball motility: A fixed stare usually indicates liver wind, for which Gastrodia and Uncaria Combination (*Tian Ma Gou Teng Yin*) is used. Treatment for lethargic or half-closed eyes is the same as that for lack of vitality described above; such tonics as Astragalus Combination (*Bu Zhong Yi Qi Tang*) can be used.

Clarity and brightness: The eyes are a reflection of health and vitality. Just as the eyes are the windows of the soul, TCM believes that they are a reflection of the *shen,* or spirit. The powers of sight and hearing are governed by the strength of the kidneys–adrenals, while the eyeball itself is the domain of the liver. Blood-shot eyes, therefore, are a sign of stagnant liver heat, which is a yang condition. Weak vision indicates liver and kidney–adrenal weakness.

Physical attributes: Narrow eyes are more yang, while large, round eyes are yin. The location of the iris is important. If the eyes tend to cross inward or the irises are situated lower in the eyes with more of the whites showing above than usual, this is a more Yang indication and can indicate a more aggressive de-meanor. Weaker, more yin individuals have what the Japanese call *sanpaku* eyes, with more of the whites of the eyes showing below the irises. The condition of the eyelids indicates the spleen, while dark areas and/or bags under the eyes indicate the condition of the kidneys–adrenals. Protruding eyes are an indi-cation of a hyperthyroid condition.

10. **Nose:** The nose is governed by the lungs. A long, pointed nose can represent a yin condition, while a short, flat nose is more yang. If the nose is enlarged and red at the tip, it can be an indication of overeating and too much alcohol. A white-tipped nose indicates deficient *qi*. A shiny nose can indicate food stag-nation. Large, flaring nostrils indicate strong lungs, while small nostrils are a sign of lung weakness. If the nose fans back and forth during breathing, it is an indication of yang heat.

11. **Mouth and lips:** A big mouth is a yang sign, while a small mouth is yin. If there is a crease between the upper lip and the nose, it is an indication of problems with the reproductive or-gans. Thick lips are a yang condition, while thin lips are yin. White, pale lips are a sign of coldness and deficiency, a yin con-dition (possible anemia). Dry, chapped lips are an indication of excess heat. Blue-green lips indicate coldness or pain. Healthy red lips represent good stomach energy. If they are bright red, it can represent stomach heat, while pale lips signify a deficiency of both *qi* and blood. If the lips are more purplish, then there is blood and *qi* stagnation. Any noticeable blackish color any-where, and in this case around the lips, represents a failing of kidney–adrenal energy. The lips generally, along with the inside of the mouth, are an indication of the digestive organs, especially the stomach. If one has dry lips, mouth sores, or gum disease, it

is an indication of excess stomach heat (avoid refined foods such as sugar and spices). Dandelion-root tea is good for this condition. A swollen upper lip indicates liver imbalance, while a swollen lower lip is an imbalance of the spleen and/or intestines. Excessive salivation is a sign of spleen dampness or stomach heat. A contorted mouth is a possible sign of hemiplegia.

12. **Ears:** In general, the ears are an indication of the kidneys–adrenals. Long earlobes have always been a sign of constitutional strength and longevity. The entire ear is a microcosmic representation of a fetus, with corresponding organ areas and points that can be used for treatment. Many people wonder what the earring on the earlobe corresponds to. It relates to the eyes and power of seeing. In years past, sailors who needed to improve their distance vision at sea would tug on their earring. Redness of the ears is a sign of kidney yin deficiency. The outer rim of the ear indicates the circulatory system. When it is wide and thick, it indicates good circulation. The inner center of the ear indicates the digestive and respiratory systems. A vertical ridge from the edge of the inner ear to the earlobe indicates the strength of the digestive system. A horizontal line on the earlobe can indicate a propensity to diabetes and heart problems; a vertical line on the tragus, in front of the opening of the ear, can indicate high blood pressure and a heart problem. One method used by acupuncturists to reduce high blood pressure is to prick a small vein at the apex of the ear to extract one or a few drops of blood.

13. **Tongue:** Along with the pulse, the tongue is considered one of the most important areas for traditional diagnosis. Before the advent of technological medicine—until about 1940 or so—both tongue and pulse diagnosis were an important part of conventional Western medicine, with Western-trained doctors basing diagnosis and treatment on their observations. In observing the tongue, there are five major areas: color of the body of the tongue, size and shape, color and thickness of the coat, moistness and dryness, and location of any abnormal signs. The quality of light where the examination is conducted is important.

Color: The first and most important feature of the tongue is the color of its body. The normal color is pinkish. In general, the redder the tongue, the more heat there is, and the paler it is, the more coldness there is. Paleness also represents deficiency of *qi* and/or blood, while redness indicates excess or congestion. A darker bluish color indicates cold stagnation, while a purplish color indicates stagnation of blood and heat. Dark red represents excess heat, while bright red is deficiency heat from yin deficiency or internal wasting. A change in the color of the tongue body can indicate the depth of the disease. If it shows more pallor, it is moving toward a more yin hypotonic state. If it is redder, it is moving toward a more yang hypertonic condition. It is important to determine whether any discoloration is caused by food.

Size and shape: The second two most important tongue indications are size and shape. If the tongue appears large, it represents an abundance of yin. If it is swollen or scalloped, it represents excess dampness and/or deficient *qi*. If it is small and thin, it indicates a lack of yin. A soft, flaccid tongue also suggests deficiency, while a hard tongue represents excess.

Color and thickness of the tongue's coat: The tongue's coat represents the body's most current state, mostly of digestion. A normal tongue has a thin white coat. During illness, a thin white tongue coat can also indicate an external condition (cold or influenza). Pathologically, the tongue coat can vary from nonexistent to white, yellow, or black. A white coat indicates coldness, while yellow, brown, or black suggests heat. A thin coat is more representative of deficiency, and a thick coat is representative of excess.

Moistness or dryness: The tongue's moistness or dryness relates to excess/deficiency and cold/heat. In general, cold is associated with dampness, while heat indicates dryness. Dryness can often indicate excess, while dampness frequently represents deficiency. Water or fluid accumulation can be seen as a more immediate condition of excess, however. A moist tongue with a greasy yellowish coat represents damp heat, but moistness with a greasy white coat indicates damp cold. Since the spleen, according to traditional Chinese physiology, is responsible for the transportation and transformation of fluids, signs of excess dampness, such as an extremely moist or greasy tongue or a swollen or scalloped tongue, can indicate spleen imbalance, usually accompanied with gastrointestinal weakness and low energy.

Abnormal signs: The fifth aspect of tongue diagnosis is the location of any abnormal signs. This corresponds with the connection of each of the twelve internal organs with specific locations of the pulse. Both represent the least certainty and the area of greatest disagreement between different schools of thought. The tip of the tongue relates to the heart. When there is a remarkable appearance of redness here, it is actually a fairly reliable indication of stress and possible insomnia. The area near the front and immediately behind the tip indicates the health of the lungs. Any unusual feature, such as a rutted stripe or discoloration down the center of the tongue, is a good indication of stomach-spleen or gastrointestinal disorder. The back of the tongue relates to the kidneys, while the sides of the tongue relate to the liver and gallbladder. Some schools diagnose the liver by the right side of the tongue and the gallbladder by the left. Others diagnose both from both sides. There are those who consider the stomach to be related more to the tongue's front and the spleen to be related more to its back. There are also those who diagnose the large intestines and kidneys by the appearance of the rear of the tongue. Determination is made when there is concordance with other signs.

14. **Bodily discharges:** In general, clear or whitish discharges represent yin and coldness, while thick yellowish discharges indicate heat.

15. **Urine:** Frequent clear urine is a sign of excess yin and deficient *qi* and yang. Scanty darker yellow urine indicates excess yang and heat.

16. **Feces:** Normal evacuation is once a day. While it is normal for individuals to occasionally experience irregularity, constipation is generally a yang condition in which there is no bowel movement for 3 or more days. Occasionally, constipation can be a yin condition when someone is too weak to void. More frequent bowel movements are usually an indication of intestinal problems. Loose stool is a sign of dampness and weak digestion and assimilation (spleen *qi*).

Listening and Smelling

The patient's voice and body odors can indicate the state of health.

1. **Voice:** A loud, overbearing voice is a yang sign of excess liver stagnation. Fast speech indicates hyperactivity of the heart–mind;

slow, reluctant, and soft speech indicates deficient *qi* and yang of the heart–mind. A soft or faint voice indicates a yin condition caused by deficient *qi*. A hollow-sounding voice is a sign of deficiency of *qi* or yin. Someone who has a singsong voice that changes pitch frequently in midsentence shows an indication of spleen-digestion imbalance. An individual who has a deep, gravelly voice may have deficient kidney-adrenal Qi.

2. **Odor:** A strong smell is a yang condition.

Interrogation

Interrogation involves asking questions that provide information not readily apparent through any other method of diagnosis. This is usually the most important aspect of diagnosis, but sometimes patients either have difficulty describing their conditions or they may not be sufficiently in touch with their bodies to provide a reliable description of their conditions. It is always best, therefore, to combine interrogation with other methods of diagnosis.

1. **Main complaint:** The practitioner asks about the main complaint and how and when the symptoms were first noticed by the patient. The patient is encouraged to describe the experience of the disease rather than guess at a diagnosis, which in terms of differential diagnosis could be either misleading or simply worthless. The practitioner also asks under what circumstances, if any, symptoms seem to worsen, lessen, or abate. This could be relevant insofar as it would corroborate other diagnostic indications.

2. **Health history:** The patient's background, including past health, previous serious illnesses or accidents, and the health of the parents, grandparents, brothers, or sisters provides information as to whether the disease is as a result of previous injury, long-standing illness, or inherited conditions that tend to affect other members of the family. This can provide some important prognostic information.

3. **Chills and fever:** When chills and fever manifest simultaneously, the condition is considered an acute pernicious influence. If cold sensitivity and chills are the stronger symptoms, the condition is considered to be related to wind/cold. If fever and hy-

persensitivity to heat are primary, then a wind/heat condition is indicated. If chills and fever alternate, then the condition is considered half external cold and half hot. When fever is aggravated in the evening (yin time), the condition is more serious. If there is deficient yin, there may be a lower fever during the day or a feeling of heat in the soles and palms that is aggravated more in the afternoon or evening.

4. **Perspiration:** Heavy sweating during the day indicates deficient *qi*; heavy sweating at night signifies deficient yin. If there is no perspiration during an illness with fever and there are other external syndrome signs, then cold has obstructed the pores. Excessive perspiration, especially during a superficial acute condition, signifies heat. When the fever breaks after perspiration, the external pernicious evil has been expunged.

5. **Pain and headaches:** Examine the area where pain is occurring. Pain in the lower back, joints, or knees signify kidney–adrenal problems. Discomfort and a full feeling in the chest indicate a liver condition. Pain on the side and/or top of the head is caused by the liver or gallbladder organ meridians. Pain in the front of the head is caused by the stomach and large intestine. If the pain is more behind the frontal hairline, it may be caused by the small intestine or bladder. Dull, aching pains are chronic and can signify kidney deficiency. Sharp pains are caused by blood stagnation. Pain with a sense of heaviness and swelling is dampness, which can also be either hot or cold, according to how it appears and feels and what aggravates it. If pain is relieved by warmth or pressure, it is a *qi* deficiency pain. If it tends to come and go or move around, then it is caused by wind.

6. **Urination:** Usually, the patient can examine his or her own urine. Frequent and/or excessive urination is caused by deficient kidney yang; clear urine indicates a cold condition, while dark or reddish urine indicates heat. Scanty urination, often regarded as damp heat in the bladder, is usually caused by an excess and can indicate inflammation.

7. **Defecation:** Infrequent, hard, or dry stools indicate heat. Depending on other findings, however, it can also denote deficient fluids (dry large intestine). Loose, watery, and/or unformed stools indicate deficient *qi*, deficient yang, or dampness. Sudden

diarrhea is considered part of an excess, while chronic diarrhea indicates spleen deficiency.

8. **Diet, Appetite, and Thirst:**

   Diet: A craving for sweets is a spleen imbalance. Usually, it is caused by overconsumption of refined carbohydrates, foods, and drinks made with white sugar or a lack of sufficiently assimilable protein. The remedy is to increase one's protein intake and to eat only complex carbohydrates, such as whole grains and beans, for several days. A bitter taste in the mouth indicates liver and gallbladder heat. A sweet, pasty taste indicates damp heat in the spleen. A foul taste usually means stomach or liver heat. A lack of taste is caused by deficient spleen *qi*.

   Appetite: Problems with appetite, either too much or not enough, is a spleen–pancreas imbalance. Another cause for constant hunger can be excess stomach heat. This is usually accompanied with halitosis and possibly a bad taste in the mouth. Lack of appetite with a bloated feeling after eating is caused by spleen dampness.

   Thirst: If there is extreme thirst, it is a yang indication of heat or yin deficiency. A lack of thirst is an excess yin condition. Thirst with no desire to drink indicates internal dampness.

9. **Sleep:** Insomnia or restless sleep is generally caused by deficient heart blood or yin. Excessive sleepiness and/or sleepiness after eating can be caused by deficient yang, deficient *qi*, or dampness.

10. **Menses and leukorrhea:** Early menstrual periods indicate heat, while late ones indicate deficient blood or cold causing stagnation. Irregular periods are caused by stagnant liver *qi*. Excessive menstruation can be a sign of heat in the blood or deficient *qi* or yang. Insufficient flow or lack of menses may indicate deficient blood, cold obstructing the blood or stagnant blood. Very dark blood indicates heat. Light-colored thin blood indicates deficiency. Purplish blood, especially if clotted, may indicate stagnant or congealed blood. Thin, clear, whitish discharges are generally a sign of dampness and deficiency. Thick yellow discharges accompanied with itching and irritation of the vagina indicate damp heat.

11. **Emotional tendencies:** The Seven Emotions (discussed in Chapter 3) are considered a primary cause of internal or chronic

disease. An excessive indulgence of these feelings can serve as both a cause of and diagnostic indication of an imbalance in the corresponding organ. Briefly, their effects are as follows:

- Anger can injure and affect the liver.
- Worry or thinking too much (pensiveness) can injure and affect the spleen–pancreas.
- Fear, fright, and insecurity can injure and affect the kidneys–adrenals.
- Joy and excessive celebration can injure and affect the heart–mind.
- Sadness and grief can injure and affect the lungs.

12. **Miscellany:** In addition, there are other questions whose answers can indicate various internal imbalances. A feeling of a lack of energy indicates deficient *qi*. This usually indicates spleen–pancreas deficiency, kidney–adrenal deficiency, or it may indicate heart–mind deficiency when there is corresponding coldness (possible low thyroid), or liver *qi* stagnation when *qi* deficiency is accompanied with fits of moodiness and depression. A reliance on coffee is also often an indication of *qi* deficiency.

Palpation

The pulse represents one of the most definitive diagnostic tools of TCM. Many skilled practitioners can use it in combination with their intuitive skills to make remarkable diagnostic determinations not only of current imbalances and past diseases but, more importantly, of ones that will occur if remedial measures are not taken in the present. Such a high level of skill and mastery comes only after many years of practice. There are some immediate pulse qualities that are really quite easy to learn, however. These are rate of speed, depth, degree of strength, and fullness.

To take your own pulse, begin by locating the radial artery on your right wrist. Place your right palm lightly against your chest. Reach around from the top with your left hand and place the index finger of your left hand just above your right wrist at the base of its thumb. Your left hand's middle finger will naturally fall on the bony protuberance felt immediately next to the index finger and your fourth ring finger will find the shallow indentation proximal to the body and next to the middle finger. There are six places to palpate on each wrist, corresponding to six different internal organs on the right wrist and six on the left.

For practice, focus more on the easier-to-feel pulse located under your middle finger. The deep pulse is located by pressing down until the pulse is hardly perceptible. Then slowly release the pressure upward a little. At this level, you feel the strength of the body's internal organs, which indicates the yin power of the body. Next, release the pressure of the middle finger so that the pulse is felt more closely on the surface of the skin. This is the yang surface pulse and indicates the body's eliminative strength to overcome such external diseases as colds, influenza, skin diseases, and minor arthritic aches and pains. Then reverse your hands' positions and compare the pulse of your left hand to that of your right. Generally, men's pulses are stronger on the left and represent qi, while women's pulses are stronger on the right and represent blood. Later, with a good deal of practice and experience, you can learn to evaluate the relative strength or weakness of the individual organs by the pulse. It often takes many years to develop a clinical proficiency at recognizing some of the pulses.

To practice pulse taking, keep a record of at least five pulses that you take each day. Note your findings, even if at first you can barely discern any differences. Eventually, you will be able to distinguish the relative strength and weakness appropriate for each position and depth. Any unusual difference in strength or fullness in any area on the wrist corresponding to one of the twelve organs can, together with other indications, confirm an imbalance in a specific organ.

Easiest to learn in pulse diagnosis is assessing the overall quality in terms of rate, emptiness or fullness, and whether the pulse is stronger on the surface or at the deeper location:

Rate: Using a timepiece with a second hand, count the number of pulse beats for 15 seconds. Multiply this times 4. If the pulse is slower than 60, it is a slow pulse that signifies yin coldness. If it is 80 or faster, it indicates yang heat.

Emptiness or fullness: Find someone who appears thinner, more yin, and timid in temperament and compare his or her pulse with that of another who appears heavier, more yang, and more outgoing and aggressive. You might have to practice on two or three sets of different individuals, but generally, you will learn to recognize the fuller pulse in the yang-type person and the more thin and empty pulse in the yin-type person.

Location: If the pulse is stronger on the surface, it indicates a yang-type imbalance, such as a cold, influenza, a skin disease, or acute rheumatic pains. If the pulse is stronger at the deep position, it indicates a more chronic yin fullness involving the emotions and the internal organs. Practice by deliberately feeling the pulse of someone with a cold or influenza and compare it to that of another who appears weaker and has a more chronic complaint.

Many times there is a combination of yin and yang pulses, such as a fast and deep pulse, a surface and empty pulse, a slow and superficial pulse, and so on. For combination pulses, memorize the following:

FAST PULSE = HEAT
SLOW PULSE = COLD
SUPERFICIAL PULSE = EXTERNAL ACUTE CONDITION
DEEP PULSE = INTERNAL CHRONIC CONDITION
EMPTY OR THIN PULSE = DEFICIENT
FULL PULSE = EXCESS

Some combinations of the above are:

DEEP, FULL, AND FAST PULSE = INTERNAL EXCESS HEAT
Therapeutic principle: Clear internal excess heat.
Possible conditions: Constipation, urinary tract infection, or other internal inflammations.
Possible dietary and herbal treatment: Lighter diet, fruit juice fast, raw or cooked vegetables, lighter vegetable proteins, laxative herbs such as cascara or rhubarb (*da huang*).

DEEP, EMPTY, AND SLOW PULSE = INTERNAL DEFICIENT COLD
Therapeutic principle: Clear internal deficient cold.
Possible conditions: Hypoadrenal, hypothyroid, digestive weakness, low energy.
Possible dietary and herbal treatment: Warm proteinaceous foods; such tonics as ginseng, codonopsis, *dang gui,* cinnamon, and prepared aconite for internal warming.

DEEP, FULL, AND SLOW PULSE = INTERNAL EXCESS COLD
Therapeutic principle: Clear internal cold excess.
Possible conditions: Hypoadrenal, hypothyroid, digestive weakness, congestion.
Possible dietary and herbal treatment: Light warm foods, meat soups, such herbs as atractylodes, ginger, cinnamon, and aconite.

SUPERFICIAL, FULL, AND FAST PULSE = EXTERNAL EXCESS HEAT
Therapeutic principle: Clear external excess heat.
Possible conditions: Influenza, meningitis, eruptive skin diseases, sore throat.
Possible dietary and herbal treatment: Lonicera and Forsythia Combination (*Yin Qiao San*).

SUPERFICIAL, FULL, AND SLOW PULSE = EXTERNAL EXCESS COLD
Therapeutic principle: Clear external excess cold.
Possible conditions: Cold, influenza, skin eruptions, acute rheumatic pain.
Possible dietary and herbal treatment: Ephedra Combination (*Ma Huang Tang*) or Pueraria Combination (*Ge Gen Tang*).

FAST AND EMPTY PULSE = DEFICIENT HEAT (YIN DEFICIENCY)
Therapeutic principle: Clear deficient heat, tonify yin.
Possible dietary and herbal treatment: More nourishing, mucilaginous foods; yin tonics.

SLOW AND SUPERFICIAL PULSE = EXTERNAL COLDNESS
Therapeutic principle: Warm external coldness.
Possible dietary and herbal treatment: Avoid cold, raw foods; have warm ginger and cinnamon tea.

SLOW AND DEEP PULSE = INTERNAL COLDNESS
Therapeutic principle: Warm internal coldness.
Possible dietary and herbal treatment: Avoid cold, raw foods; include ginger, cinnamon, and garlic in the diet; take yang herbal tonics.

SLOW AND FULL PULSE = INTERNAL EXCESS
Therapeutic principle: Clear internal excess.
Possible dietary and herbal treatment: Reduce intake of heavy, rich

foods; have less protein, less flesh foods, and little or no dairy; use internal cleansing formulas such as Triphala and foods that gently reduce excess throughout the body.

SLOW AND DEFICIENT PULSE = COLD DEFICIENCY
Therapeutic principle: Tonify and warm spleen and kidney yang.
Possible dietary and herbal treatment: Proteinaceous, cooked foods; no cold, raw foods or drinks; *qi* and yang tonics.

EMPTY AND DEEP PULSE = INTERNAL DEFICIENCY
Therapeutic principle: Blood and/or *qi* deficiency.
Possible dietary and herbal treatment: More nutritious foods and assimilable protein; Blood and *qi* tonics.

EMPTY AND FAST PULSE = DEFICIENT HEAT (YIN DEFICIENCY)
Therapeutic principle: Tonify yin.
Possible dietary and herbal treatment: No spicy foods; more nutritious foods and protein; mochi (pounded rice) and okra; yin tonics.

FULL AND DEEP PULSE = INTERNAL EXCESS
Therapeutic principle: Clear internal excess.
Possible dietary and herbal treatment: Reducing formulas and possibly laxatives.

· FIVE ·

DIAGNOSTIC SYSTEMS

While Chinese herbal medicine classifies and uses herbs from neighboring as well as more distant countries, such as American ginseng *(Panax quinquefolium)* from the eastern seaboard of the North American continent, its traditional diagnostic systems are its greatest legacy. It is the classification and diagnostic systems of traditional Chinese medicine (TCM) for the use of herbs and substances from around the world that I call planetary herbalism. If we confine ourselves to naming specific diseases, we are limited to finding specific remedies for each specific disease. Diagnosis through pattern recognition allows us to find treatments for many conditions for which there are no specific individual remedies. These can range from complex chronic and degenerative diseases to common acute diseases such as the common cold, for which TCM has many effective herbal treatments. Pattern recognition also allows us to see how one formula can be adapted to treat many diseases that share similar patterns. An example is Pueraria Combination *(Ge Gen Tang)*, which can be used to treat the common cold, coughs, stiff neck and shoulders, headaches, many gastrointestinal complaints, and in fact many diseases that result in physical injury and are caused by external physical or emotional stress. There are at least 250 to 300 Chinese herbs whose use is standard and literally thousands of treasured formulas that have been passed down through the ages. The mastery of even a single formula, such as Pueraria Combination or others described in this book, can impart great authority and produce highly effective results.

The diagnostic systems of TCM were not all created at the same time but evolved over centuries, refined in critical debates among highly revered Chinese herbalists. Currently, there are ten types of diagnostic strategies used:

- Eight Principles (*ba gang bian zheng*)
- Symptom–sign organ pattern diagnosis (*zang fu bian zheng*)
- Six stages based on the *shang han lun* (*liu jing bian zheng*)
- Four stages of heat (*wei qi ying xue bian zheng*)
- Three Heater discrimination (*san jiao bian zheng*)
- Disease discrimination (*bing yin bian zheng*)
- Qi and blood pattern discrimination (*qi xue bian zheng*)
- Three Humor diagnosis (*jin ye bian zheng*)
- Five Element discrimination (*wu xing bian zheng*)
- Meridian and connecting vessel discrimination (*jing luo bian zheng*)

These diagnostic strategies are hardly ever exclusive of each other, tending to overlap in practice. As Bob Flaws, a contemporary TCM practitioner, author and editor of numerous books published by Blue Poppy Press, so aptly describes them, each diagnostic approach is like a diagnostic tool that an experienced TCM practitioner may use according to which is better suited to the patient's condition. The practitioner can then arrive at the most appropriate diagnosis and therapeutic approach.

In this chapter we will discuss the three primary diagnostic strategies—Eight Principles, Symptom sign organ diagnosis and Three Humor diagnosis—because these embody all the others.

The Eight Principles

The Eight Principles are the most fundamental diagnostic evaluation and in most cases are sufficient to provide a complete approach to treatment. Further, the system provides an overview, while symptom–sign organ pattern diagnosis allows us to get even closer to the direct causes of a specific disease:

- External: acute diseases
- Hot: overly active metabolism
- Excess: sthenic
- Yang: hypermetabolic (sthenic)
- Internal: mostly chronic diseases
- Cold: low metabolism
- Deficient: asthenic
- Yin: hypometabolic (asthenic)

The classification of herbs as hot or cold in terms of their energies, external or internal in terms of the depth of their penetration, and eliminating or tonifying and the summation of the above as yang or yin are what make TCM highly promising and effective in treating diseases that may not be amenable to other therapeutic modalities. Because of this, it is possible to form a treatment strategy based on direct observation and diagnosis.

There are essentially two approaches to diagnosis and treatment. One is based on treating the named disease, while the other is based on treating according to pattern identification. This gives rise to the principle "one disease, many formulas, one formula, many diseases." What this means is that a specific named disease can be treated only according to a holistic differential diagnosis. It also means that a single herbal formula can be suitable for treating several diseases. The Eight Principles represent the foundation in TCM for all the diagnostic approaches. First articulated during the seventeenth century, the Eight Principles present a relatively clear approach to discerning the overall yin–yang balance of the body. This is then further elucidated, if necessary, by other diagnostic systems, including the Three Humors (blood, qi, and fluid) and symptom–sign organ classifications. The Eight Principles consist of exterior/interior, cold/heat, deficiency/excess, and yin/yang. The latter represents the overall state reflected by a preponderance of the other six principles. Because some Eight Principle symptoms can be apparent or true (sometimes called false or genuine), some practitioners consider these as important to consider in their own right. The conditions associated with the Eight Principles are shown in the table below.

THE EIGHT PRINCIPLES AND DIAGNOSIS

PRINCIPLE	CHARACTERISTICS	REPRESENTATIVE CONDITIONS
EXTERNAL	Initial stage of acute disease, chills, skin diseases. Usually contracted from exposure to one or a number of external factors such as wind, cold, or heat.	Colds, influenza, fevers, headache, respiratory congestion, eruptive skin diseases
INTERNAL	Chronic diseases involving the internal organs. Often caused by overexertion, emotional stress, imbalanced diet, and other debilitating influences.	Chronic digestive, eliminative, urinary, reproductive, and neurological diseases
HEAT	An excess of yang or a deficiency of yin will both give rise to symptoms of heat.	High fevers, inflammation, infections, sensitivity to heat and hot weather, flushed complexion, yellow or blood-tinged discharges
COLD	Either an excess of yin or a deficiency of yang will cause cold symptoms.	Chills; lack of thirst; pale complexion; cold sensitivity; any anemic, low, or "hypo-" condition, including hypothyroid and hypoadrenalism; clear or whitish discharges
EXCESS	The strong, exuberant manifestation of pathological conditions	Obesity; constipation; hypertension; high fever; severe infections; sharp, stabbing pain; mania; full, strong pulse; thick, greasy tongue "fur"
DEFICIENCY	A lack of qi, lowered immunity, weak bodily functions	Thinness, fatigue, shortness of breath, cold intolerance, anorexia, dyspepsia, loose stool, frequent and clear urine,

PRINCIPLE	CHARACTERISTICS	REPRESENTATIVE CONDITIONS
		afternoon fevers, a sensation of heat or burning of the soles and/or palms
YANG	Symptoms of external influences, heat, and excess	Diseases associated with an abhorrence of heat; fever, thirst; desire for cold drinks; hot skin, muscles, and extremities; yellow or blood-tinged discharges; constipation; concentrated, dark yellow urine; aggressive manner and loud voice; rapid, full pulse; red tongue with yellow "fur"
YIN	Symptoms of internal influences, cold, and deficiency	Diseases associated with cold intolerance; cold skin, muscles, and extremities; lack of thirst; desire for hot drinks; clear or whitish discharges; loose stools; clear or pale urine; shallow breath; timid, shy demeanor; weak, hollow, slow pulse; pale tongue with white coat

Yin and Yang, as a summation of the previous six principles, are even more important in their relationship to each other. Thus, a deficiency of yang will result in an excess of yin, which can be viewed in context either as a yin excess or a yang deficiency. A deficiency of yin can be viewed as either an apparent excess of yang or a deficiency of yin. A chronic fever or inflammatory condition arising as a result of wasting disease or severe weakness is commonly referred to as yin deficiency, but it can also be called apparent yang or false yang. A person with an excess-type overburdened body, whose systems begin to fail as a result of severe congestion or blockage and manifest, for instance, physical coldness or dampness, might be said to have yang deficiency, apparent yin or false yin. Wasting diseases, such as tuberculosis and acquired immunodeficiency syndrome (AIDS) are examples of yin deficiency, while symptoms of hypothyroid with fluid retention is an example of yang deficiency.

The Three Humors: *Qi,* Blood, and Fluid

Qi, blood, and fluid represent all basic physiological processes of the body. While they are included with much of what has been previously described in the Eight Principles, they represent another approach to arriving at an effective herbal treatment that may not be as obvious in any of the other systems. For instance, an individual who might be considered as deficient according to the Eight Principles might be seen more specifically as having *qi* or blood deficiency, according to Three Humors diagnosis. Conditions associated with *qi,* blood, or phlegm stagnation are better understood in the context of the Three Humors rather than of the Eight Principles. To understand a given condition, according to TCM, specifically means that it allows one to efficiently arrive at an effective herbal and dietary treatment strategy.

Qi Diseases

Qi imbalances can manifest in seven ways.

QI DEFICIENCY

Symptoms of *qi* deficiency include low energy, physical weakness, shortness of breath, timidity, soft-spokenness, pale complexion, dizziness, tinnitus, palpitations, easy perspiration during the slightest physical exertion. Because *qi* is considered the "commander of blood," there may also be bleeding disorders, such as menstrual flooding or blood in the nose, sputum, urine, stool, and so on. Herbs that treat *qi* deficiency include ginseng *(ren shen),* astragalus root *(huang qi),* and dioscorea *(shan yao).* Formulas are usually based on Four Major Herbs (*Si Jun Zi Tang*).

WEAK DIGESTION, GAS, AND BLOATING CAUSED BY QI DEFICIENCY

Other symptoms of *qi* deficiency are abdominal bloating, gas, weak digestion, lack of appetite, pale complexion and lips, desire for warmth and pressure on the abdomen, white and moist tongue coat, and a pulse that is weak, large, slippery, and/or hollow. Herbs that treat *qi* deficiency are those that clear abdominal fluid, such as pinellia *(ban xia),* and carminative or *qi*-regulating herbs, such as citrus peel *(chen pi),* cardamon (sha ren), saussurea root (mu xiang), or fresh ginger (sheng jiang). Representative formulas include Six Major Herbs Combination (Liu Jun Zi Tang) and Six Major Herbs with Saussurea and Cardamon (Xiang Sha Liu Jun Zi Tang).

SINKING OF SPLEEN QI OR COLLAPSE OF QI

Symptoms of spleen qi deficiency are loose stools, diarrhea, frequent urination, and a downward feeling in the abdomen. These symptoms are often associated with prolapse of the internal organs of the stomach, intestines, and uterus. Qi tonics mentioned above are indicated, as are other herbs that have an upward energy, such as astragalus root (huang qi) and bupleurum root (chai hu). A representative formula for this condition is Ginseng and Astragalus Combination (Bu Zhong Yi Qi Tang), also called Elixir of Life in the Planetary Formulas line.

QI STAGNATION

Qi stagnation is characterized by local pain and distension. Herbs that promote qi circulation include citrus peel (chen pi), cyperus (xiang fu), Cardamon (sha ren), saussurea root (mu xiang), and medicated leaven (shen qu). A representative formula for this condition would be Pills to Relieve Stagnation of All Kinds (Yue Qu Wan).

QI DEPRESSION

Qi depression is characterized by emotional depression and is frequently seen in the premenstrual phase of the menstrual cycle and during menopause. Herbs such as bupleurum (chai hu) and cyperus (xiang fu) are used to regulate and open liver qi, which is responsible for the smooth flow of qi. The most representative formula is Bupleurum and Dang Gui Combination (Xiao Yao Wan), also known as Bupleurum Calmative in Planetary Formulas.

UPRISING QI

Uprising qi refers to imbalances that are mostly associated with the lung and stomach. If the lung adversely rebels or uprises, symptoms include shortness of breath and cough. When the stomach adversely rebels, symptoms include belching, hiccups, nausea, and vomiting. Herbs that have a downward energy are indicated according to the organ(s) involved. For the lung, pinellia *(ban xia)* is used. For the stomach, black bamboo shavings *(zhu ru)* and the calyx of the persimmon (especially good for hiccups) are used. Representative formulas are Pinellia and Magnolia Combination *(Ban Xia Hou Po Tang)* and Citrus Peel and Bamboo Shavings Combination *(Ju Pi Zhu Ru Tang)*.

FEVER CAUSED BY *QI* DEFICIENCY

Low energy is usually associated with cold; however, in some conditions, this can lead to heat and fever. Because the underlying cause is *qi* deficiency, it can be associated with perspiration, shortness of breath, extreme fatigue, thirst, and a desire for warm drinks. Ginseng *(ren shen)* or American ginseng *(xi yang shen)*, which are usually contraindicated for fevers and inflammations, can be effectively used for this condition.

Blood Diseases

BLOOD DEFICIENCY

Symptoms of blood deficiency reflect anemia and include pale complexion and lips, dizziness, insomnia, numbness of the extremities, and thready, weak pulse. Because blood is considered the "mother of *qi*," blood deficiency is often accompanied with either or both *qi* and yang deficiency. Blood deficiency can also be the underlying cause of an anemic fever that is accompanied with a flushed face, thirst, and other anemic symptoms described above. Treatment of blood deficiency requires herbs and substances that enrich blood, such as rehmannia *(shu di huang)*, *dang gui (Angelica sinensis)*, and lycii berries *(gou qi zi)*, and blood tonic formulas, such as Dang Gui Four *(Si Wu Tang)*.

BLOOD STAGNATION

Blood stagnation can be the result of blood deficiency, *qi* deficiency, or internal coldness. It can manifest in various areas of the body with symptoms such as irregular, painful menstruation and abdominal and chest pains. Various formulas can be used, but again, the representative formula is Dang Gui Four *(Si Wu Tang)*, with ginseng *(ren shen)* added if there is *qi* deficiency and cinnamon bark *(rou gui)* and prepared aconite *(fu zi)* added if there is internal coldness. Herbs that invigorate the blood are also used.

Fluid Conditions

FLUID DEFICIENCY

The primary characteristic of fluid deficiency is dryness, which can manifest on the skin or lips or in the throat or reproductive organs. There may also be dry constipation or dry tongue with a thready, rapid pulse. Demulcent and lubricating herbs, such as apricot seed (xing ren) and tiger lily bulb (bai he) for the lungs and flax or psyllium seeds for the intestines, are used. Representative formulas include Apricot Seed and Perilla Formula (Xing Su San) and Lily Bulb Decoction to Consolidate the Lungs (Bai He Gu Jin Tang).

EXCESS DAMPNESS

Fluid retention or edema is the most characteristic symptom of excess dampness. Herbs such as poria cocos (fu ling) and polyporus mushrooms (zhu ling) are used to drain dampness. The representative formula is Poria Five Herb Combination (Wu Ling San).

PHLEGM

In Chinese herbalism, phlegm has two general forms, visible and invisible. Visible phlegm is associated with the upper-respiratory system of the lungs, bronchioles, and sinuses and can be heated (inflamed) or cold. Invisible phlegm can have many serious manifestations, including enlarged thyroid, swollen glands, impaired consciousness, epilepsy, and stroke. Symptoms include a greasy tongue coat and a slippery or gliding pulse. Pinellia and ginger are two major herbs used for phlegm. The representative formula for phlegm conditions is Citrus and Pinellia Combination (Er Chen Tang, or Two Cured Decoction). There are countless variations of this formula, making it suitable for all conditions associated with phlegm. In its unaltered form, however, it is primarily useful for treating cold phlegm. For heated phlegm, such herbs as black bamboo shavings (zhu ru) and a cool-natured formula such as Bamboo and Poria Combination (Wen Dan Tang) are used. For swollen thyroid or goiter, kelp laminaria (kun bu) and/or sargassum seaweeds (hai zao) are used. The representative formula is Seaweed Decoction (Hai Zao Yu Wu Tang).

Organ Syndromes

The organ syndromes represent twelve organ meridians to which the Eight Principles may be applied to identify pathological change. Despite the fact that the organs are identified according to Western anatomical names, their meaning includes and often extends far beyond localized somatic structures. The yin and yang organs represent not only specific organ functions and processes but also territories or terrains, called meridians, which form the basis of TCM acupuncture. In TCM herbalism, the functional processes of the organs are of far greater importance than their relation to the accompanying meridians. For the beginner, the use of Western anatomical organ names and the fact that only twelve organs are delineated may pose some confusion. Always pragmatic, the ancient Chinese included only as much factual information in their calculations as was necessary to arrive at an effective treatment. For this reason, many of the symptomatic correspondences associated with each TCM organ, such as the ears and hearing with the kidneys, the mental faculties with the heart, and the skin with the lungs, may not be immediately apparent from a Western anatomical consideration. In fact, these relationships represent profound observations by the ancient Chinese, who in different periods were specifically prohibited from dissecting the bodies of the dead. When we subject even the most minute correspondences to the most rigorous physiological scrutiny using contemporary standards, it is amazing how the Chinese were able to closely define the correspondences through empirical observation.

As an example, the relation of the ears with the strength of the TCM kidneys has to do with the hormonal relationship governing calcium metabolism and the fact that the ears contain the finest bones of the body (called the incus and the stapes). If the kidney–adrenal function is diminished, these bones are most likely to become weakened as a result of poor calcium assimilation. All traditional cultures postulate a relationship between the mind and the heart. Only in the most advanced reasoning of Western physiology have such relationships been recognized on the hormonal level, but only because the preponderance of blood required by the brain for normal function necessitates a strong heart impulse to sufficiently regulate its presence in that part of the body. Thus, a lack of heart blood in TCM terms is in fact accompanied by forgetfulness. These are only a few of the TCM correspondences that can be corroborated in Western physiology.

The twelve TCM organs form an interior–exterior relationship in the body as shown in the table below.

ॐ

INTERNAL–EXTERNAL RELATIONSHIPS OF ORGANS

YIN ORGAN	YANG ORGAN
Heart	Small intestine
Pericardium	Triple Warmer
Lungs	Stomach
Spleen	Large intestine
Liver	Gallbladder
Kidneys	Urinary bladder

ॐ

The twelve organs of Chinese medicine, divided as the six yin organs of transformation and the six yang organs of transportation, refer to a functional matrix of interdependent processes that extend beyond the meaning of their specific physiological structures. Following is a description of the twelve TCM Organs.

Yin Organs

HEART

The heart is the king or chief of all the organs because it regulates them by controlling the circulation of blood. Its main functions are to govern blood and blood vessels and to house the spirit, or mind (shen). The heart coordinates the processes of the mind, which are emotions and sensations. Symptoms of heart disharmonies include palpitations, insomnia, chest pains, excessive chatter, mental confusion, and panic. The heart is particularly vulnerable to heat. TCM imbalances of the heart include basic heart symptoms plus the following:

- Deficient heart qi with low energy and coldness
- Deficient heart blood with paleness, insomnia, forgetfulness, dizziness, and thin pulse
- Deficient heart yin with deficient heart blood symptoms plus red tongue, night sweats, warm palms and soles, and malar flush

- Congealed heart blood with palpitations; purple face, lips, and nails; irregular pulse; and stabbing pains
- Cold mucus confusing the heart openings, with abnormal behavior, coma, muttering to oneself, and thick white tongue "moss"
- Hot mucus confusing the heart openings, with incessant talking; abnormal, irrational behavior; agitated manner; and yellow, thick tongue "moss"
- Hyperactivity of the heart's fire with dark yellow urine, red tongue, rapid pulse, flushed face, and swelling and pain of the mouth and tongue

PERICARDIUM

The pericardium is the sac, or outer shield, surrounding the heart. It protects the heart—thus the term *heart protector*. It is considered the sixth yin organ, although in theory, it is not distinguished from the heart except as the first line of defense against external pernicious influences. Thus, rather than heat attacking the heart, the high fever, coma, and red tongue in febrile diseases are described as the attack on the pericardium by pathogenic heat. Other than this, there are no patterns of disharmony given for the pericardium.

LUNGS

The lungs control vital energy in the body. They extract *qi* from the air during respiration and transfer it through the respiratory passages to the blood, with which it is then circulated throughout the body. The lungs also have direct contact with the outer environment through breathing, so they are considered to be directly related to the skin. Because of this, they are the most prone to external pernicious influences and thus are often called a delicate organ, or the "princess" of the organs. The lungs are also the uppermost organ in the body and consequently are often termed a "lid" on the other organs. They are particularly susceptible to wind and coldness. Symptoms of lung disharmonies include cough; mucus in the sinuses, throat, bronchioles, and lungs; shortness of breath; vulnerability to colds and influenza; melancholy (sadness); and skin eruptions. TCM imbalances of the lungs include the following:

- Coldness in the lungs with chills, clear phlegm and sputum, body aches, and stuffy, runny nose

- Heat in the lungs with high fever, thirst, perspiration, constipation, shortness of breath, and yellow or blood-tinged sputum
- External wind in the lungs with an itchy throat and possibly fever and chills. Symptoms of wind with cold include coldness and chills, thin white tongue coat, clear sputum and mucus, and thin white nasal discharge. Symptoms of wind with heat include high fever, yellow tongue coat, sore throat, and yellow purulent phlegm
- Deficient lung *qi* with low energy, lowered resistance to colds and influenza, and weak cough
- Deficient lung yin with wasting and emaciation; bloody sputum; thin, rapid pulse; red cheeks and malar flush; night sweats; afternoon fever; red tongue with dry "moss"; dry, unproductive cough; and feverish sensation on the palms and the soles
- Damp phlegm in the lungs with a lot of phlegm; wheezing or asthma; increased difficulty breathing when reclining; thick, greasy, or sticky tongue "moss"; and slippery pulse

SPLEEN

The spleen is the primary organ for digestion in the body. It rules transformation and transportation, which can be loosely translated as metabolism and absorption. It is the crucial link between the transformation of food and drink into *qi* and blood for the entire body. The spleen, together with the stomach, is considered the root of postheaven *qi*, or the source of all *qi* produced by the body after birth. Thus, it is of central importance in the health of the body. The spleen is particularly injured by dampness, which means humid environment or highly moist foods. Symptoms of spleen disharmonies include digestive problems, appetite irregularities (too much or too little), abdominal distension, excessive weight gain or inability to gain weight, diarrhea, a tendency to dwell too long on things, and a feeling of heaviness and laziness. TCM imbalances of the spleen include basic spleen symptoms plus the following:

- Deficient spleen *qi* with low energy, loose stools, lack of appetite, and lassitude. The symptoms of deficient spleen *qi* with prolapse include prolapsed uterus, intestines, or other internal organs; hemorrhage; urinary incontinence; and chronic diarrhea
- Deficient spleen yang with cold extremities; edema; swollen, moist,

pale tongue; leukorrhea; loose stools; and abdominal distension that responds positively to heat

- Dampness of the spleen with lack of appetite, nausea, lack of taste sensation, loose stools, general lassitude, lack of thirst, abdominal fullness and pain, slippery pulse, and wet, swollen tongue with scalloped edges
- Damp heat of the spleen has the symptoms of inflammation, jaundice, and bitter taste in the mouth

LIVER

The main function of the liver is to regulate the smooth flow and proper direction of qi and blood throughout the body. Because of this, it is likened to an army general, as it is responsible for the overall planning (or strategy) of the body's functions. Further, it stores blood and regulates the amount of blood circulated by the heart. Liver stagnation and excess cause feelings of anger and depression. A balanced liver and gallbladder are responsible for courage. Symptoms of liver imbalance are depression, moodiness, pain or discomfort in the chest, anger, and the stagnation symptoms of pain, gas, belching, intestinal rumbling, and diarrhea. TCM imbalances of the liver include the following:

- Deficient liver blood with pale, lusterless face; blurred vision; pale fingernails; dizziness; dryness of the eyes; thin pulse; and dry tongue
- Deficient liver yin with depression, reddish tongue, muddled vision, red cheeks, afternoon fever, hot palms and soles, hypertension, red tongue, and thin, quick pulse
- Liver fire rising with hypertension, splitting headaches, red face and eyes, insomnia, irritability, frequent and sudden bursts of anger, feeling of discomfort in the head, dizziness, tinnitus, and epistaxis
- Arrogant liver yang with symptoms of both liver fire with deficient yin and throbbing headache, periodic hot flushes in the head and face, anger, and depression
- Constrained or stagnant liver qi with belching; gas; chest discomfort; depression; feeling of something (like a pit) stuck in the throat; irregular menses; distension or lumps in the breast, groin, or neck; and wiry or tight pulse
- Liver invading the spleen has the above symptoms plus digestive upset, nausea, vomiting, abdominal pain, and sour belching

- Internal liver wind with spasms, tetany, epilepsy, Parkinson's syndrome, poststroke syndrome, convulsions, Bell's palsy, and coma
- Cold in the liver with pain and distension in the lower side and groin or testicles (hernia) that is relieved by heat; deep, slow, and wiry pulse; and pale, moist tongue "moss"

KIDNEYS

The kidneys store preheaven essence, or *jing,* the refined aspect that represents our essential "inherited" constitutional strength and that forms the material foundation for yin and yang. Thus, the kidneys are considered to be the root of yin and yang for the entire body. Kidney yin provides the material foundation for kidney yang, while kidney yang provides the heat and movement for kidney yin. Because they have the same source, they are interdependent: a depletion of one creates a deficiency in the other and vice versa. Thus, when strengthening kidney yin, one also tonifies kidney yang, and vice versa. Further, the kidneys are the source of water and fire in the body: water because of essence and being part of the water element; fire because the kidneys house the life gate fire of the body. Symptoms of kidney imbalance include lower back pain, joint pains, knee pains, retarded growth, poor hearing, urinary problems, paranoia, apathy, and despair. TCM imbalances of the kidneys include basic kidney symptoms plus the following:

- Deficient kidney *qi* with low energy, frequent urination, infertility, dribbling of urine after urination, and possibly asthma caused by weakness of the kidneys
- Deficient kidney yang with kidney deficiency plus coldness, coldness of the lower back and waist, impotence, frigidity, and sterility
- Deficient kidney yin with emaciation; night sweats; hot palms and soles; forgetfulness; constipation; malar flush; dizziness; dry throat; dark yellow urine; thin, rapid pulse; and ringing in the ears or hearing loss

Yang Organs

While the yin organs, responsible for transforming energy, are the most frequently used in TCM diagnosis and treatment, the yang organs are also important. The yang organs of transport are responsible for receiving, digesting, excreting, rotting, ripening, transforming, transporting, and waste management. With all the yang organs, except the gallbladder, this has to do with food and drink and their waste products. Yang organs include the small intestine, triple warmer, stomach, large intestine, gallbladder, and urinary bladder. Of all the yang organs, the stomach, sharing the responsibility for digestion with the spleen, is the most important. Together with the spleen, it is known as the "root of postheaven *qi*" because the essence of the digested food and fluids ultimately is transformed into the *qi* and blood of the body. Thus, proper digestion is essential for the production of *qi* and blood and the subsequent nourishment of all the organs in the body.

SMALL INTESTINE

The small intestine receives the partially decomposed food from the stomach and further digests and absorbs it by separating the pure part from the waste. According to the TCM model, the pure part is sent to the spleen, which then transports and distributes it throughout the body. The impure part is sent down to the large intestine, where it is further separated into pure and impure portions before the waste is excreted. The impure waters are sent from the small intestine to the urinary bladder to be excreted from the body. In normal function, this results in smooth urination and normal elimination of feces. With disharmony, water is mixed with waste, leading to dysuria, loose stools, constipation, diarrhea, intestinal rumblings, and abdominal distension and pain.

TRIPLE WARMER

The Triple Warmer, also known as the Three Heater or Triple Burner, is more of an organic function rather than a specific organ. It is a perspective involving the coordination of three bodily areas: Upper Warmer, which is the heart, lung, pericardium, throat, and head; the Middle Warmer, which extends from the diaphragm to the umbilicus and houses the spleen, stomach, and gallbladder; and the Lower Warmer, which comprises the lower abdominal area below the umbilicus, housing the liver, kidney, urinary bladder, intestines, and uterus. The liver is included in the Lower Warmer because of its close relationship with the kidney rather than because of its physiological placement in the body. Pathologically, diseases of the Upper, Middle, or Lower

Warmer are considered to involve a dysfunction of the organs contained within that warmer.

STOMACH

It is in the stomach that the important process of ripening and rotting occurs. The impure portion of foods and beverages is sent to the small intestine for further digestion, while the pure portion goes to the spleen. Of course, this is not anatomically correct, since we know that both the spleen and the liver secrete important digestive enzymes to aid assimilation in the small intestine, so the TCM description describes an energetic relationship between the stomach and the spleen. Both organs receive energy but the TCM spleen goes to a deeper cellular level of assimilation. Unlike the spleen, the stomach does not like to be hot or dry and prefers moisture.

Improper diet is the main cause of stomach disorders. Foods that are heating, drying, greasy, spicy, or cold and iced upset the stomach. Poor eating habits, such as working, driving, or standing while eating, eating at irregular times, and over- or undereating, also disrupt stomach functions. Excessive worry or thinking either stagnates or depletes stomach *qi*. A disturbance of stomach functions results in poor appetite, indigestion, food retention, and epigastric distension and pain. If stomach *qi* does not properly descend, belching, burping, hiccuping, nausea, or vomiting occur.

LARGE INTESTINE

The large intestine receives the contents of the small intestine, where it reabsorbs the moisture from food and discharges the waste from the body. Dysfunctions have to do with disturbances in bowel movements, including the substance and amount of feces and the frequency of defecation.

Large-intestine imbalances can have both external and internal causes. First, the large intestine can be directly invaded by exterior cold, which passes through the exterior layers of the body. This occurs as a result of prolonged exposure to cold weather or of sitting on something cold, such as concrete. Internally, excessive consumption of cold, damp foods and drinks such as iced drinks, ice cream, popsicles, raw vegetables, and certain fruits causes coldness in the large intestine, while prolonged eating of greasy, fatty, and spicy foods produces dampness and heat. Just as sadness, grief, and worry affect the lungs, they also can affect the large intestine and cause *qi* stagnation.

GALLBLADDER

Of all the yang organs, the gallbladder alone stores a pure fluid, which is bile. It is a bitter fluid produced by the liver that is then stored in the gallbladder for secretion into the small intestine. With this comes important digestive liver enzymes that are also important for the further breakdown and digestion of food. If liver *qi* is stagnant, bile from the gallbladder does not flow smoothly, resulting in poor digestion and absorption, loss of appetite, diarrhea, nausea, and belching. The gallbladder is the "officer" in charge of making decisions. Since bile is a pure substance, it is said to give the ability to judge clearly and purely. This capacity to make decisions links well to the liver's capacity to plan one's life. The gallbladder also is the source of initiative to make decisions and the bravery to carry them out. Thus, timidity, indecisiveness, lack of drive to make decisions, and being easily discouraged reflect a gallbladder disharmony.

URINARY BLADDER

The bladder receives, stores, and excretes urine. Fluids are dispersed to keep the body adequately lubricated. After this, they accumulate in the kidneys, where urine is produced from the final portions of impure fluids sent down from the lungs and small and large intestines. This impure fluid is then sent down to the bladder, where it is stored until excreted. This function requires *qi* and heat provided by kidney yang. Dysfunctions of the bladder involve urinary problems such as frequent or infrequent urination and cystitis. On an emotional level, the bladder relates to jealousy, suspicion, and holding grudges. It also reacts to anger over time, which can result in bladder infections.

· SIX ·

FOOD THERAPY

It was Hippocrates, the revered Greek doctor of antiquity regarded as the father of Western medicine, who once said, "Let your medicine be your food and your food, your medicine." Who today would think of having a plate of antibiotics for lunch, perhaps with a serving of cortisone pills for dessert? Who would snack on a handful of Tylenol or aspirin periodically through the day? How about the many cancer patients who are taking weekly chemotherapy cocktails? These images show how far we have come from our origins. But is it truly possible to cure ourselves of diseases solely from diet alone? Traditional Chinese medicine (TCM) maintains that in most cases, it is not only possible but desirable.

Food therapy involves following a specific dietary program based on what the Chinese call the *qing dan* diet. The diet integrates wholesome, simple foods, including whole grains; beans and legumes; lightly cooked vegetables; seasonal fruits; small amounts of organic, lean meat; and eggs with a complement of special therapeutic foods and herbs, such as sea vegetables, nuts, various fungi, and special herbs.

Traditional Chinese herbalists have always emphasized the importance of diet. Despite this fact, too many in the West visit even very experienced Chinese doctors and receive little or no dietary guidance.

Why is this so? The reason is that the Chinese generally are not very direct in their communication. Many traditional practitioners consider interfering with someone's dietary preferences invasive and rude. Among their own people, proper diet is not so much of an issue because there is a cultural appreciation for the customary foods—rice, tofu, and so forth—which makes it easier to offer only a few suggestions. Another factor is that Chinese medical practitioners still feel they are perceived as foreigners and outcasts in Western society, so it is not common for a Chinese TCM practitioner to put forth his or her views, even to his or her own patients. The fact remains, however, that the Chinese regard diet to be of primary importance for good health. As Dr. Henry C. Lu, M.D., states in his book, *Chinese Foods for Longevity* (Sterling, 1990), "Today, a prevailing belief among the Chinese people is that one should eat the right foods to maintain good health before trying to take natural herbs for the same purpose, that one should take natural herbs to maintain good health before resorting to chemical drugs, and that one should take chemical drugs to maintain good health before undergoing surgical operations, which should be the last resort." This is in total agreement with another sage assertion by Hippocrates: "Above all else, do no harm."

Isn't this the reason increasing numbers of us are so avidly interested in alternative medicine? For many, it is not a complete rejection of conventional medicine but a recognition of its limits. It is probably true that conventional medicine may be appropriate for only 15% to 20% of the instances in which it is used. I feel, as do growing numbers of forward-thinking medical doctors and health-care practitioners, that various alternative methods, such as herbal medicine, should therefore be used for the remaining 80% to 85% of cases. Given 15% to 20% for conventional medical therapeutics, herbs might be used for another 20% to 30% of cases, but food therapy would be appropriate for 50% or more. This does not include the use of herbs as special foods. Such herbs as astragalus root, lycii berries, codonopsis root, dioscorea root, ophiopogon, burdock, nettles, lamb's quarters, seaweeds, dandelion, watercress and purslane should be part of everyone's weekly diet. Herbs used in this way can provide a significant contribution in maintaining the immune system and overall health.

However far we venture into the realm of natural healing, we should always begin with diet and food if our lifestyle changes are to be of any lasting value. This is because all of life is sustained from the energy of food. By food, I do refer not only to that which we take by mouth but also to all that nourishes and sustains our physical, emotional, and spiritual life. No matter how pure the quality of our "food," if it emanates from a fanatical, one-sided mental viewpoint, it will reflect the limitations of a thought process that perpetuates the underlying sickness of our emotional and spiritual being. An individual who is unable to achieve a balance of physical exercise, creative expression, and introspective soulful enjoyment will find it difficult to achieve a healing balance with food alone. A life of denial and reaction can breed only the fruits of narrowness and rigidity, which in terms of food, becomes like a poison of imbalance.

In the West, the Chinese *qing dan* diet is also known as the Japanese macrobiotic diet. Personally, I have always admired the macrobiotic diet—not necessarily the way that it is expounded or practiced by many, but for its fundamental principles of balance and wholeness. I still think that carefully prepared macrobiotic food is the most deeply satisfying. Macrobiotics, devoid of its "shoulds and shouldn'ts," has its origins in all traditional cultures. It should never be denigrated to the simplistic level of whether one should or should not include meat, dairy, fruit, or spices, because for some people and under certain circumstances, these may or may not be beneficial. Too often, I have met macrobiotic followers who choose their food based on the dictates of their heads rather than on the needs of their bodies. Consequently, many of the individuals I have counseled at macrobiotic centers in different parts of the world were some of the most malnourished, chronically sick, emotionally unstable group of patients I have ever counseled. I remember too well one woman at an overseas macrobiotic center who came to me with a full range of weird physical and emotional symptoms, probably expecting a definitive facial or palm diagnosis with appropriate admonitions such as "too much (or not enough) salt," "more seaweed," "a daily dose of kuzu-root tea" (one of the few medicinal herbs for which macrobiotics encourages regular use), "*Oops!* You've been eating too many umeboshi plums," or some other finicky thing. I saw her skinny, kidney yin–deficient body, and along with giving her a heavy dose of philosophy, which she didn't seem to appreciate at all, I recommended that she eat pork daily to tonify her kidneys. I had spent a long, hard hour with this woman, but in the end, she became so incensed that she was the only patient to ever physically accost me with an umbrella. Fortunately the extent of my injury was only to my patience and frustrated good intentions.

One of the things we learn from TCM is that the whole is reflected in all of its parts. Besides referring to zone-oriented foot or ear therapy, in which there are corresponding points that affect all parts of our bodies, this belief also implies that the choice we make concerning food is also a reflection of our prevailing imbalance. Therefore, it may not be the food that is the problem, but the eater. So how can one change? Is change ever really possible? These are two of the least asked but certainly more profound questions of inquiry, especially in the light of various inherited and acquired propensities and destiny. I think the answer is that change is certainly possible, but for some, at least, not without considerable difficulty.

Food Cravings: An Energetics Perspective

Let us move from the realms of the highest to the most mundane of considerations: "What do I eat today?" The answer is fundamental. Eat simply and more bland for a while, at least until your taste and judgment are sufficiently restored so that what you crave is closer to what you truly need. People are amazed at how good a simple bowl of brown rice and aduki beans can be, especially when they are suitably hungry and that is all there is to eat. Behind every craving is a genuine need. For many, Chinese herbs can be among the strangest and least desirable taste experiences. While herbs usually fall far short of being absolutely delectable, many find that a particular herbal brew that may at first seem repugnant becomes somewhat strangely acceptable because of their bodies' ability to recognize in it something that is needed and beneficial. In the ancient Upanishads of India, it is said repeatedly, "We are made from food." Since what we eat will always be both the cause as well as the reflection of our disease imbalance, it seems important to look at some of the other reasons we eat—why we crave foods with refined carbohydrates such as sugar; overly strong spicy foods; fried, fatty foods; alcohol, coffee, and other stimulants and depressants; too little food; too much food; dairy products, salty or sweet foods; and so forth.

Launched into life, this little boat of our physical being has only its five senses, including its sense of smell and taste, to help it determine what it needs to survive. Why does it so often seem that we are betrayed by our senses and desires? This is another question with profound implications. The philosophy of the ancient Chinese seems so different from some of the contemporary Eastern religious sects and puritanical ideals that are based on sin, negation, and denial. A study of the Chinese Five Elements, with their corresponding flavors and foods, reveals a positive, life-affirming perspective that even today can help unveil the true underlying need behind many of our cravings. In the theory of the Five Elements, Chinese medicine teaches that somehow behind the flavors we most crave lies what we most need. How different this news is from that of certain puritanical Eastern sects and a sin-oriented philosophy. One is life-giving and the other is life-denying.

A Journey Through the Five Flavors

EARTH: A CRAVING FOR SWEETS

You might ask what it is that you really need when you crave sweets. From the TCM Five Element perspective, our earth-element (grounding) spleen energy is deficient because sweet flavors go to the earth spleen. So how does chocolate fit into that reasoning? Sugar and chocolate are strong sweets and may reflect any number of physical or emotional deficits, such as a lack of protein, reassurance, love, centeredness, carbohydrates, sense of self, mother's affection, security, satisfaction, feeling connected—a strange mixture of things that have been missing or long denied. When a patient complains of cravings for sweets, we realize from the above that the sweet flavor corresponds to earth, which represents a grounded feeling of centeredness. The sweet flavor is not just refined sweets, such as sugar, but also such so-called mildly sweet foods as whole grains and all other proteinaceous foods. It therefore represents the essence of all nutrition and our need for better nutrition.

Overindulgence in strong sweets overstimulates the adrenal glands and pancreas, which results in a sudden secretion of insulin that burns off all available blood sugar. This in turn causes sudden fatigue and negativity associated with low blood sugar and a feeling of being chronically tired and deprived. If the patient craving sweets is a vegetarian, he or she probably could use more vegetable protein in the form of beans and tofu, or animal protein (if these foods can be tolerated), at least a little more cooked dairy (which is far less mucus-forming), or some eggs. For individuals who maintain that they already have sufficient daily amounts of protein in their diet, the problem could be more one of yang excess, where overindulgence in refined carbohydrates overloads and overworks their system and becomes a major contributor to the development of degenerative disease.

METAL: A CRAVING FOR SPICES

What if what I crave most is strong, spicy food? Spiciness belongs to metal–lungs–large intestine, the organs of letting go, moving on, needing a new experience, stimulating bodily warmth and circulation, clearing mucus, clearing congestion out of my life, being conscientious, being open, releasing the old to make room for the new, obtaining clarity and detachment.

WATER: A CRAVING FOR SALT

What if what I most crave is excess salt? Salty flavors belong to water kidneys–adrenals–bladder, the element of storage and reserve, the need to retain moisture to keep our bodily tissues soft and youthful, willpower, focus, tolerance, endurance, the need for minerals, drive, motivation, hormonal reserve, determination, libido.

WOOD: A CRAVING FOR SOUR FLAVORS

What if I crave sourness? Sour flavors belong to wood–liver–gallbladder, the element of regulation and control. Sourness astringes, helps to retain essence, engenders greater courage, prevents us from losing too much of ourselves to others. Sour flavors include vitamin C, citrus, and fermented foods, for instance. As with fermented foods, the sour flavor, in balance, engenders new growth and creativity. At the same time, a strong sensation of sourness, such as with a lemon, causes us to wince and contract, limiting our ability to absorb inappropriate stimuli. From this, we can see that the sour flavor upholds the general function of the liver to regulate the way we use our energy, our creativity, the way we stand up for ourselves; we take sour inside so we don't become sour on life outside.

FIRE: A CRAVING FOR BITTERNESS

What if I crave bitterness? Such a craving is not too likely, but the bitter flavor does belong to fire–heart–small intestine and in fact can be of real assistance to the function of these organs. This is perhaps the most paradoxical association, deserving of a lengthier consideration, since bitterness is also allied to the emotion of joy. The bitter flavor represents alkaloids, the flavor of something that is roasted or burned. Bitter herbs are used to clear evil fire and thereby restore normal heat and life energy. They are also used to detoxify, dry, stimulate the secretion of bile, purify the blood, remove parasites, promote bowel movement, and clear excess cholesterol and blood lipids. From an herbalist's perspective, a bitter flavor is probably what most people need. The saying of olden times is that after a period of pleasure and overindulgence, we must drink our bitter brew. Considering that the fire element quintessentially represents heat, it is the pure fire of life that is exalted rather than the heat of stagnation and congestion. One of the functions associated with the small intestine applies to the bitter flavor—to separate the pure from the impure. The heart represents the mind and thoughts. Consider how the purity of our mind and thoughts can enhance our ability to more deeply love another, freeing our heart of unnecessary obstacles as the bitter taste clears obstruction from our circulatory system. There are those who, unable to govern their desires, seem committed to dangerously playing them out in order to get beyond them. For these, experience becomes a bitter learning. Again, on the most mundane levels, it may be that if we avoid the intake of even a small amount of bitter taste in our food each day, bitterness in the form of ill health and disease may visit us too frequently.

Whole Grains and the 10-Day Brown Rice Diet

With all the physiological and resulting emotional imbalances created by such dietary imbalances, most people require a short period of nutritional rest to allow their bodies to naturally fall back into balance. Many traditional healing cultures recommend following a bland diet for a period of 10 days or so to reinstate balance. An exclusive 10-day diet of brown rice and azuki beans or some other combination of a whole grain and beans, such as the Ayurvedic kichari diet (mung beans and rice), has never failed, after the first 1 or 2 days of adjustment, to induce a sense of inner calm and centeredness.

Why does this work? Essentially, it does because it encourages a normal process of detoxification of acid wastes from the various layers of the body, including the blood and lymphatic system. Acids represent the metabolic wastes of food and other substances that are no longer needed. They are produced in all living organisms, regardless of whether the food that is eaten is of the best quality. Acid toxins are neutralized by various buffers in the blood as a consequence of the natural presence of alkaline minerals. These mineral compounds are also present in abundance in green and sea vegetables as well as in all the herbs classified as blood purifiers or alteratives in Western herbalism, or herbs that clear heat (heat represents acids) in Chinese herbology. The normal systems of discharge and elimination include the lungs, which discharge metabolic acids that have been transformed into carbon dioxide, as well as urine, sweat, and feces. Eating foods that are mostly alkaline forming, such as whole grains and most vegetables, helps to maintain a normal pH balance of between 7.3 and 7.45.

In the complex physiological processes of the body, it is never a question of what is eaten but what is ultimately digested and transformed that matters. Body chemistry is always a matter of a series of actions and reactions that represent these profound physiological processes. Often, such foods as cereal grains, which are slightly acid before eaten because of the presence of phosphorus compounds, are changed to a more alkaline state in the body. Vegetables, which are alkaline, remain alkaline. Sugar, which is alkaline, produces acid. Meat and other animal foods, as well as fats and oils, which are acid, remain acid. Such complex chemical reactions are difficult to understand in practice and are better understood as yin and yang. An excess of yin and yang foods will cause an acid condition, while a balanced diet, working with the body's innate normalizing processes, generates a balanced alkaline condition. Whole grains and beans are classified as neutral because they contain all aspects of the life cycle, which provide an energetic balance of yin and yang. The effect of a diet based on whole grains, especially rice, is balance. Another reason that traditional herbalists from around the world tend to espouse such a simple program for recovery is that it creates a nutritional program that will not neutralize or compromise the effects of the herbs that are given. In fact, it will optimize their effects, because with the grains and beans representing neutral balance, the herbs will be more strongly yin or yang and thus able to effect change more quickly.

WHITE OR BROWN RICE?

Unpolished grains, such as whole, organic brown rice, are the richest in nutrition and fiber. It has long been known that an exclusive diet of white rice will cause vitamin B deficiency. In addition, there are many factors in unpolished grains that reduce the risk of colon cancer, effectively prevent and treat high blood pressure, reduce cholesterol, and prevent diabetes. Chinese energetics considers brown rice to be a yin tonic, effective for symptoms of excessive perspiration, night sweats, diarrhea, diabetes, and other problems associated with yin deficiency. Brown rice makes one stronger. During World War II, the Chinese Communists demonstrated exceptional endurance and strength against the Japanese onslaught. They had many victories, but after they proudly positioned themselves in the cities, they weakened considerably. The Chinese claimed that the difference was that while they were sequestered in the mountains, they ate only unpolished brown rice, but after taking over the cities, their health and subsequent strength was compromised by their indulgence in refined white rice.

Ever since the advent of TCM in the West, there has been controversy over whether brown rice is nutritionally better than white. Many Chinese practitioners maintain that white rice is easier to digest—which it is—and that eating even a small amount of meat with it will more than compensate for the loss of B vitamins. All of this is true, but the fact that a food is easier to digest can be both positive as well as negative. It is positive for those who have very weak digestion and must improve their assimilation to regain their strength. It is negative in that without any digestive challenges, the digestive system, like any muscle or bodily function, becomes weaker with the pampering. As people grow older, their digestion tends to weaken. In Japan, people traditionally took their unpolished grains to the miller, specifically requesting varying amounts of polishing to leave as much of the fiber with the grains as possible. Lacking this high level of appreciation for whole grains in the West, we must content ourselves with either mixing proportions of brown and white rice together or being sure to eat them at different times. One thing is certain: the body will ultimately be much stronger and healthier if we can accustom ourselves to the use of organically grown brown rather than white rice.

The answer to the question of how to deal with difficulty digesting brown rice is chewing, which can make a difference in anyone's digestion. Some of the most important processes of digestion begin in the mouth with the thorough mastication of food. The saliva begins the process of converting acid-based food to a more alkaline state, which

greatly assists digestion in the stomach. The process of digestion is literally a yin–yang miracle of chemical transmutation that begins with alkaline substances in the mouth changing to acid in the stomach and back
to alkaline in the small intestine. It is through this alternation of acid
and alkaline that important nutrients are converted and released for
assimilation.

Occasionally eating white rice, especially the delicious white basmati
rice, will not deter from the value of the 10-day brown rice diet. However, it is far more preferable to use brown rather than the refined white
rice in any healing program. There may be occasions when brown rice
is simply not available; under such circumstances, white rice is an acceptable choice. Fanatical adherence to anything, especially regarding
diet, can become its own disease. Furthermore, it is possible and sometimes even preferable to integrate a variety of other foods, especially
whole grains with no added yeast or sugar, during the 10-day diet.
These include a wide variety of simple ethnic combinations that may
include whole-grain pastas, East Indian chapatis, Mexican whole-wheat
flour or corn tortillas (little or no fat, please), Mediterranean pocket
bread (pita bread), and so forth. A garnish of dry toasted, ground sesame seeds will help fulfill protein, calcium, and other mineral requirements and contribute wonderful flavor. In Japan, a mixture of 7 to 10
parts dry toasted sesame seeds and 1 part dechlorinated sea salt (made
by preroasting the sea salt in a hot skillet), carefully ground together, is
used as a healthful condiment on many foods, including grains and
vegetables. Chinese food therapy regards black sesame seeds as having
superior health value as a yin and blood tonic. Regular intake of black
sesame seeds will restore normal hair color in premature graying. Its
disadvantage is the possibility of having unsightly little pieces of black
sesame seeds stuck on one's teeth. Black sesame seeds are also slightly
more bitter than the yellow varieties. Other additions to a rice diet can
be small garnishes of sautéed onions, garlic, ginger, freshly chopped
parsley, coriander, sweet basil, oregano, and a basic nonoverspiced
curry mixture consisting of fresh finely ground coriander, cumin seeds,
turmeric root. These foods all have their unique healing attributes and
will contribute to flavor immensely. A simple and healthful sauce can
be made with equal parts sesame tahini butter, miso paste, and water.
Variations of this include the addition of curry powder, grated lemon or
orange peel, cooking wine, garlic, and other things with which one

might experiment. This sauce added to the rice or any dish is one of the secrets for making simple healthful food delicious.

KICHARI: THE FOOD OF THE GODS

In all my books, I include the recipe for kichari because I think it is the safest and most healing food. I recall having lunch with Dr. Vasant Lad, M.D., an Ayurvedic doctor and author of many books on Ayurveda. On being served a bowl of kichari, he gratefully exclaimed, "This is not food; this is medicine!" Indeed, kichari has been celebrated as such throughout India for centuries and has been routinely prescribed by Ayurvedic herbalists to patients for all diseases. There is a saying in India that kichari taken for 3 weeks will cure all curable diseases.

The use of the kichari diet in India is similar to that of the 10-day brown rice diet of Japan and China. I have found that kichari does everything and perhaps more than the more austere macrobiotic 10-day brown rice. I have personally met at least one yogi (Dyan Yogi), who in his nineties could outstride any of his more youthful followers. He claimed to eat, as one of his austerities, an exclusive diet of kichari with the addition of some cooked vegetables three times daily for years and had no apparent nutritional deficiencies. The only herbal supplement he took was Triphala.

So what is it about kichari that at least for the Indians makes it the most perfect food? The combination of brown rice and mung beans in kichari represents a perfect combination of life-sustaining protein and carbohydrates. Secondly, the addition of whole rock salt supplies added trace minerals the body needs to properly use other nutrients. Third, but not least, the three essential spices, coriander, cumin, and turmeric, the basis of curry mixtures, each have unique therapeutic properties that aid digestion and prevent food and other stagnations from occurring. Traditional nutrition beliefs of both China and India seem to imply that it is the subtle combination of the five flavors, which activates each of the internal organic processes, and this may be more important even than the nutritional content of food. Let's look at these. Coriander and cumin seeds have warm, spicy energy and benefit the lungs and spleen for better assimilation and transformation of food into energy. Turmeric, with its bitter and spicy flavors, is well known in TCM for its liver-detoxifying and blood- and qi-circulating properties that help to prevent stagnation and relieve pain. Now that you know some of the many values of kichari, here is the basic recipe:

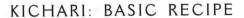

KICHARI: BASIC RECIPE

Mung beans: 1 cup
Brown rice: 1 cup
Rock or dechlorinated sea salt: ½–1 teaspoon
Coriander seeds (finely ground): 1 tablespoon
Cumin seeds (finely ground): 1 tablespoon
Turmeric root powder: 1 tablespoon
Ghee* sesame oil: 1 tablespoon
Water: 3–4 cups, depending on desired thickness

Cook the mung beans and rice together. Sauté the salt and spices in ghee (clarified butter) or sesame oil until they achieve a fine odor and flavor. Stir in the mung beans and rice and serve.

The basic kichari, also called *mung dahl* and rice in East Indian restaurants, is itself very versatile. There are innumerable variations that can further alter and possibly contribute to its therapeutic value. The first and most obvious choice is to have it thick or more like a thin soup or porridge. Next, one can add a variety of vegetables, such as green leafy vegetables, carrots, tomatoes, potatoes, and so forth, to make more of a stew. One or 2 tablespoons of yogurt can also be added when it is served and has cooled down a bit. The yogurt adds flavor and texture, as well as important nutrients, such as calcium. Yogurt, the fermented food of India, is a more easily assimilated form of milk and supplements calcium and important beneficial intestinal bacteria. If there is a need for more yang warmth and pungency, one can add a dash of red or black pepper, ginger, or a slice of dried galangal root cooked with the rice and beans or sautéed with the spices. One can be very creative with the basic kichari recipe and still preserve its essential therapeutic value.

MUNG BEANS AND DETOXIFICATION

We have discussed the value of brown rice as the most balanced food because it supplies a well-balanced complex carbohydrate for sustained balanced energy. Mung beans are unique in that they supply the necessary amino acids, which, with the brown rice, help enrich the overall

---

*See page 92 for how to prepare ghee.

protein value. Another important and unique aspect of mung beans is that because they have a cool energy, they are detoxifying and help neutralize acids. Mung beans are even recommended as one of the substances to treat toxicity symptoms of aconite poisoning. Mung beans are therefore a proteinaceous, highly nutritious blood purifier. By neutralizing toxins throughout the body, they are able to calm the mind, relieve hypertension, clear the accumulation of excess cholesterol and other lipids from the veins and arteries of the body, and promote the healing of all diseases. Unlike fruit or vegetable juice fasts, which are also cooling but lack the denser nutrients, a diet high in mung beans, especially a kichari and mung bean diet, achieves a more balanced detoxification without aggravating any nutritional deficiencies.

GHEE (CLARIFIED BUTTER) AND THE IMPORTANCE OF FATS AND OILS

One of the other ingredients in kichari is ghee, or what is called clarified butter in the West. This is becoming increasingly more available from natural-food stores throughout the country. In one sense, this is too bad, since it is good to spend a part of each day doing the menial tasks necessary for survival, and making ghee is one of the easiest things to do in the kitchen. Simply place a pound of unsalted butter in a skillet over low heat, low enough to melt the butter but not so high as to burn it. Gradually, you will notice how the saturated fats of the butter separate out from the pure unsaturated butter fat. White solids may form and float to the surface, then eventually settle to the bottom. The pure golden oil, called ghee, is carefully poured off from the settlings at the bottom of the pan, which are probably best discarded. Ghee is one of the few oils that will not become rancid even without refrigeration. We have all heard about the importance of essential fatty acids from fats and oils. We also know how easy it is to ingest certain vegetable oils that can contain cancer-causing free radicals because of their almost invisible rancidity. The most stable of all vegetable oils are sesame and olive oils, which is why these have become the staples of so many great cultures throughout the world. Ghee adds tremendous flavor to foods and will keep indefinitely without losing any of its nutritional value. In fact, the Tibetans are famous for having a warm drink called *sampah* (disgusting to many Westerners unaccustomed to its distinct flavor), simply made of old ghee dissolved in hot water. It so happens that this has probably the same nutritional importance to the Tibetans living in the cold, high Himalayas as whale and seal blubber have to the Eskimo. In both of these traditional societies, as well as in France, where wine and butter are commonly used in the cuisine, neither high cholesterol nor heart disease is a problem to the extent that it is in North America. This may indicate that stress, which is particularly high in North America, is most likely the biggest culprit in these circulatory diseases and that the use of certain oils and fats in the diet is far less likely to cause high cholesterol than many presently believe.

According to Ayurvedic theory, 1 or 2 teaspoons of ghee each day is important for the health of the whole body. It aids circulation and digestion, adds softness and luster to the skin, and is also one of the recommended ingredients in kichari. From the TCM perspective, ghee, along with all other oils, is a yin tonic. Besides ghee, sesame and olive oils are the best of all vegetable oils to use because of their greater resistance to oxidation and rancidity.

A Balanced Diet

Most of us will not, and perhaps many should not, eat only brown rice and beans as an exclusive diet for the rest of our lives. First, doing so will probably not satisfy most of our emotional or experiential food needs, which can be important. Second, it may not be, in the long run, as completely healthy a sole diet for everyone as it was for Dyan Yogi.

From the perspective of TCM, a balanced diet is one that uses foods energetically. It incorporates more foods with a neutral to cool and neutral to warm energy and a little less food with warm or cool energies and uses sparingly those foods with extreme hot and cold energies. If these energies are placed on a continuum, it is easier to visualize how they affect us:

hot   warm   neutral–warm   neutral–cool   cool   cold

It is unfortunate but true that the beginning of all good diets seems to involve informing us what we should avoid. The problem is that an excess of certain foods, such as sugar, can so utterly sabotage an otherwise great diet. It is also useful for us to know what foods and substances can deprive us of our healing goals. Do not feel overwhelmed. The foods and substances that can weaken and compromise our health are shown in the table below.

FOODS AND SUBSTANCES TO AVOID

INJURIOUS SUBSTANCE	GENERAL EFFECTS
Refined sugar, including various sweets, chocolate, pastries, and sodas; refined flour and flour products generally	Robs and depletes our nutritional reserves, weakens our immune system, and makes us weak
Excess of alcoholic beverages	Puts too much heat in the blood; injures the liver
Excess of coffee	Aggravates nervousness and hypertension; stagnates liver *qi;* depletes our adrenals
Tobacco	Causes chronic upper-respiratory problems and lung cancer
MSG (monosodium glutamate)	Weakens the immune system; is a known carcinogen; causes acute yin deficiency reactions in some, manifested as "Chinese restaurant" syndrome
Carbonated drinks	Overstimulates the stomach; can cause bloating and digestive problems
Ice-cold drinks and cold foods	Injures stomach *qi;* weakens digestion
Excess of fruit and fruit juices	Causes bloating and gas, especially when consumed in conjunction with protein and complex carbohydrates
Meat and dairy products from inorganically raised animals	Ingestion of residual drugs in the form of steroids given to animals to make them fatter, antibiotics to cure them of infections, and other toxic material to make them more commercially viable; these weaken the immune system and increase vulnerability to chronic degenerative diseases
Artificial chemical food coloring and preservatives	Most are toxic and carcinogenic and can accumulate in the body
The abusive use of various recreational drugs, including marijuana	Can destroy brain cells and distort judgment, thus adversely affecting everything in life

Whenever it is possible, I try to offer substitutes for each of these foods. Do not think of these as replacements but as healthful alternatives.

Injurious Foods and Substances

REFINED SUGAR

In order to be metabolized, refined sugar draws from our nutritional reserves of important vitamins, minerals, and other nutrients, thereby making us weaker. Of all the food taboos, refined sugar is the worst. For many, it will be a major challenge to overcome the addiction because sugar is so entwined in our lives at all levels. Physically, it will aggravate blood sugar, either high or low. Mentally, it will create instability, a tendency to depression, and negativity as a result of liver *qi* stagnation. Acceptable substitutes should be used to eventually completely eliminate all craving for sweets, even the substitutes. Begin by substituting the following: fruit juice and foods sweetened with fruit juice, honey, barley, or rice malt syrup; maple syrup; whole, unrefined sugar, such as Sucanat.

REFINED FLOUR PRODUCTS

Milled flour quickly oxidizes and is a deadening food. It greatly contributes to obesity, stagnation, formation of mucus, and congestion. Wheat is nutritionally the densest grain. When taken as flour in bread or pastries, wheat can cause all types of allergic reactions in many people; it should be completely avoided. I have never seen such aggravations caused by foods made with sprouted whole wheat or whole-wheat berry seeds. An important vegetarian high-protein food made from wheat gluten, called seitan, is a wonderfully proteinaceous food and can be substituted for animal products, dairy, cheese, or tofu whenever desired. It is a staple protein source for vegetarian Seventh Day Adventists. It is happily becoming more commonly available in many quality natural-food stores. Flour products made with yeast seem to be another source of aggravation and digestive upset for many. Perhaps this is why traditional cultures often use various forms of unleavened freshly ground flour products, such as the chapatis of India, the tortillas of Central America, the pasta of Italy, and the unleavened pita or pocket bread of the Mediterranean region. If you must have flour products, try to use freshly milled grains, which are far superior to much of the oxi-dized flour that occupies the bins and shelves of mainstream grocery stores for weeks or even months. An optimally healthy weight-regulat-ing diet should limit use of flour products, oils, fats, and dairy products.

ALCOHOL

A single glass of pure, high-quality wine, rice wine (such as sake), or beer is actually beneficial for health. The problem is that many cannot stop with one glass and form a dependency that causes sickness and imbalance. I have found that nonalcoholic wines and beers, many of which are very delicious, are increasingly available and can be used for those special occasions of indulgence.

COFFEE

People with high levels of anxiety and stress in their lives should avoid coffee. It can contribute to hypertension, insomnia, and an acid condition. At least 85% of patients who tell me that they regularly drink coffee are suffering from unnatural fatigue. There is a time and place for most things, however. An occasional cup of coffee should not do any harm and may even be beneficial. Good alternatives are the many toasted barley– and grain-based drinks that are on the market. These often include roasted dandelion or chicory roots in their ingredients, which are quite good for the blood and liver. Green tea contains only a fraction of the caffeine of coffee and black tea and has some important health benefits. Studies have found that green tea neutralizes cancer-causing free radicals and reduces cholesterol and fat buildup in the veins and arteries. Green tea is good to drink after a meal to aid diges-tion and counteract the negative effects of oils or fats.

ICED DRINKS

Iced drinks and even cold foods injure the stomach and negatively affect digestion. In the summer, they reactively increase thirst. It is bet-ter to take drinks at room temperature or warm.

CARBONATED DRINKS

Carbonation is overstimulating and detrimental to the stomach and digestion. Drink only noncarbonated drinks.

DAIRY PRODUCTS

For many, all dairy products are mucus forming, predisposing them to upper-respiratory allergies, lymphatic congestion, and skin diseases. It must be remembered, however, that many people—perhaps the majority—who practice a strict nondairy vegetarian diet may after months or years, manifest nutritional diseases. For this reason, even the vegetarian Hindus of India recommend the addition of some dairy products to the diet, especially yogurt. This may be no more than a few tablespoons a day. For sick babies, we give herbs to the mothers and the babies retroactively receive the value of the medicine through their mothers' milk. Likewise, it is critical to avoid inorganic dairy products that contain traces of the drugs and hormones given to the cows from which the products are made. Whatever happened to the milkman who daily delivered fresh milk from "contented cows"? Cow's milk is much more assimilable if it is taken scalded and warm, but the best-quality milk is unpasteurized. You may ask, however, if we should take it scalded and warm, what the difference is between this and pasteurized milk. The problem, according to Dr. Rudolf Ballentine, M.D. (*Diet and Nutrition,* 1978 Himalayan Institute), is that the milk is only flash-heated, and the temperature is not high enough to sufficiently break down the long protein chain of cow's milk that has trouble passing through the liver. Substitutes, therefore, should have smaller protein molecules than cow's milk, as found in an unpasteurized, warm, scalded cow's milk; yogurt; or goat or sheep's milk.

From a TCM perspective, milk enters the lungs. This is why it can easily cause mucus. For individuals with dryness of the lungs, however, or wasting diseases such as tuberculosis (TB) or acquired immuno deficiency syndrome (AIDS), boiled warm milk with ginger and a little honey is a tonic remedy. In India, one of the most delicious Ayurvedic tonics is called *chyavanprash,* which consists of fifty or more herbs, honey, sugar, and ghee. The combination of these is exceptionally fortifying. Over 50% of *chyavanprash* consists of amla (*Emblica myrobalans*), which is one of the three ingredients of triphala. Amla has the highest known levels of natural vitamin C, second to acerola berries. However, it is also uniquely impervious to both aging and heat.

INORGANIC MEAT

For many, meat is important for health. It is considered a first-class protein, which essentially means that it is more easily assimilated than vegetable-based foods. As a class, all flesh foods are easier for the spleen to assimilate and digest, but beef is specifically a spleen tonic. It has a neutral energy. The assignment of various flesh foods is according to the Five Elements, so that lamb is warmer and better for the heart and circulation; chicken, for the liver; pork, for the kidneys; and horsemeat (eaten in some countries, such as France), for the lungs. Fish is considered to have a cold energy because it lives in water; nevertheless, it is also easier to metabolize and digest for individuals with a weak spleen and stomach *qi*. It is very good to have fish rich in essential fatty acids, such as salmon, at least once a week.

THE HIGH-PROTEIN DIET

Protein, normally regarded as an essential building nutrient needed for growth and repair, is also important to maintain normal rates of metabolism. For some individuals, obesity is the result of long-term protein-deficient diets. Many of these people are descended from Northern European ancestors, whose hunter-gatherer native diets historically were high in meat protein, in contrast to Asian and Mediterranean peoples, whose more agrarian background mandated less meat protein. For those who seem to require higher percentages of animal protein, the diet should also include a high percentage of vegetables (especially green leafy vegetables), to help neutralize the acids, and a somewhat lower percentage of complex carbohydrates in the form of whole grains. While some complex carbohydrates should be eaten, they must be in lesser ratio to the meat that is consumed. The reason that vegetable protein does not work as well for many is that it requires a considerably larger amount to equal the protein value of meat. Concentrated vegetable protein, such as tofu, tempeh, and seitan, as well as some eggs and dairy, can be used to satisfy a considerable amount of the protein requirements for this diet, however.

There are various theories as to the basis of such a diet. As mentioned above, some think that individuals of Northern European stock, specifically with type O blood, have a greater need for protein because of their ancestral hunter-gatherer eating patterns, while individuals whose ancestors have had a longer agricultural ancestry, such as Asian and Mediterranean people with type A blood, can tolerate more complex carbohydrates. At this time, this may be another theory that needs to be proven through years of study. I have observed how high-protein diets, at least for a limited time, can be of particular benefit for individuals who have an accumulated protein deficiency resulting in chronic spleen *qi* deficiency and weakness. These individuals, formerly unable to drop a pound of weight with dieting and exercise but then advised to follow a high-protein diet, were able to rapidly shed water weight even while eating four and five times the quantity of foods that they might normally consume. I have found that for others, however, a diet high in animal protein causes greater congestion, circulatory problems, and even gout. What we can learn from this is that protein is extremely important and perhaps the most important element in our diet. Certain individuals who may be genetically predisposed to eat protein and those with chronic long-term deficiencies may require animal protein to effect a balance, because of the ability of animal protein to powerfully stimulate spleen metabolism.

FOOD ADDITIVES

Food additives are insidious substances, added to prepackaged foods either to maintain their color, add color to them, or serve as preservatives. Most of these have been found to be carcinogenic but are still added to lengthen products' shelf life and to heighten desirable appearance. Monosodium glutamate (MSG) is often added to Asian dishes to destroy the superficial cells on the surface of the tongue so as to increase taste sensitivity. Many people are extremely sensitive to this substance, experiencing a combination of symptoms known as "Chinese restaurant" syndrome.

Food as Medicine

Following are some food recipes for treating specific conditions.

AMARANTH (THREE-COLORED; *AMARANTHUS MANGOSTANUS*)

Three-colored amaranth has a characteristic pinkish red blush at the extremities of its leaves. It is a wonderful green vegetable that, once introduced, will commonly continue to grow as a weed. It has a sweet flavor with a slightly cool nature. It clears heat, induces urination, removes dampness, and promotes bowel elimination. It can be served as a sautéed vegetable to relieve dysentery as well as constipation.

ARTICHOKE LEAVES

A tea of artichoke leaves is an excellent source of the bitter flavor. It can be used to treat all liver and gallbladder problems as well as lower cholesterol.

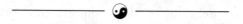

BARLEY

Barley is used for edema, fluid retention, obesity, cancer, and arthritic and rheumatic conditions. For edema and swelling of the body, make a soup with pearl barley and azuki beans. Boil the soup and reduce 10 cups of it down to 1 cup, then drink only the liquid. For weeping eczema, drink a tea of mung beans and pearl barley. Wash the skin with the tea as well.

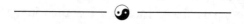

CUCUMBERS

For excessive thirst, eat cucumbers. For edema and difficult urination, cut 1 cucumber in half, boil in equal amounts of water and apple-cider vinegar until it is soft and well cooked, and drink the juice at mealtimes. Cucumber juice is also good for any heat condition: for eczema and other inflamed skin problems, cucumber juice applied topically will give great relief.

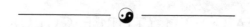

EGG OIL

Egg oil is an excellent remedy for a weak heart. Roast the yolks of 5 eggs in a skillet until black. At this stage, the oil will become apparent. Take 1/2 teaspoon once or twice a day for 1–3 months.

EGGPLANT

Eggplant moves blood, relieves pain caused by blood stagnation, detoxifies, and promotes urination. It can be used for high blood pressure and skin eruptions. For frostbite, make a tea of sliced eggplant and soak the affected part. To promote urination to relieve swelling and edema, pound dried eggplant to powder and take 1 teaspoon in a glass of warm water 3 times a day.

GINGER (FRESH)

Fresh ginger is one of the most versatile spices. For mucus and the first sign of a cold, steep 3 or 4 slices of ginger in 1 cup of boiling water. Add honey to taste. For dysentery with diarrhea, burn dry ginger to charcoal. Take 1 teaspoonful with rice that has been preroasted to a brownish color. For the common cold with chills and fever but no perspiration, drink a tea of ginger and sweet basil. If the cold is a wind heat type and you have high fever, slight chills, sweating, and sore throat, drink cabbage and fresh ginger broth freely.

MOLASSES

Molasses has a warm energy and a sweet flavor. It tonifies *qi*, strengthens the spleen, lubricates the lungs, and stops coughs. For cough caused by weakness or *qi* deficiency, dice carrots and mix them with molasses. This is left overnight. The dose is 2 tablespoons 3 or more times daily. For acute stomach pains as well as the pain of duodenal ulcers, take 2 tablespoons of molasses mixed with warm water as often as needed.

MUSTARD GREENS

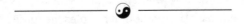

Mustard greens have a spicy flavor and a warm energy that affect the lungs and stomach. They benefit and warm the stomach and relieve exterior cold conditions, such as phlegm and cough. They can be served sautéed or juiced.

For cold stomach with nausea, vomiting, and loss of appetite, make mustard green soup, adding fresh ginger and brown sugar.

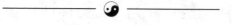

ONION

Onions are used for cold phlegm with cough and congestion in the chest, pleurisy, bronchitis, asthma, emphysema, angina, stomach pains, dysentery, and diarrhea. For severe croup, bronchitis and chest congestion, make an onion poultice by wrapping finely chopped fresh onions in a cloth wide enough to cover the chest or upper back. This is then lightly steamed and applied to the chest while it is as warm as possible. For colds, make a strong onion soup, but do not overcook the onions, as this will diminish their effectiveness. Sauté ¹/₂ cup white onions, ¹/₂ cup red onions, and 2 cloves fresh garlic with a little butter, then add 1¹/₂ cups tomato juice.

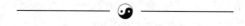

OX-TAIL SOUP

Ox-tail soup is a good treatment for hypoglycemia. It is made by cracking open the tail bones of a cow to expose the marrow. This is then cooked with some root vegetables, such as onions and carrots, and made into a soup. To add to the tonic properties, add 6 grams of codonopsis, ginseng, or jujube dates.

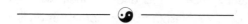

PAPAYA

Papaya has a neutral energy with sweet and sour flavors. It strengthens the stomach and spleen, assists digestion, lubricates the lungs, stops cough, kills worms, and increases the quantity of mother's milk. For worms, pound sun-dried green papaya to a powder. Take 2 teaspoons on an empty stomach, morning and evening. For indigestion, eat cooked or raw papaya with or after meals. To increase the quantity of mother's milk, eat fresh papaya with fish soup.

PEARS

Pears are good for heat and dryness of the lungs. To expectorate mucus from the bronchioles and/or lungs, remove the core of a fresh pear. Stuff it with raisins and rock sugar and bake it in the oven. These can be eaten throughout the day for the treatment of bronchitis.

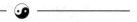

SESAME SEEDS (BLACK)

Black sesame seeds are a blood and yin tonic. Their regular use will tonify the liver and kidneys, restore hair color, and cure dizziness, tinnitus, and aching soreness of the lower back and knees. They can be cooked with rice congee. For premature balding or gray hair, grind together *he shou wou (Polygonum multiflorum)* and black sesame seeds. Mix together with honey and take 2 tablespoons each morning with brown rice porridge.

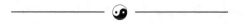

WALNUTS

Walnuts are a yang tonic with some yin lubricating properties. As a brain tonic and for male impotence and lower back pain from yang deficiency, eat 20 walnuts a day for at least 1–2 months. For chronic cough and constipation, grind walnuts to a meal and mix them with honey; take 2 tablespoons once or twice daily. This is both delicious and a very good remedy for constipation in the elderly.

The Balanced Diet Continued

A balanced diet is based upon many factors, especially a proper ratio of complex carbohydrates to protein and vegetables. Other factors are also important, however, including availability of various foods, climate, level of physical activity, genetic predisposition, and so forth. Thus, these ratios must be flexible. In general, one should try to eat lighter foods in the spring and summer, such as vegetables and seasonally available fruits, and eat denser, heavier foods in the fall and winter, including a higher percentage of grains, protein, and root vegetables.

Because Americans have more sedentary habits and longer life spans today than in earlier centuries, their digestive capabilities lessen with age as their metabolisms become lower. As a result, it is best to eat predominantly lightly cooked foods to improve assimilation. In all systems of traditional medicine, one who is weak and unable to digest food is given thin rice porridge, ideally with the addition of ginseng. Meat soups, such as chicken soup, are also good. The weaker one is, the longer the food should be cooked. Rice porridge, called congee, cooked with jujube dates and other herbs according to the condition of the patient, is ideal during illness.

Pressed Salad

Salads are not considered an important part of diet in traditional cultures. One of the reasons is because of the very real apprehension of contracting parasites or germs because of poor sanitation. The major reason from the TCM perspective, however, is that raw food weakens digestion and causes coldness and dampness of the stomach and spleen. For these reasons, salads are not a traditional part of the cuisine of China, Japan, and India, though they are a popular health food in the West. In Japan, a method of achieving a balance with the coolness of a raw salad is a pressed salad. To make a pressed salad, finely chop green lettuce leaves and other vegetables. Sprinkle some organic salt on them and wrap them into a porous cotton cloth. Place the cloth-enclosed salad on a plate and under a weight, such as a rock or brick. Within 30 minutes, the salt extracts much of the fluid in the salad, making it softer and wilted. The water is then poured off with the dissolved salt and the salad is ready to serve. Add a little oil and lemon or some other favorite dressing. Most people who like raw salads are often delighted to find that a pressed salad can be both delicious as well as quite pleasantly filling.

Primary Foods

Whole grains: Thirty percent of a healthy diet should be whole grains. This includes brown and white rice, wheat, millet, rye, oatmeal, barley, corn, amaranth, and quinoa.

Protein: Twenty percent of a healthy diet should be protein. This includes beans (azuki, mung, black, garbanzo, kidney, and lentil), tofu and tempeh (made from soybeans), and seitan (made from wheat). Besides being the highest vegetable source of protein, soybeans contain genistein, an estrogen precursor that has been found to both prevent and inhibit the growth of estrogen-sensitive cancers and tumors, such as breast cancer and cervical and ovarian tumors. Soy has also been found to help prevent osteoporosis by regulating estrogen, especially in postmenopausal women, and bone calcium density in turn. Because of this property, many believe that the significantly lower incidence of breast cancer and abnormal menopausal symptoms, including osteoporosis, in Japanese women is at least partially due to the regular use of soybean products. Protein also means the inclusion of animal food products in the form of organic meat, fowl, fish, eggs, and dairy products. As stated previously, animal protein may be essential for the health of more people than has been previously thought. Approximately 2 to 4 ounces of animal protein can be eaten daily. There is certainly something to the Jewish tradition of kosher slaughtering of animals by bleeding them: the toxins of the animal, including the fear hormones, are discharged with the blood. Taoists similarly recommend detoxifying red meat by first soaking it for a half hour or so in cool water, which will leech out much of the blood.

Secondary Foods

Vegetables: Thirty percent of a balanced diet should be vegetables. This includes a variety of root vegetables, such as carrots, yams, potatoes, radishes (including the white daikon radish that helps reduce fat), turnips, burdock, and dioscorea (Asian yam), and leafy greens, such as collards, Swiss chard, watercress, broccoli, cabbage, green lettuce (not iceberg), arugula, nettles, purslane, chicory, and dandelion leaves. Other vegetables that should be included are eggplant, peppers, tomatoes (actually a fruit and possibly not good for individuals with arthritis), cauliflower, artichoke, and the different varieties of squash.

Tertiary Foods

Fruits: Five percent to 10% of a balanced diet should be fruits. Ideally, these should be eaten seasonally. Oranges are high in fruit sugar (fructose) and seem to aggravate conditions of yin dampness, causing excess mucus, increased susceptibility to colds and influenza in the winter, and lower back and joint pains. Grapefruits have a similar but much less negative effect. Lemons and limes seem to be excellent vitamin-rich foods, and it is a good idea to have the juice of one lime or lemon in water daily. Bananas are high in potassium; one banana daily is a good tonic for the kidneys. Most peeled fruits are better digested if a piece of the peel, which is usually more yang, being warm or hot and dry, is eaten along with the fruit. This helps counteract the cold dampness of the internal part of the fruit. Apples are considered to be half vegetable and half fruit, perhaps because of a comparatively high starch content compared to other fruits. It seems that any stewed or baked fruits are more balanced even when out of season. Melons are another fruit of which only the sweet, watery inner parts are eaten, so they should be limited for those with spleen dampness.

Important Whole-Food Supplements

Seaweed: The Japanese eat a wider variety of sea vegetables regularly than any other people. Certain seaweeds are also regarded as a delicacy by coastal northwest Native Americans, who once dried them and traded them to inland tribes. Nutritionally, seaweed is rich in important trace minerals, including organic iodine, which has been depleted from the soil by erosion and overcultivation. Considering the numbers of people who seem to be experiencing symptoms of either high or low thyroid, the iodine found in various seaweeds is an important addition to the diet.

Miso paste: Miso paste, made with fermented soybeans and various grains and commonly found in natural-food stores throughout the country, is a delicious and valuable, healthful food supplement. Its anaerobic bacteria is beneficial for the intestines. The soybeans, from which it is made, are predigested, making them easily bioavailable. Miso can be used in a variety of ways, but the most common is in miso soup. This soup is served before or with Japanese-style meals because it aids digestion. Miso soup can be made with various seaweeds, such as wakame, and/or with one or two vegetables added. Soba (buckwheat) noodles can be added and cooked in the broth. Because of the live beneficial bacteria, miso should never be boiled. Simply add 1 level tablespoon of miso paste to 1 cup of hot water for each serving of soup. Another favorite use for miso is as a sauce. Mix together equal amounts of miso paste, sesame butter, and water and stir to a sauce consistency. A little grated garlic, grated lemon, or curry spices make a delicious variation. Almond butter or peanut butter can also be occasionally substituted for the sesame butter.

Umeboshi plum: Umeboshi plum is another Japanese fermented food that offers many health benefits; it is known as mume plum to the Chinese. As a salt-fermented fruit, it neutralizes acidity. Only a small amount needs to be used in any particular dish, imparting an interesting salty-sweet-sour flavor to various foods. Umeboshi is considered the very best acid neutralizer and can be taken in teas at the beginning of colds, influenza, or simple stomach upset. Umeboshi plum is delicious lightly mixed with rice.

Fermented vegetables: Most cultures have a tradition of fermented foods, such as pickles made from fermented cucumbers. The German people are famous for sauerkraut made from shredded cabbage. Any vegetable can be fermented. The most beneficial anaerobic bacteria result from salt-cured fermented foods. Fermented food made with vinegar generates aerobic bacteria, which are not as compatible with our intestinal flora. Yogurt is a fermented food. Those who must take antibiotics or any other drugs or undergo chemotherapy are likely to suffer ill effects from the imbalance of intestinal flora. For these, it is a good idea to incorporate more fermented foods, such as miso, sauerkraut, or plain yogurt (without added sugar) as part of the regular diet, because fermented foods are powerful digestive aids and boosters of immune strength.

Cooked versus Raw Food

We have already discussed eating cooked versus raw food, but there is a point that must be stressed here. The argument is often made that food loses nutrients, such as a certain amount of vitamins and raw enzymes, when it is cooked. While this is true, the question is never about what one eats but what is absorbed and used. By lightly cooking food, we do lose some nutrients, but what is there our bodies can better assimilate. The regular use of vitamins is based on the notion that they are lacking in our diet. Again it is a question of what we assimilate. Vitamins are commonly found in minuscule amounts in all foods except those that are over-refined or processed, such as white flour, white rice, white cornmeal, and white sugar. Those who regularly eat processed and refined foods may do better by taking a vitamin supplement. As David Reuben, M.D., states (in *Everything You Always Wanted to Know about Nutrition,* 1978 Simon & Schuster), "If you heaped up all the vitamins you need each day in a pile, that pile would be smaller than the period at the end of this sentence." The problem is not so much a lack of vitamins but the overconsumption of refined foods that inhibits their manufacture and use or otherwise destroys them through imbalance.

The Energetics of Food According to Traditional Chinese Medicine

Chinese herbology and food therapy are closely related to each other. Most foods, when used in a special way, become medicine, and many Chinese herbs used as medicine are also used as foods or with food to enhance flavor and therapeutic value. The difference between what we call a food and what we regard as a medicine is that foods have milder qualities and energies. That is why in most cases when food is the primary therapeutic modality, concentrated quantities of certain foods must be taken to achieve a result. Herbs, on the other hand, including substances from the plant, mineral, and animal kingdoms, have stronger qualities and flavors that must be used in prescribed dosage— usually less than that of comparable foods—to effect positive change.

From the aspect of TCM, foods and herbs are classified according to their healing properties along the same energetic continuum. All foods have an inherent cooling or warming energy, as do all herbs and diseases. They also possess the therapeutic properties embodied by the Five Flavors (sweet, spicy, salty, sour, and bitter, as well as the curious sixth nonflavor, bland) and the qualities of dryness or dampness. Other qualities of food, reflected by their textures and colors, also have therapeutic value. From the Western nutritional perspective, nutrients are quantified as to their protein, carbohydrate, vitamin, mineral, and other content, but from the perspective of traditional Chinese nutrition, the energetic qualities described above are considered at least as important and probably more important for healing.

In order to achieve a state of balanced well being, one must learn the energies and qualities of food as well as their grosser nutritional components. An individual complaining of heat in the form of an infection or inflammation will have difficulty fully recovering from the condition if he or she continues to eat warming and heating foods, such as refined sugar, fried onions, fatty foods, and alcohol. This is because these tend to engender more heat and further aggravate the condition. An individual with coldness who complains of lower back stiffness and pain or poor circulation but who ingests such cold-natured items as cold milk, ice cream, and iced drinks will further aggravate their deficient yang and cold damp condition.

While an herbalist can help the person with heat and inflammation recover with such mild-natured herbs as echinacea, lonicera, or coptis, a medical doctor might also achieve similar success with strong antibiotic drugs. This may clear the disease, but further weaken and injure the body's immune system, making it more vulnerable to either recurrence of the same disease or onset of a completely different set of symptoms and diseases. When an individual undergoing herbal therapy eats in a way that energetically opposes what the body needs and what the herbs are intended to do, then the herbal treatment will either be less effective, take longer to have an effect, or have no effect at all. Even when a patient's disease is correctly diagnosed and the proper herbal treatment is prescribed, the body of a patient eating contraindicated foods may not respond favorably or healing may generally progress too slowly. If, on the other hand, an herbalist specifically recommends foods with the correct energies and properties—however mild they may be, they can greatly assist the healing process. Thus, diet can either undermine or contribute to healing, depending on one's condition. Food can tonify and nourish yang, qi, yin, or blood, called the Four Treasures. However, it can also cause coldness, dampness, dryness, heat, or stagnation. Because most people eat two to three times a day, food is a vital part of healing, and "You are what you eat" is not such a strange adage from this perspective.

Therapeutic Foods

Following is a description of the energies, flavors, Five Element organ correspondences, and therapeutic uses of some of the most common foods.

ADUKI OR AZUKI BEANS

Energy; flavors; organs affected: Neutral; sweet, sour; heart, small intestines.

Properties: Reduce weight.

Conditions for which used: Edema, beriberi, mumps, jaundice, diarrhea, discharge of blood from anus.

Avoid under these conditions: Dryness or emaciation.

ALMONDS

Energy; flavors; organs affected: Neutral; sweet; lungs, spleen–pancreas.

Properties: Relieve cough, resolve phlegm, lubricate lungs, tonify *qi* and blood.

APPLES

Energy; flavors; organs affected: Cool; sweet; spleen–pancreas.

Properties: Lubricate, clear heat, counteract depression.

Conditions for which used: Low blood sugar, indigestion, morning sickness, chronic enteritis.

ASPARAGUS

Energy; flavors; organs affected: Cool; sweet, bitter; lungs, kidneys.

Properties: Clears heat and dampness, lubricates dryness, tonifies yin.

Conditions for which used: Cough, mucous discharge, swelling, various kinds of skin eruptions, shortage of mother's milk, diabetes, TB, wasting heat disease.

Avoid under these conditions: Deficiency cold diarrhea, wind cold cough.

BANANAS

Energy; flavors; organs affected: Cold; sweet; spleen, stomach.

Properties: Demulcent, clear heat, counteract toxins, lubricate intestines, tonify yin.

Conditions for which used: Constipation, bleeding piles, hemorrhoids, alcoholism.

Avoid under these conditions: Cold damp conditions.

BARLEY

Energy; flavors; organs affected: Cool; sweet, salty; spleen, stomach.

Properties: Regulates stomach, promotes urination, clears heat, lubricates dryness, expands intestines.

Conditions for which used: Edema, dysuria, indigestion, burns, diarrhea.

BEEF
Energy; flavors; organs affected: Neutral; sweet; spleen, stomach, large
    intestine.
Properties: Tonifies *qi*, blood, and yin; strengthens tendons and bones;
    tonifies stomach and spleen.
Conditions for which used: Emaciation, edema, diabetes, weak knees,
    and low back pain with emaciation; various parts are good for corre-
    sponding organs.

BEETS
Energy; flavors; organs affected: Neutral; sweet; spleen.
Properties: Tonify *qi* and nourish blood, fluids; open meridians; expels
    cold.
Conditions for which used: Rheumatic pains, poor circulation.

BLACK PEPPER
Energy; flavors; organs affected: Hot; sweet; lungs, spleen, stomach,
    large intestine.
Properties: Regulates *qi*, warms the body, is carminative, removes blood
    stagnation and coldness, dries mucus.
Conditions for which used: Vomiting of clear liquid, diarrhea from cold-
    ness, food poisoning, toothache (relieved through topical applica-
    tion).
Avoid under these conditions: Yin deficiency, internal heat.

BLACK SESAME SEEDS
Energy; flavors; organs affected: Neutral; sweet; kidneys, liver.
Properties: Tonifies liver and kidneys, lubricates the organs.
Conditions for which used: Vertigo, constipation, gray hair, weak knees,
    rheumatism, dry skin, shortage of mother's milk; black sesame seeds
    are better for the kidneys–adrenals, while the yellow seeds are better
    for the spleen–pancreas.
Avoid under these conditions: Spleen dampness and watery stools.

BLACK SOYA BEANS
Energy; flavors; organs affected: Neutral; sweet; spleen, kidneys.
Properties: Promote blood circulation and urination, detoxify, nourish
    kidney and liver blood, expel wind.
Conditions for which used: Lower back and knee pains, infertility, invol-

untary seminal emission, premature ejaculation, blurred vision, difficulty urinating, edema, jaundice, rheumatism, muscular cramps, lockjaw, drug poisoning, arthritic and rheumatic conditions.

BUCKWHEAT

Energy; flavors; organs affected: Cool; sweet; large intestine, stomach, spleen.

Properties: Clears heat, lowers rebellious *qi,* improves appetite, eliminates swelling and accumulations.

Conditions for which used: Boils, chronic diarrhea, dysentery, skin lesions and eruptions.

Avoid under these conditions: Vertigo, indigestion, or wind or heat diseases.

BUTTER

Energy; flavors; organs affected: Warm; sweet; spleen, stomach.

Properties: Removes stagnant blood, expels coldness.

Conditions for which used: Scabies, skin eruptions, body odor.

CABBAGE

Energy; flavors; organs affected: Neutral; sweet; spleen, stomach, large intestine.

Properties: Promotes urination, beneficial to kidneys and brain after long consumption.

Conditions for which used: Constipation, thirst due to intoxication, ulcers, depression, coughs and colds, hot flashes.

Avoid under these conditions: Qi deficiency, spleen/stomach yang deficiency, nausea.

CARROTS

Energy; flavors; organs affected: Neutral; sweet; lung, spleen.

Properties: Act as diuretic and digestive, improve eyes, remove swellings and tumors.

Conditions for which used: Indigestion, cough, dysentery, difficult urination, skin eruptions, chronic diarrhea.

CAYENNE

Energy; flavors; organs affected: Hot; pungent; spleen, heart.

Properties: Warms, removes blood stagnation, disperses congestion, expels cold.

Conditions for which used: Poor appetite, cold abdominal pains, diarrhea, vomiting.

Avoid under these conditions: Yin deficiency, excess fire, cough, eye disease.

CELERY

Energy; flavors; organs affected: Cool; bitter, sweet; stomach, liver, kidneys.

Properties: Clears heat, dries damp, calms liver, expels wind, promotes urination.

Conditions for which used: Hypertension, headache, dizziness, discharge of blood in urine, conjunctivitis, carbuncles.

Avoid under these conditions: Scabies.

CHEESE

Energy; flavors; organs affected: Neutral; sour, sweet; liver, lungs, spleen.

Properties: Tonifies *qi*, blood, and yin; quenches thirst.

Conditions for which used: Deficiency fever, dryness, constipation, skin eruptions, itchy skin.

Avoid under these conditions: Weak digestion or conditions involving overproduction of mucus.

CHERRIES

Energy; flavors; organs affected: Warm; sweet; heart, spleen.

Properties: Move blood in lower half of body, expel cold and wind damp.

Conditions for which used: Rheumatism, arthritis, lumbago, paralysis, numbness, frostbite.

CHICKEN

Energy; flavors; organs affected: Warm; sweet; spleen, stomach.

Properties: Tonifies *qi*, moves blood, expels cold, tonifies *jing*.

Conditions for which used: Underweight, diarrhea, edema, poor appetite, vaginal bleeding and discharge, lack of mother's milk, general weakness, frequent urination, weakness after childbirth, diarrhea, dysentery, diabetes, edema, anorexia.

Avoid under these conditions: Excess conditions, external diseases.

CLAMS

Energy; flavors; organs affected: Cold; salty; stomach.
Properties: Clears heat, lubricates dryness, tonifies yin, softens hardness.
Conditions for which used: Diabetes, edema, scrofula, leukorrhea, hemorrhoids, vaginal bleeding.

COCONUT MEAT

Energy; flavors; organs affected: Neutral; sweet; spleen, stomach.
Properties: Tonifies *qi* and blood, expels wind.
Conditions for which used: Malnutrition in children.

COCONUT MILK

Energy; flavors; organs affected: Warm; sweet; spleen, stomach.
Properties: Tonifies *qi* and blood, expels cold, moves blood, quenches thirst.
Conditions for which used: Diabetes.

CORN

Energy; flavors; organs affected: Neutral; sweet; stomach, spleen, large intestine.
Properties: Regulates digestive organs.
Conditions for which used: Weak heart, difficulty urinating, sexual weakness, including lack of libido, frigidity, impotence and infertility.

CRABMEAT

Energy; flavors; organs affected: Cold; salty; stomach.
Properties: Clears heat, moistens dryness, tonifies yin, moves blood.
Conditions for which used: Fractures, poison ivy, burns.
Avoid under these conditions: Wind disease, spleen/stomach yang deficiency; do not overconsume crabmeat.

CUCUMBER

Energy; flavors; organs affected: Cool; sweet; stomach, spleen, large intestine.
Properties: Detoxifies, clears heat, promotes urination, quenches thirst.
Conditions for which used: Sore throat, pink eyes, inflammation, burns.

DATES (RED JUJUBE DATES)

Energy; flavors; organs affected: Warm; sweet; spleen, stomach.
Properties: Tonifies *qi* and blood.
Conditions for which used: Weak stomach, palpitations, nervousness, hysteria from weakness.

DUCK

Energy; flavors; organs affected: Neutral; sweet, salty; lungs, kidneys.
Properties: Tonifies *qi,* blood, and yin; lubricates dryness.
Conditions for which used: Swelling and edema, hot sensations, cough.
Avoid under these conditions: Spleen deficiency, stagnant *qi,* symptoms of hemorrhage.

EGGPLANT

Energy; flavors; organs affected: Cool; sweet; large intestine, spleen, stomach.
Properties: Clears heat, removes stagnant blood, relieves pain and swelling; prevents strokes.
Conditions for which used: Dysentery, bleeding from anus and in urine, boils, skin ulcers, mastitis.
Avoid under these conditions: Women without stagnant blood in the uterus should avoid overconsumption.

FIGS

Energy; flavors; organs affected: Neutral; sweet; large intestine.
Properties: Detoxifies, tonifies stomach, heals swelling.
Conditions for which used: Constipation, hemorrhoids, sore throat, diarrhea, dysentery.

GARLIC

Energy; flavors; organs affected: Warm; pungent; lungs, stomach, spleen.
Properties: Warms, expels cold, promotes *qi* and blood circulation, destroys worms and kills parasites, acts as antiviral and antibacterial.
Conditions for which used: Arthritis, cold abdominal pain, edema, diarrhea, dysentery, whooping cough, tuberculosis (TB), pneumonia, hepatitis.
Avoid under these conditions: Yin deficiency with false fire rising; canker sores.

GINGER (DRIED)

Energy; flavors; organs affected: Hot; pungent; lungs, stomach, spleen.

Properties: Warms, acts as a carminative, expels cold, moves blood, benefits digestion, relieves cramps. Fresh ginger is warm and is best for colds and flus and indigestion.

Conditions for which used: Colds, coughs, cold limbs, diarrhea, vomiting, nausea, mucus, rheumatism, cold abdominal pain.

Avoid under these conditions: Yin deficiency, internal heat, hot blood hemorrhage.

GLUTEN, WHEAT (SEITAN)

Energy; flavors; organs affected: Cool; sweet; stomach, spleen, liver.

Properties: Tonifies *qi,* clears heat, reduces fever, lowers hypertension, quenches thirst.

GOOSE

Energy; flavors; organs affected: Neutral; sweet; lungs, spleen.

Properties: Tonifies *qi,* harmonizes stomach.

Conditions for which used: Diarrhea, diabetes.

Avoid under these conditions: Damp heat conditions.

GRAPES

Energy; flavors; organs affected: Neutral; sweet, sour; lungs, spleen, kidneys.

Properties: Red variety is tonifying to *qi* and blood, strengthens bones and tendons, promotes urination, harmonizes stomach, relieves anger and irritability.

Conditions for which used: Blood and *qi* deficiency, cough, palpitations, night sweats, rheumatism, difficulty urinating, edema.

HERRING

Energy; flavors; organs affected: Neutral; sweet; lungs, spleen.

Properties: Tonifies deficiency, moistens dryness.

Conditions for which used: Deficiency fatigue.

Avoid under these conditions: Skin eruptions or when recovering from chronic diseases.

HONEY

Energy; flavors; organs affected: Neutral; sweet; lungs, spleen, large intestine.

Properties: Tonifies *qi* and blood, lubricates dryness, relieves pain.

Conditions for which used: Dry cough, constipation, stomach ache, sinusitis, mouth cankers, burns, neurasthenia, hypertension, TB, heart disease, liver disease, aconite poisoning.

KELP

Energy; flavors; organs affected: Cold; salty; stomach, spleen.

Properties: Clears heat, moistens dryness, tonifies yin, softens hardness.

Conditions for which used: Scrofula, goiter, edema, leukorrhea, orchitis.

Avoid under these conditions: Stomach and spleen yang deficiency and/or dampness.

KIDNEY BEANS

Energy; flavors; organs affected: Neutral; sweet; spleen, kidney.

Properties: Tonifies yin, promotes urination, clears heat, acts as a diuretic, reduces swelling.

Conditions for which used: Edema.

KUDZU ROOT POWDER

Energy; flavors; organs affected: Cool; sweet; stomach, large intestines.

Properties: Clears heat, tonifies yin, quenches thirst.

Conditions for which used: Stomach and intestinal influenza, hangover, toothache, hot skin eruptions, stiff neck and shoulders.

LAMB (MUTTON)

Energy; flavors; organs affected: Warm; sweet; spleen, kidneys.

Properties: Tonifies *qi*, warms and expels coldness, removes blood stagnation, strengthens sexual power and penile erection.

Conditions for which used: Indigestion, fatigue, emaciation, coldness, lumbago, general weakness, underweight, abdominal pain, postpartum cold sensations, sore loins.

Avoid under these conditions: Cold external diseases, internal heat.

LEMON

Energy; flavors; and organs affected: Cool; sour; liver.

Properties: Produces fluid, considered good for pregnancy.

Conditions for which used: Cough with mucous discharge, diabetes, indigestion, laryngitis, fat reduction.

LETTUCE

Energy; flavors; organs affected: Cool; sweet, bitter; large intestine.

Properties: Clears heat, dries damp, promotes urination and milk secretion, calms, inhibits bleeding.

Avoid under these conditions: Eye disease; overconsumption can cause dizziness and blurred vision.

LOTUS ROOT

Energy; flavors; organs affected: Cool; sweet; stomach, spleen, heart.

Properties: Cools blood, tonifies yin, clears heat, strengthens appetite, tones spleen, increases muscle strength.

Conditions for which used: Thirst, dryness, weakness, bleeding; cooked root is used for anorexia, diarrhea, and lung ailments.

LOQUAT

Energy; flavors; organs affected: Neutral; sour, sweet; spleen, liver, lungs.

Properties: Lubricates dryness of the throat, and lungs, quenches thirst.

Conditions for which used: Cough, constipation, laryngitis.

MANGO

Energy; flavors; organs affected: Cold; sweet, sour; stomach.

Properties: Quenches thirst, strengthens stomach, relieves vomiting, promotes urination.

Conditions for which used: Cough, indigestion, bleeding from gums.

Avoid under these conditions: Common cold, indigestion, during convalescence; overconsumption can cause itching or skin eruptions.

MILK

Energy; flavors; organs affected: Neutral; sweet; lungs, stomach, heart.

Properties: Tonifies blood and qi, produces fluids, lubricates dryness of the intestines, tonifies deficiencies.

Conditions for which used: Indigestion (take scalded and warm), upset stomach, difficulty swallowing, diabetes, constipation.

Avoid under these conditions: Weak spleen–stomach with dampness.

MILLET

Energy; flavors; organs affected: Cool; sweet, salty; stomach, spleen, kidneys.

Properties: Tonifies *qi,* clears heat, benefits kidneys and Middle Warmer, lubricates dryness associated with wasting and yin deficiency.

Conditions for which used: Indigestion, counteraction of toxins, diabetes, vomiting, diarrhea.

Avoid under these conditions: Undigested food in stools, spleen and stomach yang deficiency.

MUNG BEANS

Energy; flavors; organs affected: Cool; sweet; stomach, heart.

Properties: Promotes urination, clears heat, detoxifies, relieves hypertension and summer heat.

Conditions for which used: Diarrhea, dysentery, diabetes, boils, edema, burns, lead and drug poisoning; sprouts are good for alcoholism.

MUSHROOMS, COMMON BUTTON

Energy; flavors; organs affected: Cool; sweet; lungs, large intestine, stomach, spleen.

Properties: Clear heat; calm spirit; reduce tumors, edema, mucous discharge.

Conditions for which used: Vomiting, diarrhea.

Avoid under these conditions: Cold stomach, skin problems, allergies.

MUSHROOMS, SHIITAKE

Energy; flavors; organs affected: Neutral; sweet; stomach, liver.

Properties: Tonify blood, benefit the stomach, act as an anti-inflammatory.

Conditions for which used: High cholesterol levels, hypertension, common colds, chickenpox, cancer, kidney problems, gallstones, hemorrhoids, lack of vitamin D, softening of the bones, cataracts, pyorrhea, ulcers, neuralgia, anemia, measles.

MUSTARD GREENS

Energy; flavors; organs affected: Warm; pungent; lungs.

Properties: Act as a carminative, regulate *qi,* remove blood stagnation, expel cold, dry up mucus.

Conditions for which used: Cough, mucous discharge, chest congestion.

Avoid under these conditions: Skin eruptions, eye disease, hemorrhoids, anal hemorrhage, heat conditions, bleeding, pink eye.

NORI

Energy; flavors; organs affected: Cold; sweet, salty; lungs.
Properties: Clears heat, tonifies yin, softens hardness, acts as a diuretic.
Conditions for which used: Goiter, beriberi, edema, dysuria, hypertension.

OLIVES

Energy; flavors; organs affected: Neutral; sweet, sour; lungs, stomach.
Properties: Moisten, clear lungs.
Conditions for which used: Sore throat, coughing blood, alcoholism.

ONIONS

Energy; flavors; organs affected: Warm; pungent; lungs, stomach.
Properties: Tonify and regulate *qi,* remove blood stagnation, expel cold, act as a diaphoretic, counteract toxins, act as a diuretic, act as an expectorant.
Conditions for which used: Pneumonia, common cold, headache, constipation, cold abdominal pain, dysuria, dysentery, mastitis, nasal congestion, facial edema; externally, used for *Trichomonas* vaginitis and for ulcers.

OYSTERS

Energy; flavors; organs affected: Neutral; sweet, salty; kidneys, liver.
Properties: Tonify blood, yin, and hormones.
Conditions for which used: Stress, insomnia, nervousness.
Avoid under these conditions: Skin diseases.

PAPAYAS

Energy; flavors; organs affected: Neutral; sweet; spleen, heart.
Properties: Promote digestion, destroy intestinal worms.
Conditions for which used: Stomachache, dysentery, difficult bowel movements, rheumatism, rheumatic conditions.

PEAS

Energy; flavors; organs affected: Neutral; sweet; stomach, spleen.
Properties: Lowers rebellious *qi,* act as a diuretic, induce bowel movements.
Conditions for which used: Spasms, carbuncles, skin eruptions.

PEACHES

Energy; flavors; organs affected: Warm; sour, sweet; spleen.
Properties: Promote blood circulation, remove blood stagnation, expel cold, lubricate intestines.
Conditions for which used: Dry cough, hernial pain, excessive perspiration, indigestion.
Avoid: Excess intake—can produce internal heat.

PEANUTS

Energy; flavors; organs affected: Neutral; sweet; lung, spleen.
Properties: Lubricate lungs, promote lactation.
Conditions for which used: Stomachache, dry cough, upset stomach.
Avoid under these conditions: Damp conditions, *qi* stagnation.

PEARS

Energy; flavors; organs affected: Cool; sweet; lungs, stomach.
Properties: Clear heat, produce fluids, lubricate dryness, eliminates phlegm.
Conditions for which used: Hot cough with mucus, constipation, alcoholism, indigestion, difficulty swallowing, difficulty urinating, diabetes.

PERSIMMONS

Energy; flavors; organs affected: Cold; sweet; lung, heart, large intestine.
Properties: Clear heat, tonify yin, lubricate lungs, quench thirst.
Conditions for which used: Cough, canker sores, chronic bronchitis.
Avoid under these conditions: Spleen/stomach yang deficiency, diarrhea, malaria.

PINEAPPLES

Energy; flavors; organs affected: Neutral; sweet; spleen.
Properties: Quench thirst, promote digestion, relieve diarrhea.
Conditions for which used: Anorexia, edema, thirst, sunstroke, oliguria.
Avoid under these conditions: Damp and/or cold conditions.

PINE NUTS

Energy; flavors; organs affected: Warm; sweet; lung, liver, large intestine.

Properties: Tonify *qi*, remove blood stagnation, expel cold, demulcent, expel wind.

Conditions for which used: Wind *bi* (rheumatism), vertigo, dry cough, constipation.

PLANTAINS

Energy; flavors; organs affected: Cold; sweet; large and small intestines.

Properties: Clear heat, tonify yin, expel sputum, sharpen vision.

Conditions for which used: Anuria, dysuria, leukorrhea, hematuria, pertussis, jaundice, edema, dysentery, epistaxis, conjunctivitis, eye pain, skin ulcers.

Avoid under these conditions: Spermatorrhea.

PLUMS

Energy; flavors; organs affected: Neutral; sweet, sour; kidneys, liver.

Properties: Clear liver and heat, moisten intestines and promote urination and digestion.

Conditions for which used: Liver disease, diabetes, fatigue.

Avoid: Excess intake—can cause bloating and gas.

PORK

Energy; flavors; organs affected: Neutral; salty, sweet; kidneys, stomach, spleen.

Properties: Lubricates dryness, tonifies yin.

Conditions for which used: Diabetes, weakness, emaciation, dry cough, constipation.

Avoid under these conditions: Hot sputum or *qi* stagnation.

POTATOES, WHITE

Energy; flavors; organs affected: Neutral; sweet; spleen, stomach.

Properties: Heal inflammation, tonify *qi* and the spleen.

Conditions for which used: Lack of energy, mumps, burns.

POTATOES, SWEET

Energy; flavors; organs affected: Neutral; sweet; spleen, kidneys.

Properties: Tonify *qi* and spleen, remove blood stagnation, expel coldness, produce fluid, induce bowel movements.

Conditions for which used: Jaundice, emaciation, skin eruptions, stomach and kidney weakness, premature ejaculation.

Avoid under these conditions: Qi and food stagnation.

PUMPKINS
Energy; flavors; organs affected: Neutral; sweet; spleen, stomach.
Properties: Dry dampness, tonify *qi,* induce sweating.
Conditions for which used: Bronchial asthma.

RADISHES
Energy; flavors; organs affected: Cool; sweet, pungent; lungs, stomach.
Properties: Detoxify, promote digestion, eliminate hot mucous discharge, expel cold.
Conditions for which used: Abdominal swelling due to indigestion, laryngitis due to continual cough with mucous discharge, vomiting of blood, nosebleed, dysentery, headache, bloating, hoarseness, diabetes, occipital headache, epistaxis, dysentery, *Trichomonas* vaginitis.
Avoid under these conditions: Coldness from deficiency.

RASPBERRIES
Energy; flavors; organs affected: Neutral; sweet, sour; liver, kidneys.
Properties: Tonify liver and kidneys, check frequent urination, sharpen vision.
Conditions for which used: Impotence, dizziness, spermatorrhea, polyuria, enuresis, deficiency fatigue, blurred vision.
Avoid under these conditions: Painful or difficult urination.

RICE, BROWN
Energy; flavors; organs affected: Neutral; sweet; spleen, stomach.
Properties: Tonifies *qi* and spleen, harmonizes stomach, relieves depression, quenches thirst.
Conditions for which used: Diarrhea, morning sickness, thirst.

RICE, SWEET
Energy; flavors; organs affected: Warm; sweet; lungs.
Properties: Tonifies *qi* and assists yang, expels cold, moves stagnant blood.
Conditions for which used: Diabetes, polyuria, diarrhea, excessive sweating.
Avoid under these conditions: Stomach/spleen *qi* deficiency, sputum heat, wind disease.

RICE, WHITE

Energy; flavors; organs affected: Slightly cool; sweet; spleen, stomach.
Properties and uses: Similar to those for brown rice but clears heat from acidity.

RYE

Energy; flavors; organs affected: Neutral; bitter; heart.
Properties: Dries dampness, acts as a diuretic.
Conditions for which used: Postpartum hemorrhage, migraine; can be toxic.

SALT

Energy; flavors; organs affected: Cold; salty; large and small intestines, stomach, kidneys.
Properties: Detoxifies, lubricates dryness, induces vomiting, cools blood.
Conditions for which used: Abdominal swelling and pain, difficulty moving bowels, dysuria, pyorrhea, sore throat, toothaches, corneal opacity, skin eruptions, constipation, bleeding from gums, cataracts.
Avoid: Fluid retention high blood pressure.

SARDINES

Energy; flavors; organs affected: Neutral; sweet, salty; spleen, stomach.
Properties: Demulcent, tonify yin, warm Middle Burner, strengthen tendons and bones, activate blood, act as a diuretic, act as a digestant.
Conditions for which used: Urinary strain.
Avoid: Overconsumption—can cause fire and sputum.

SEAWEED

Energy; flavors; organs affected: Cold; salty; kidneys, stomach.
Properties: Lubricates dryness, softens hardness (lumps and tumors), tonifies yin, eliminates mucus, promotes water passage.
Conditions for which used: Goiter, abdominal swelling and obstruction, edema, beriberi.

SESAME OIL

Energy; flavors; organs affected: Cool; sweet; stomach.
Properties: Detoxifies, lubricates dryness, promotes bowel movements, clears heat, increases muscle strength.

Conditions for which used: Constipation, abdominal pain caused by indigestion, roundworms, skin eruptions, ulcers, tinea, scabies, dry and cracked skin.

Avoid under these conditions: Diarrhea with deficiency of spleen *qi*.

SHRIMP

Energy; flavors; organs affected: Warm; sweet; spleen, stomach.

Properties: Tonifies *qi* and yang, removes blood stagnation, expels cold, eliminates wind, expels sputum, promotes lactation, destroys worms.

Avoid under these conditions: Hot skin diseases, period of recuperation from chronic illness.

SOYBEANS

Energy; flavors; organs affected: Cool; sweet; large intestine, spleen.

Properties: Clear heat, sedate yang, strengthen spleen, moisten dryness.

Conditions for which used: Diarrhea, emaciation, skin eruptions, hemorrhage from trauma, *qi* stagnation, cough and/or heavy sensations in the body.

SPINACH

Energy; flavors; organs affected: Cool; sweet; large and small intestine.

Properties: Lubricates dryness, arrests bleeding, clears heat, acts as a hemostatic.

Conditions for which used: Nosebleed, discharge of blood from anus, thirst in diabetes, constipation, alcoholism, scurvy, hemorrhoids.

Avoid under these conditions: Spermatorrhea.

SQUASH, WINTER

Energy; flavors; organs affected: Warm; sweet; stomach, spleen.

Properties: Tonifies *qi* and blood, assists yang, heals inflammation, relieves pain, moves blood, expels cold.

Conditions for which used: Pulmonary abscess, roundworms.

Avoid under these conditions: Dampness and/or *qi* stagnation.

STRAWBERRIES

Energy; flavors; organs affected: Warm; sweet, sour; liver, kidneys.

Properties: Remove blood stagnation, expel cold.

Conditions for which used: Polyuria, vertigo, motion sickness.

STRING BEANS

Energy; flavors; organs affected: Neutral; sweet; spleen, kidneys.

Properties: Tonify yin and kidneys, strengthen spleen.

Conditions for which used: Polyuria, diarrhea, diabetes, spermatorrhea, leukorrhea.

Avoid under these conditions: Qi stagnation, constipation.

SWISS CHARD

Energy; flavors; organs affected: Cool; sweet; large intestine, lungs, stomach.

Properties: Clears heat, detoxifies, acts as a hemostatic.

Conditions for which used: Delayed eruptions of measles, dysentery, amenorrhea, carbuncles.

TANGERINES

Energy; flavors; organs affected: Cool; sour, sweet; lungs, kidneys, stomach.

Properties: Regulate *qi,* clear heat, quench thirst, lubricate lungs, relieve coughing, stimulates appetite.

Conditions for which used: Chest congestion, vomiting, hiccuping, diabetes.

Avoid under these conditions: Cough and sputum from external wind and cold.

TOMATOES

Energy; flavors; organs affected: Cold; sweet, sour; stomach, liver.

Properties: Clear heat, tonify yin, quench thirst, promote digestion.

Conditions for which used: Thirst and anorexia.

TROUT

Energy; flavors; organs affected: Hot; sour; liver, gallbladder, stomach.

Properties: Assists yang, expels cold, regulates *qi,* harmonizes Middle Warmer, warms stomach.

Avoid: Overconsumption—can aggravate scabies and skin eruptions.

TUNA

Energy; flavors; organs affected: Neutral; sweet; stomach.

Properties: Tonifies *qi* and blood, transforms damp.

Conditions for which used: Beriberi, damp *bi* (arthritic and rheumatic conditions).

VINEGAR
Energy; flavors; organs affected: Warm; sour, bitter; stomach, liver.
Properties: Disperses coagulation, removes blood stagnation, detoxifies, arrests bleeding, dries dampness, induces perspiration, expels cold, acts as a hemostatic and vermifuge.
Conditions for which used: Postpartum syncope, genital itching, abdominal swelling and obstruction, jaundice, food poisoning.
Avoid under these conditions: Spleen/stomach yang deficiency, muscular atrophy, rheumatism, tendon trauma, at the beginning of a common cold.

WALNUTS
Energy; flavors; organs affected: Warm; sweet; lungs, kidneys.
Properties: Tonify kidneys, lubricate intestines, check seminal emission, expel cold, solidify sperm, warm lungs, calm.
Conditions for which used: Asthma, cough, lumbago, impotence, spermatorrhea, frequent urination, dry stools, kidney and bladder stones, constipation.
Avoid under these conditions: Yin deficiency with false fire rising.

WATER CHESTNUTS
Energy; flavors; organs affected: Cold; sweet; lungs, stomach.
Properties: Clear heat, relieve fever and indigestion, promote urination, disperse accumulations.
Conditions for which used: Hypertension, diabetes, jaundice, conjunctivitis, measles, dysentery with bloody stools, smoker's sore throat.
Avoid under these conditions: Anemia, coldness or blood deficiency.

WATERCRESS
Energy; flavors; organs affected: Cool; pungent; lungs, stomach.
Properties: Removes blood stagnation, clears heat, benefits fluids.
Conditions for which used: Jaundice, edema, urinary strain, leukorrhea, mumps, oliguria.
Avoid under these conditions: Spleen/stomach deficiency or frequent urination.

WATERMELON

Energy; flavors; organs affected: Cold; sweet; stomach, heart, bladder.
Properties: Clears heat, lubricates intestines, relieves summer heat, relieves mental depression, quenches thirst, acts as a diuretic.
Conditions for which used: Oliguria, sore throat, canker sores, diminished urination.
Avoid under these conditions: Excess dampness, anemia, frequent urination, coldness in the Middle Warmer.

WHEAT

Energy; flavors; organs affected: Cool; sweet; spleen, heart, kidneys.
Properties: Nourishes heart, calms spirit, clears heat, quenches thirst.
Conditions for which used: Insomnia, nervousness, irritability, thirst.

WHITEFISH

Energy; flavors; organs affected: Neutral, sweet; lungs, stomach, liver.
Properties: Tonifies spleen, relieves indigestion, promotes water flow.

YAMS

Energy; flavors; organs affected: Neutral; sweet; lungs, spleen, kidneys.
Properties: Tonify spleen, lungs, kidneys; benefit semen.
Conditions for which used: Diarrhea, dysentery, diabetes, leukorrhea, spermatorrhea, polyuria, cough.
Avoid under these conditions: Diseases caused by excess.

SEVEN

EIGHT METHODS OF
HERBAL TREATMENT

Chinese herbalism outlines eight methods of herbal treatment, most of which correlate to Western therapeutic properties: vomiting, purging, harmonizing, warming, cooling, supplementing, and reducing. From a broader perspective, each of the eight methods can be placed into one of four categories: eliminating, regenerating, inhibiting, or moving. Nature seems to defy any attempts at developing definitive simplistic classifications. Even a single herb may possess two or more properties. In general, an herb with only one outstanding property tends to be milder, while an herb with many paradoxically opposite properties is often more therapeutic. The way that it is described and classified reflects its predominant usage, but often, the secondary properties of an herb reflect its unique therapeutic identity. For instance, pueraria is used to induce perspiration in the treatment of colds and influenza, but it is used in the treatment of muscle spasms and colitis because of its nourishing, lubricating, and antispasmodic properties.

The following table defines the most common properties of herbs, based on Western classifications and subclassified into the Chinese eight methods and the four categories under which they may be understood.

PROPERTIES AND CLASSIFICATIONS OF HERBS

PROPERTY	DEFINITION	METHOD	CATEGORY
ABORTIFACIENT	Induces abortion	Cooling, warming, moving	Eliminating
ALTERATIVE	Detoxifies by chemical reaction or the promotion of a normal detoxifying or eliminative function, restoring normal bodily functions	Cooling, harmonizing, purging	Eliminating
ANALGESIC	Relieves pain when taken internally	cooling, harmonizing, purging, reducing, vomiting, warming	Eliminating, moving
ANHYDROTIC	Stops sweating	Reducing, cooling, tonifying, harmonizing	Inhibiting
ANODYNE	Relieves pain when applied externally	Warming, cooling, reducing	Moving, eliminating
ANTHELMINTIC	Eliminates and/or destroys internal parasites	Cooling, purging	Eliminating, inhibiting, moving
ANTIBIOTIC	Destroys or stops the growth of bacteria	Cooling, reducing	eliminating, inhibiting, moving
ANTIEMETIC	Lessens nausea, stops vomiting	Harmonizing, warming	Inhibiting
ANTI-INFLAMMATORY/ ANTIPHLOGISTIC	Counteracts inflammation	Cooling, reducing, purging, harmonizing	Eliminating, inhibiting, moving
ANTIPYRETIC	Relieves fever	Sweating, purging, harmonizing, cooling, reducing	Eliminating, inhibiting

PROPERTY	DEFINITION	METHOD	CATEGORY
ANTISPASMODIC	Relieves spasms	Sweating, purging, harmonizing, warming, cooling, reducing	Moving, eliminating, inhibiting
ANTITUSSIVE	Prevents or stops coughing	Vomiting, harmonizing, supplementing, cooling, warming	Inhibiting, eliminating, tonifying, moving
APERIENT	Mild laxative	Purging, cooling, reducing	Eliminating, moving
AROMATIC	Contains odorous volatile oils	Sweating, warming, cooling	Eliminative, inhibiting, moving
ASTRINGENT	Firms tissues and organs, reduces discharges and secretions	Reducing, cooling, drying, warming	eliminative
CALMATIVE	Soothes, sedates	Warming, cooling, sweating, purging, reducing	Inhibiting, eliminating
CARDIAC	Assists the heart	Supplementing, cooling, reducing, harmonizing, warming	Moving, regenerating, eliminating
CARMINATIVE	Relieves intestinal gas, promotes peristalsis	Warming, reducing, purging, supplementing	Moving, inhibiting, eliminating, tonifying
CATHARTIC	Violent purgative	Purging, reducing, cooling, warming	Eliminating, moving
CHOLAGOGUE	Promotes bile secretion	Purging, cooling, reducing	Eliminating, moving
DEMULCENT	Lubricates tissues	Cooling, harmonizing, supplementing	Regenerating

PROPERTY	DEFINITION	METHOD	CATEGORY
DEPURATIVE	Purifies blood	Reducing, purging, cooling, harmonizing	Eliminating
DIAPHORETIC	Causes perspiration	Sweating, reducing, cooling, warming	Eliminating, moving
DIGESTANT	Promotes digestion	Warming, supplementing, cooling	Regenerating
DIURETIC	Causes urination	Reducing, cooling, warming	Eliminating, moving
EMMENAGOGUE	Promotes menstrual periods, stimulates blood circulation	Cooling, warming	Moving, eliminating
EMOLLIENT	Softens tissue	Harmonizing, cooling, supplementing	Regenerating
FEBRIFUGE	Clears fevers	Cooling, reducing	Eliminating
GALACTAGOGUE	Promotes milk secretion	Supplementing, harmonizing	Regenerating
HEMOSTATIC	Stops bleeding	Reducing, cooling	Inhibiting
HYPNOTIC	Acts as powerful sedative	Harmonizing, warming, cooling	Inhibiting
LAXATIVE	Promotes bowel movement	Purging, reducing, cooling	Eliminating, moving
LITHOTRIPTIC	Dissolves or discharges urinary and biliary stones	Cooling, reducing	Eliminating, moving
NERVINE	Strengthens functional activity of the nervous system, generally calming	Supplementing, harmonizing, reducing, cooling, warming	Regenerating
NUTRITIVE	Nourishes the body	Supplementing, harmonizing, warming	Regenerating

PROPERTY	DEFINITION	METHOD	CATEGORY
OPHTHALMIC	Treats the eyes	Cooling, reducing	Eliminating
PARTURIENT	Assists or induces labor	Reducing, warming, cooling	Moving, supplementing
PECTORAL	Affects the bronchopulmonary area	Warming, cooling, reducing, harmonizing, supplementing	Eliminating, regenerating, inhibiting, moving
PROPHYLACTIC	Prevents disease	Supplementing, warming, harmonizing	Regenerating, eliminating
PURGATIVE	Causes a strong bowel evacuation	Purging, cooling, warming, reducing	Eliminating, moving
REFRIGERANT	Reduces temperature	Cooling, reducing	Eliminating, inhibiting
RUBEFACIENT	Dilates the capillaries and causes a red, flushed appearance when topically applied	Warming, reducing, moving, eliminating	Moving, eliminating
SEDATIVE	Induces sleep	Cooling, warming, harmonizing, sweating, supplementing	Tonifying, eliminating, moving
SIALAGOGUE	Promotes the secretion of saliva	Reducing, cooling, supplementing	Regenerating, moving
SPECIFIC	Has a curative effect for a specific organ or disease	All	All
STIMULANT	Increases internal heat and organ functions	Warming	Moving
STOMACHIC	Relieves stomach problems, strengthens digestion	Cooling, purging, reducing, supplementing	Eliminating, moving, regenerating
STYPTIC	Stops bleeding when externally applied	Reducing	Inhibiting

PROPERTY	DEFINITION	METHOD	CATEGORY
SUDORIFIC	Increases perspiration	Sweating, warming	Moving, eliminating
TONIC	Strengthens vital functions	Supplementing	Regenerating
VASODILATOR	Dilates the blood vessels	Cooling, warming, harmonizing	Moving
VERMICIDE	Destroys worms	Cooling, purging, reducing	Eliminating
VERMIFUGE	Expels or repels intestinal worms	Cooling, purging, reducing	Eliminating
VULNERARY	Promotes the healing of wounds, stimulates agglutination and cell proliferation	Supplementing, harmonizing	Regenerating

A Further Examination of the Eight Methods

Sweating

Sweating, or diaphoretic therapy, is used for treating external wind cold or external wind heat. (*Wind* in this sense refers to the spreading or proliferating nature of the condition.) Symptoms for external wind cold are chills, fever, headache, aching stiffness (especially of the neck and shoulders), thirst, a white-coated tongue, and a floating and tense pulse. Warming diaphoretic formulas, including Ephedra Combination (*Ma Huang Tang*), Pueraria Combination (*Ge Gen Tang*), and Cinnamon Combination (*Gui Zhi Tang*), are used. External wind heat exhibits symptoms of high fever, chills, thirst, red tongue with a thin yellow coat, and a rapid pulse. Representative formulas for this are Lonicera and Forsythia Combination (*Yin Qiao San*) or Morus and Chrysanthemum Combination (*Sang Ju Yin*).

Contraindications: Sweating therapy should not be used when there is anemia, a severe loss of bodily fluids from vomiting and diarrhea, or a deficiency of blood and/or yin.

Vomiting

Vomiting (emetic) therapy is primarily used in traditional Chinese medicine (TCM) for treating food and narcotic poisoning. The most convenient substance, ipecac, from South America, is available at pharmacies through the West.

Contraindications: Vomiting should never be induced when caustic substances, such as lye or various other petroleum or chemical poisons, have been ingested. In such a case, the safest approach is to dilute the poisonous substance with a protecting demulcent substance such as licorice tea, marshmallow root, or slippery elm gruel. For such serious poisoning, proper medical assistance should be obtained as soon as possible.

Purgation

Purgation is used to eliminate a buildup of waste and toxins through the colon. Purgatives are used for excess patterns with gastric and intestinal pains, constipation, dry stools, and stagnant blood in the lower abdomen with possible lower abdominal pain. Purgative formulas containing rhubarb are characteristically bitter, cold, and detoxifying. Chinese purgative formulas include Major and Minor Rhubarb Combination (*Da Cheng Qi Tang* and *Xiao Cheng Qi Tang*) and Rhubarb and Moutan Combination (*Da Huang Mu Dan Pi Tang*). In East Indian Ayurvedic medicine, the safest and mildest purgative is triphala, made from *Terminalia emblica, T. belerica, and T. chebula.* This formula will not cause laxative dependency, and it can be used for both excess and mild deficiency conditions to aid internal cleansing and detoxification.

Contraindications: Purgatives are generally not used in the presence of any surface conformation, since purgatives can weaken and cool the internal and drive the external disease inward. They also should not be used for half-external, half-internal conditions (which require harmonizing therapy instead). In general they are not for individuals with fluid loss, for those in delicate health, or for those who lack vitality. Purgatives should be avoided during menstruation, pregnancy, and the postpartum period.

Harmonizing

Harmonizing therapy is used for diseases involving the liver, gallbladder, or stomach. Being the most commonly indicated therapy, it is used for diseases of mixed conformation, commonly involving the liver and gallbladder, such as hepatitis, liver *qi* stagnation with chest and abdominal discomfort, depression, moodiness, nausea, intermittent fever (such as malaria), and premenstrual syndrome in women. It is also indicated for lingering colds and fevers in which the symptoms are mixed external, internal, hot, cold, excess, and deficiency. Some of the most commonly used harmonizing formulas are Minor Bupleurum Combination *Xiao Chai Hu Tang)*, Bupleurum and Cinnamon Combination (*Chai Hu Gui Zhi Tang*), and Major Bupleurum Combination (*Da Chai Hu Tang*).

Contraindications: Harmonizing therapy is contraindicated for individuals with a clear external, internal, or excess conformation.

Warming

Warming therapy is used to supplement and strengthen yang *qi*. It is therefore used for coldness, vomiting, abdominal pain, weak pulse, and a general cold, weak conformation. Symptoms of coldness are digestive weakness, loose stools, clear urine, weakness of body and spirit, cold extremities, poor appetite, abdominal distension, and stomach pains. Biomedically, it is often associated with such conditions as hypoglycemia, hypothyroidism, and hypoadrenalism. For this, internal warming stimulants, such as red and black pepper, dried ginger, cinnamon, cloves, galangal root, and prepared aconite are used. For general coldness and hypofunction, one can use Aconite, Ginger, and Licorice Combination (*Si Ni Tang*). For cold, yang-deficient digestion (deficient spleen yang), use Vitality Combination (*Zhen Wu Tang*) or Ginseng and Ginger Combination (*Li Zhong Tang*). For deficient kidneys–adrenals, use Rehmannia Eight Combination (*Ba Wei Di Huang Tang*).

Contraindications: Do not use warming therapy where there is internal excess heat or internal heat with external chills, in individuals with yin deficiency and symptoms of false yang, when there is spitting up of blood or blood in the stools, or during diarrhea with fever.

Cooling

Cooling therapy is used to counteract inflammation and fevers caused by bacteria and viruses. Formulas such as Lonicera and Forsythia Combination (*Yin Qiao San*) are used for external wind heat conformation with symptoms of high fever, mild chills, sore throat, headache, thirst, pink tongue with a yellow coat, and a floating, rapid pulse. White Tiger Combination (Bai Hu Tang), Coptis and Scutellaria Combination (Huang Lian Jie Du Tang) and Gentiana Combination (Long Dan Xie Gan Tang) are used for inflammatory symptoms when there are high fever; no chills; irritability; excess perspiration; great thirst; constipation; abdominal pain; flushed face; abhorrence of heat; cough with yellow phlegm; dark concentrated urine; red tongue with a yellow coat; and a strong, full pulse. Anemarrhena and Philodendron Combination (Zhi Bai Di Huang Wan) is used for yin deficiency and inflammations with symptoms of late afternoon and evening fever; insomnia; irritability; delirium; dry, scarlet tongue; and rapid, thin pulse. A fourth stage of blood heat, which requires the use of unprepared rehmannia, scrophularia, and water buffalo horn, has symptoms of high fever, delirium or unconsciousness, coma, insomnia; signs of bleeding, such as vomiting of blood, bleeding from the nose, blood in the stool, and easy bruising underneath the skin; and symptoms of spasms from heat and exhaustion. The tongue is dark red with prickles and the pulse is thready and rapid.

Contraindications: Cooling therapy is contraindicated for individuals with delicate health who have cold extremities, loose stools, diarrhea, low energy, blood deficiency, and anemia.

Tonification

Tonification therapy is indicated for individuals who are weak and are in need of some level of nutritional supplementation. In Chinese herbalism, there are four kinds of deficiencies—qi, blood, yin, and yang, with tonics for each.

Qi deficiency is accompanied with such symptoms as low energy, weakness, prolapse, shallow breath, timidity, and soft-spokenness. Such herbs as ginseng, astragalus, and atractylodes are indicated. The basic formula for qi deficiency is Four Major Herb Combination (Si Jun Zi Tang).

Blood deficiency is diagnosed in individuals with pale complexion, weakness, dizziness, thirst, palpitations, and scanty or stopped menstruation. Dang Gui Four (Si Wu Tang) is the base formula indicated.

Yin deficiency presents with a thin, emaciated appearance, possible night sweats, insomnia, dizziness, exhaustion, excessive palpitations, five burning spaces (a sensation of heat on the soles of the feet, hands, and chest), nocturnal emissions, and spitting of blood. Rehmannia Six Combination (Liu Wei Di Huang Wan) is commonly used for kidney and liver yin deficiency.

Yang deficiency is indicated by feelings of coldness and chills, especially of the lower body, knee pains, aching lower back pain, irregular bowel movements, lower abdominal pains, frequent urination, impotence, frigidity, and diarrhea. Rehmannia Eight Combination (Ba Wei Di Huang Tang) is commonly used.

Since food is considered the supreme tonic, appropriate tonic foods (rice or proteinaceous foods) are most effective if they are prepared with corresponding tonic herbs. An example of this is to precook the herbs, such as ginseng, astragalus, dang gui, lycii berries, and jujube dates, according to the needs of the individual and then to cook rice in the resultant tea or use the tea as a stock for soup. Herbs cooked with sweet glutinous rice is called congee; eating congee is superior to taking only the food or the herbs by themselves.

Contraindications: Tonification is contraindicated for individuals with an excess conformation or stagnation of qi.

Reducing

Reducing therapy is used to remove stagnation of qi, blood, or phlegm. Unlike purgation therapy, reducing therapy dissolves or breaks up such accumulations as cysts, tumors, abnormal swellings, fat (obesity), ulcers, blood clots, and extravasated blood. Unlike purging, reducing therapy tends to be slower and more gradual; it may be weeks or months before results are noticed. Such formulas as Cinnamon and Poria Combination (Gui Zhi Fu Ling Tang) and the patented Yunnan Paiyao are used for blood stagnation; Stephania and Astragalus Combination (Fang Ji Huang Qi Tang) together with Siler and Platycodon Combination (Fang Feng Tung Shen San) are given to reduce obesity; Crataegus and Citrus Combination (Bao He Wan) is used for food stagnation; and Bupleurum and Chih Shih Combination is given for qi stagnation.

Contraindications: Do not use the reducing method when there is weakness of qi with abdominal distension, low-grade fever, thirst, loss of appetite, diarrhea, weak digestion, and gynecological problems with loss of blood and amenorrhea.

Combining Methods

Because contemporary diseases are often quite complex, different combinations of the eight methods of treatment are often used:

• Sweating and purging are used when chills, fever, headaches, and stiffness are associated with constipation. The rule is first sweat, then purge.
• Warming and cooling are used when there are upper- or lower-body chills or fever following infectious diseases. Warming herbs are combined with cooling herbs to offset side effects and prevent loss of vitality.
• Attacking and supplementing are used when the disease causes signs of both weakness and excess congestion. If one gives only supplementing therapy, the disease might not be uprooted; if one gives only purging therapy, further prostration could occur. In these cases, a combination of ginseng and similar tonics can be given along with purgatives.

Treatment Principles

The principles of the eight methods of treatment are as follows:

1. Supplement weakness before purging and eliminating. This is done to protect the righteous energy from degenerating.
2. Treat external diseases first before treating extravasated blood.
3. Treat the outer stem before treating the root. Treat external diseases before working on internal weaknesses. Even for those who experience weakness and deficiency, cool-natured, antibiotic herbs should be given to resolve inflammatory conditions either before or simultaneous with the use of appropriate tonics. This approach can be used for about 3 days to 1 week. If this doesn't work, then the treatment principle should be reversed. Some formulas, such as Minor Bupleurum Combination, can treat both inside and outside conformations at the same time.
4. Always treat cautiously at first to be sure that the condition is one of either excess or deficiency, or hot or cold. If there is any question, begin treating as if it were a deficient disease so as not to aggravate the illness.
5. If during the course of treating an internal chronic disease the

patient develops an acute condition, treatment for the chronic condition should be suspended and the acute condition should be treated instead. When the acute condition is alleviated, then resume treatment of the chronic one.

6. Most often, an appropriate herbal treatment exhibits its positive effects within 3 days, in which case it should be continued. If no improvement is noted, it may, however, still be the right treatment and so should be continued anyway. A healing crisis syndrome can occur at this point. If so, treatment can be temporarily suspended or the dosage can be lowered for a time. A healing crisis is always accompanied by signs of improvement. It is also characterized by a shortened retracing of earlier disease syndromes.

7. Because conditions change, especially in acute diseases, it is important to have regular follow-up evaluations. This may be necessary during the 2 or 3 days acute disease stages last or once or twice monthly during certain chronic conditions. A patient taking a reducing formula should be reevaluated weekly or every other week.

8. It is often a part of good herbal strategy to first prescribe a purgative formula, such as one of the rhubarb formulas, for anywhere from 3 days to 1 week before or while giving the primary formula that seems indicated. In most cases, such an eliminative formula can be tolerated without any significant imbalance, by most, except the very deficient. If this strategy is followed, the primary tonic formula will be more effective than if it were taken immediately. Alternatively, a balanced eliminative formula, such as the Ayurvedic triphala, is very safe and can be safely prescribed as a single dose each evening throughout the primary course of treatment.

9. Patients' bodies often respond more effectively with more than one formula is taken simultaneously. This can be prescribed by taking the more tonic formula 20 to 30 minutes before eating and the more eliminative formula after meals. This is especially effective if one uses pills or extracts, but teas are equally effective when taken in this way.

10. Foods and drinks of contrary energies and properties should be avoided during herbal therapy. For instance, foods with strong cooling properties should be avoided if one is taking warming

tonic herbs and formulas. Conversely, strong heating foods, such as sugar, coffee, and alcohol should be avoided if one is taking cooling herbs and formulas. Stimulating foods and drinks should be avoided while taking sedative herbs, and greasy or oily foods should be avoided while taking digestives.

11. Herbs with strong moving properties, such as blood- or *qi*-regulating herbs (strong carminatives or emmenagogues), are contraindicated during pregnancy. Similarly, highly toxic herbs should be avoided by pregnant or nursing women. There is only one molecule of difference between mother's milk and blood: because mother's milk is manufactured by the body from the mother's blood, anything the mother ingests carries over into her milk. Therefore, the safety of anything for a nursing child must be considered before the mother takes it. Consider whether there is an indication that either individual could benefit by a particular herb or formula. Strong or toxic herbs are contraindicated for children, the very weak, and the aged.

· EIGHT ·

MATERIA MEDICA

Chinese herbalism classifies herbs according to the Four Energies, the Five Flavors, the Four Directions, and their relationship to the twelve internal organs. While the majority of the substances used consist of plants, substances from the animal and mineral kingdoms are also used, but to a lesser extent. Herbs are also classified as foodlike, mildly toxic, or very toxic.

The Four Energies

The Four Energies are cold, cool, warm, and hot. Sickness is also classified as cold or hot in nature, so herbs have the ability to oppose or counterbalance a cold or hot disease. Herbs that have a cold energy are used to treat inflammatory and toxic heat conditions. Examples of these are lonicera, forsythia blossoms, and gentian root. In Western herbalism, these might be classified as alterative, blood purifying, or detoxifying. Herbs such as dried ginger or cinnamon bark have a warm energy and counteract cold, hypotonic conditions, promoting digestion and circulation. One characteristic of a cold-natured disease is the presence of clear or white mucus. A tea of fresh or dried ginger is a simple and effective treatment for these conditions. Warm- or cool-natured herbs are a lesser degree of cold or hot and are used accordingly. There is actually a fifth, or neutral, energy, which is commonly found in whole grains and seeds.

The Five Flavors

The Five Flavors are spicy, sweet, sour, bitter, and salty. Herbs may possess a complex of more than one flavor. This organoleptic classification represents the way Chinese herbalism uses herbs according to their biochemical actions. In Chinese herbalism, the flavors of herbs do not always relate to their actual perceived tastes but are used to indicate the actions of specific herbs.

Spicy flavor: Herbs classified as spicy include cinnamon, pepper, ginger, mint, and cardamon. These are used to promote diaphoresis, disperse external pathogenic influences, promote circulation, and restore energy. Commonly, the spicy flavor indicates the presence of volatile oils. This means that such herbs are usually not boiled or decocted but are steeped for 10 or 20 minutes after first preparing the other herbs in the formula.

Sweet flavor: Sweet herbs include many that are tonic or nourishing, such as ginseng, codonopsis, astragalus root, rehmannia root, and jujube dates. Herbs with this flavor have nourishing and tonifying properties. They also serve to normalize the functions of the stomach and spleen, harmonize the effects of different herbs in formulas, and relieve spasm and pain. They are generally used to treat symptoms of deficiency, including dry cough, constipation caused by dryness of the intestines, malnutrition, and low energy. Some sweet-flavored herbs also have detoxifying properties. The sweet flavor usually indicates the presence of carbohydrates, proteins, various sugars, and glycosides.

Sour flavor: Sour herbs include citrus, schisandra, and dogwood berries and are used to induce astringency and arrest sweating and various discharges. They are used for perspiration caused by weakness, chronic cough, chronic diarrhea, spermatorrhea, enuresis, frequent urination, chronic leukorrhea, metrorrhagia, and so on. They may contain acid compounds and tannins.

Bitter flavor: Bitter herbs include coptis, gentian, phellodendron, lonicera, rhubarb, and many others. Herbs with this flavor are generally used for clearing heat, inflammation, infections, toxicity, purgation, discharging dampness, cough, and vomiting. Herbs with this flavor may have many different chemical constituents, but most characteristic is the presence of alkaloids.

Salty flavor: Salty herbs include various seaweeds, such as kelp or dulse; certain mineral salts such as sodium sulfate (Glauber's salts), and certain plants. Herbs with this flavor are often used to lubricate, soften hard masses, and relieve constipation by purgation. In many cases, herbs with the same flavor have similar properties, while those of different flavors often have different properties. Some herbs, however, may have similar flavors but different properties or different properties with similar flavors. Because of this, both the nature and flavor of an herb are jointly taken into consideration.

The Four Directions

Herbs have upward, downward, outward, or inward directions in terms of their ability to influence physiological processes.

Lifting refers to herbs that stimulate yang *qi*. *Lowering* or *inward* means to sedate or penetrate more deeply. *Dispersing* means to extend outward to the surface and usually includes diaphoretic properties. *Downward* means to purge or treat the lower part of the body.

Lifting: Herbs with a lifting energy are used for diseases associated with a collapse of *qi*, prolapse of various internal organs, coldness, depression, low energy, and fatigue. These may include warm tonic herbs, such as astragalus root, but may also include bupleurum and cimicifuga, which, while having a cool energy, are used to raise the *qi*. Mint is also used because it has the ability to direct the *qi* upward to the mind and relieve depression.

Dispersing: Herbs with a dispersing energy have diaphoretic (perspiration-inducing) properties and are used for the initial stages of colds, influenza, fevers, and eruptive skin diseases. Examples of herbs with this property are numerous and include ephedra (*Ma huang*), cinnamon twigs, mint, and schizonepeta.

Descending: Herbs with a descending or downward energy are used to treat diseases whose symptoms express themselves upward, including symptoms of cough, vomiting, and asthma. Two examples of herbs in this category include pinellia and perilla. Herbs whose energy is downward have the ability to purge or promote circulation in the lower part of the body. Examples are rhubarb root, angelica (*du huo*) and achyranthes.

Inward: Herbs that are tonics, such as ginseng, codonopsis, lycii berries, ophiopogon and many others. They are used to tonify and nourish the internal organs.

Herbs also have heavy or light qualities. In general, flowers or leaves are light while roots, seeds, and fruits are heavy. For this reason, light herbs are commonly used for treating acute, feverish diseases, while heavy herbs are used for deeper, more chronic conditions.

The Twelve Internal Organs

In more recent Chinese medical history, herbs have been classified as entering or affecting one or more of the twelve internal organs. Since the internal organs in Chinese medicine refer not only to the specific organ but to the acupuncture channel or meridian that belongs to that organ, specific herbs are known to have a more or less specific effect on the corresponding organ meridian. Many of the relationships are obvious and correspond, with some exceptions, to the relationship of the flavors to the Five Elements.

Herbs with a sweet flavor typically belong to the earth element and therefore enter the spleen–pancreas and stomach organ meridians. These commonly have a nutritive and tonifying energy. Those with a spicy flavor belong to the lungs and large intestine, which are part of the metal element. At least in terms of the lungs, these have the ability to promote diaphoresis and decrease production of mucus. Herbs with a salty energy belong to the kidneys–adrenals and bladder, which belong to the water element. These herbs have the effect of lubricating and moistening bodily tissues. Herbs that are sour enter the liver and gallbladder meridians, which belong to the wood element, and aid in inhibiting and regulating bodily secretions. Finally, herbs that are bitter belong to the fire element, which includes the heart, pericardium, small intestine, and Triple Warmer. These are detoxifying and help to clear heat and congestion in the form of fatty buildup in the veins and arteries.

As stated previously, there are exceptions to the relationships of the flavors with their corresponding organs and acupuncture meridians. Because herbs often have complex biochemical properties, they may have more than one flavor and thus affect and enter more than one organ meridian.

A somewhat minor theory based on Five Element correspondence is the use of herbs according to their colors. Green herbs enter the liver, red-colored substances enter the heart, yellow-colored herbs enter the spleen, white-colored herbs enter the lungs, and black-colored herbs enter the kidneys. The Chinese even go to the trouble of coloring sugar-coated pills according to the particular organ that is primarily affected.

Toxic and Nontoxic Herbs and Diet

The Chinese materia medica clearly indicates when an herb has reputed toxicity, indicating this as "toxic" or "slightly toxic." Herbs that are toxic have a much more narrow margin of safety in dosage, and they are usually taken for a short period, ranging from 1 to 5 days at a time.

Contraindications

A *contraindication* is when there is the possibility that an herb might aggravate a preexisting condition or imbalance. There are classically contraindicated and incompatible herbs, listed in the next section below, as well as herbs contraindicated during pregnancy. Other contraindicated uses of herbs include use of drying or warm-natured herbs for conditions associated with yin deficiency or heat, moistening herbs for conditions of dampness, tonifying herbs for conditions of excess, and cold-natured herbs associated with conditions of coldness.

One may encounter contraindications with herbs if they are prescribed too heavily for a specific disease. Nearly all diseases have at least two faces and often more, based on the Eight Principles. Most diseases can have underlying excess or deficiency, coldness or heat, or yin or yang, or be chronic or acute, and require different herbal approaches accordingly.

In spite of all this, herbs are relatively safe. In fact, in terms of many physiological propensities, they have amphoteric or regulating properties. It is wise to take herbs carefully, beginning with a lower dosage and periodically being reevaluated (at least weekly).

THE NINETEEN ANTAGONISMS AND EIGHTEEN INCOMPATIBLES

Following is the list of the classically incompatible or antagonistic herbs that one should generally avoid combining together. They involve

combinations of herbs that one never finds together in traditional formulas or they have properties that are directly opposite or antagonistic
to each other.

Nineteen antagonisms:

- Sulfur (liu huang) is antagonistic with *Sal glauberis (po xiao)*.
- Hydrargyrum (shui yin) is antagonistic with arsenicum (pi shuang).
- *Radix euphorbiae* (lang du) is antagonistic with lithargyrum (mi tuo seng).
- *Semen Croton tiglii (ba dou)* is antagonistic with *Semen pharbitidis (qian niu zi)*.
- Nitrum (ya xiao) is antagonistic with *Rhizoma sparganii (san leng)*.
- *Flos caryophylli (Ding xiang)* is antagonistic with *Tuber curcumae (yu jin)* and *Radix curcumae (jiang huang)*.
- *Radix aconiti (wu tou)* is antagonistic with *Cornu rhinoceri (xi jiao) and/or water buffalo horn*.
- *Radix ginseng (ren shen)* is antagonistic with *Excrementum trogopteri seu pteromi (wu ling zhi)*.
- *Cortex cinnamomi (rou gui)* is antagonistic with *Halloysitum rubrum*.

Eighteen incompatibles:

- *Radix Glycyrrhizae uralensis (gan cao)* is incompatible with:
  - *Radix euphorbiae kansui (gan sui)*
  - *Radix euphorbiae seu knoxiae (da ji)*
  - *Flos daphne genkwa (yuan hua)*
  - *Herba sargassi (hai zao)*

- *Radix aconiti (wu tou)* is incompatible with:
  - *Bulbus fritillariae (bei mu)*
  - *Fructus trichosanthes (gua lou)*
  - *Rhizoma pinelliae ternatae (ban xia)*
  - *Radix ampelopsis (bai lian)*
  - *Rhizoma bletillae striatae (Bai ji)*

- *Rhizoma et radix veratri (li lu) is incompatible with:*
  - *Radix ginseng (ren shen)*
  - *Radix adenophorae seu glehniae (sha shen)*
  - *Radix salviae miltiorrhizae (dan shen)*
  - *Radix sophorae flavescentis (ku shen)*
  - *Herba cum radice asari (xi xin)*
  - *Herba paeoniae lactiflorae (bai shao)*

To put things in perspective, in a world that finds the plethora of adverse drug reactions and side effects an acceptable risk in not only prescriptions but also over-the-counter drugs, it may be worth noting that contemporary Chinese research has found no serious side effects for most of the above combinations.

CONTRAINDICATIONS DURING PREGNANCY

Certain substances can induce miscarriage or damage the fetus. These are generally herbs that have strong blood- and qi-moving properties, purgatives and those that are toxic or have strong heating properties. The following representative group of herbs are prohibited during pregnancy: croton (*ba dou*), pharbitidis (*qian niu zi*), euphorbiae (*da ji*), mylabris (*ban mao*), phytolaccae (*shang lu*), moschus (*she xiang*), cyperii (*xiang fu*), zedoariae (*e zhu*) and hirudo (*shui zhi*). The following representative herbs should be used with great care during pregnancy: rhubarb root (*da huang*), aconite (*fu zi*), Ginger (*gan jiang*), pinellia (*ban xia*), cinnamon bark (*rou gui*), abutili (*dong kui zi*), carthami (*hong hua*), persicae (*tao ren*).

Dietary Restrictions

Certain foods tend to be contraindicated with some herbs and formulas. In most cases, this means the avoidance of foods that could aggravate a previous imbalance. For example, raw, cold foods are contraindicated for conditions of coldness. Hot, spicy foods; heavy, sweet foods; and richly nutritious animal protein foods are contraindicated for conditions of excess. Greasy and mucilaginous foods are contraindicated for conditions of dampness, and foods that are heavy and hard to digest are contraindicated for conditions of food stagnation and digestive weakness. In addition, there are certain herbs that should not be taken simultaneously with various foods. For instance, neither licorice (*gan cao*), coptis (*huang lian*), platycodon (*jie geng*), nor mume (*wu mei*) should be taken with pork. Mint should not be taken with turtle meat, and poria mushroom should not be taken with vinegar.

Principles of Herbal Formulation

Chinese herbalism is primarily formula based. Herbs represent an energy composed of complex biochemical constituents that are enhanced and/or altered when they are combined together. Formulations can be classified as follows:

- **Mutually synergistic:** When two or more herbs with similar characteristics are combined to amplify the original effect, the formulation is mutually synergistic. Examples are the combination of *Angelica sinensis (dang gui)* and ligusticum *(chuan xiong)*, which together promote blood circulation; rhubarb and sodium sulfate, which together promote purgation; and gypsum and *anemarrhena*, which together reduce fevers and inflammation.

- **Mutual assistance:** If one herb is used as the major herb, the others are subordinately used to bring out the properties of the major herb. Examples are the use of ephedra *(ma huang)* and pueraria root to induce perspiration and release the surface or rhubarb root and scutellaria to purge and detoxify.

- **Mutually enhancing:** Sometimes herbs with different properties are combined to mutually enhance each other's actions. Examples are the combination of poria cocos and astragalus root for treating edema and deficient *qi* and the combination of rhubarb root and coptis for purging and detoxifying.

- **Mutually pacifying:** It is possible to combine two herbs together so that one eliminates the toxicity of the other. Examples are the combination of pinellia and ginger—in fact, pinellia is commonly pretreated with ginger to eliminate its toxic properties—and the combination of licorice with prepared aconite to counteract its toxicity.

- **Mutually antagonistic:** By combining certain herbs together, one will cause the other to lose all or part of its therapeutic effect. Classically, Chinese herbalism delineates Nineteen Antagonisms. Examples are the use of ginseng and green tea and the combination of ginseng with radish seeds.

- **Mutually incompatible:** A small number of herbs, when used together, can create toxicity or strong side effects.

- **Herbs that are best used alone:** Some herbs work best when used alone, such as deer antler.

Standard Pharmaceutical Principles of Formulation

Principles of organizing an herbal formula are the same in both traditional Western pharmacy and Chinese medicine. The Chinese, however, organize their formulas to reflect Confucian ideals expressed in the ancient political organization of the state, as follows:

- **Emperor or sovereign herbs:** Ingredients in emperor category represent the primary therapeutic action of the formula.
- **Minister herbs:** Ingredients in the minister category are added to assist the primary effect.
- **Assistant herbs:** Ingredients in the assistant category added to treat accompanying symptoms or to lessen the toxicity or harshness of the primary substances. These can also serve as counterassistants, in that they may have a property opposite to that of the main herb. For example, they may be cooling to lessen the heating properties of the primary herbs or warming to control or lessen the cooling properties.
- **Messenger herbs:** Ingredients in the messenger category used either to direct and guide the primary herbs or smooth the way for their use.

Two examples of these principles are as follows:

Major Four Herb Formula (Four Nobles):
- Ginseng or codonopsis (emperor or sovereign herb; *qi* tonic)
- Atractylodes (deputy herb; complements the *qi* tonic effect of ginseng)
- Poria (assistant herb; clears dampness and helps *qi* tonification)
- Licorice (messenger herb; harmonizes the formula)

This is the basic formula for *qi* tonification and strengthening digestion.

Dang Gui Four Combination:
- *Dang gui* (sovereign herb; blood tonic)
- Ligusticum (assistant herb; promotes blood circulation with *dang gui*)
- White peony root (assistant herb; aids in tonifying blood)
- Rehmannia root (assistant herb; nourishes blood and yin)

This is the basic formula for blood tonification used in most gynecological formulas.

Processing Herbs

Many Chinese herbs are standardly processed before use to enhance their therapeutic properties. Some of these include (*Angelica sinensis* and *Rehmannia glutinosa,* which are presoaked in rice wine and dried for use;

Pinellia ternata, which is fried in fresh ginger juice to detoxify it; and prepared aconite, for which there are several methods of preparation that are used to neutralize its toxicity. In addition, herbs can be stir-fried in honey to make them warmer and more tonifying, such as prepared or baked licorice root. They are also commonly calcined, or burned, to enhance their astringent properties. Chinese herbs are each methodically sliced, tied together, or cosmetically presented to prevent adulteration as well as to grade their quality. Because of this, one may find several grades of a single herb available in a traditional pharmacy. As with many imported herbs and foods, some Chinese herbs are fumigated to preserve their color and fresh appearance as well as to prevent insect infestation. To date, I have never witnessed or heard of any adverse reaction to this processing. It must be remembered that Chinese herbs represent a relatively small part of one's dietary intake and are ingested on a limited basis to achieve a specific therapeutic objective. Pills, tablets and extracts taken over a longer period are unprocessed. Furthermore, not all Chinese herbs are fumigated, and increasingly, there are importers who are making unfumigated Chinese herbs commercially available. The problem is that the consumer may not always be aware that cosmetically fumigated Chinese herbs present a better appearance that does not necessarily attest to any therapeutic superiority.

Dosage and Preparation of Herbs

As previously stated, the range of safe dosage for the majority of Chinese herbs is wide, while those that are classified as toxic have a more restricted range of dosage and preparation requirements.

Metric weights are used throughout this book for Western readers; however, Chinese herbal dosage is customarily given according to the Chinese standard of weights and measures. The table below shows approximate quivalents.

CHINESE WEIGHTS AND MEASURES AND WESTERN EQUIVALENTS

CHINESE UNITS	WESTERN EQUIVALENTS
1 fen	0.3 grams (approximately)
10 fen = 1 qian	3 grams (approximately)
10 qian = 1 liang	30 grams (approximately)
16 liang = 1 jin	480 grams (approximately)

Decoctions and Teas

The most common forms of Chinese herbal preparations are decoctions and teas. Traditionally, these are prepared in a clay pot, but they can also be prepared in glass, unchipped enamel, or high-quality stainless steel containers without interfering with their properties. They should not be prepared in iron, copper, aluminum, or any type of metal containers that can alter the chemistry of the herbs. The herbs should be soaked for 30 to 60 minutes in 4 cups of water before exposing them to heat. They are then quickly brought to a boil and simmered until the fluid is reduced by half. This is then strained and the original liquor is set aside for use. The same batch of herbs can be similarly cooked to make two or three further decoctions. The usual dose is 1 cup twice a day.

Herbs with volatile oils, often diaphoretics, are usually prepared in less water and cooked for only 5 or 10 minutes. Tonics are simmered in more water for a longer period of time, usually 45 to 60 minutes.

Certain herbs should receive individual extractive consideration based on their constituents. Minerals and shells, such as gypsum, oyster shell, abalone shell, turtle shell, or dragon bone are boiled for 15 minutes before other herbs are added. Aromatic herbs, such as mint, cardamon, citrus peel, or saussurea, are added during the last 5 to 10 minutes in order to prevent the volatilization of their active constituents. This also applies to some purgative herbs, such as rhubarb and senna leaf. Herbs that are particularly precious should be decocted separately. This may include high-grade ginseng and deer antler. They can be taken separately or added to the decoction.

Certain herbs and substances, including amber and pseudoginseng, are unsuitable for decoction. These are finely powdered and infused in warm boiled water or added to the decoction. Some herbs, such as donkey-hide gelatin and malt sugar, are dissolved in boiling water or in the finished decoction.

One cup or dose is taken twice a day or as often as every 4 hours for more acute diseases. Tonics are taken before meals, while herbs that are bitter and might adversely effect digestion are given after (though not immediately after) meals. Anthelmintics and purgatives should be taken on an empty stomach. Sedatives and tranquilizers should be taken a half hour before bedtime. Antimalarial herbs should be taken profilactically in small doses to prevent malaria and in larger doses at the beginning of an attack.

In most cases, herbs are taken warm, but for inflammatory or heat diseases, they can be taken cool. For yin deficiency with heat signs, the herbs should be taken cool, while in yang deficiency with cold signs, the herbs are taken in a warm decoction.

Pills should be taken with warm boiled water. Liquid alcoholic extracts are either 1:5 tinctures or concentrated 6:1 extracts. The tinctures are taken in prescribed 10- to 60-drop doses, while extracts are taken in single- to 10-drop doses because of their greater concentration. If one desires to nearly eliminate the alcohol, the prescribed alcoholic extract can be placed in a cup of boiling water, which will volatize most of the alcohol.

Dried extracts are fast becoming the most popular and convenient form of Chinese herbs to take. These are presently manufactured by a handful of companies based mostly in Taiwan, Hong Kong, or mainland China. They are usually 5:1 in potency, and the average adult dose is ½ to 1 teaspoon twice daily. These can be put into gelatin capsules, if desired. Children take less according to their age. Dried extracts can be taken in hot water or placed in gelatin capsules as desired. Note that all dosages given throughout this book are average daily amounts, divided in two or three portions daily.

Classical Herbal Formulas

Herbal formulas represent the heart of traditional Chinese herbalism. Many of them date back well over 2,000 years and have had the benefit of scrutiny and revision by some of the greatest Chinese herbalists down through the ages. Many of these are available in various forms, such as teas, patented commercial pills, and liquid and dried extracts. For the beginning student of Chinese herbalism, it is a good principle to first use the traditional formulas and then branch out to learn basic methods to modify them according to the individual. With more experience, an herbalist learns to extract the most salient principle of various formulas to create combinations appropriate for each individual.

Herbal Names

In the sections that follow, the most commonly used name is first presented, followed by the traditional Chinese name. Underneath is the full Latin binomial (genus and species), the common name, the pharmaceutical name that uses the Latin name, and the part or parts of the plant that are used. The following table defines some of the most common Latin plant parts used in the Chinese materia medica:

☯

PLANT PARTS USED IN HERBAL PREPARATIONS

LATIN	MEANING
Folium	Leaf
Flora or flos	Flower
Semen	Seed
Fructus	Fruit
Pericarpium	Peel
Caulis	Stem
Cortex	Bark
Ramulus	Twig or branch
Rhizoma	Rhizome

☯

Materia Medica

Herbs That Open and Release the Exterior: Diaphoretics

Herbs in diaphoretic category are among the most widely used because they treat common acute symptoms, ranging from colds and influenza to upper-respiratory diseases, skin diseases, and rheumatic symptoms. They characteristically have a spicy or pungent flavor (sometimes called acrid) and stimulate diaphoresis (sweating). They are further subdivided into the categories of warm-spicy and cool-spicy. The warm-spicy herbs produce diaphoresis by increasing and stimulating circulation to the surface of the body. They are used to treat external-Cool diseases. The cool-spicy surface-relieving herbs generally produce diaphoresis by relaxing the surface tension and pores of the skin to facilitate perspiration. These are used to treat external-heat diseases.

The active constituents of most of these herbs are their volatile oils. When ingested in a warm tea, these are released either through the pores of the skin, if they are taken in a warm infusion, or through the urine, if they are taken as a cool infusion. The volatile oils of these plants give them their characteristic pungent odor. The function of these volatile oils, is thought to be to protect the plants from invading air-borne pathogens, just as the oils help to expel and protect our bodies from invading pathogens. A pungent odoriferous herb that possesses volatile oils should never be subjected to prolonged decoction or boiling, as this will cause the oils to vaporize their active constituents. Instead, such herbs are added after all other ingredients of the formula have been properly boiled. The mixture is then steeped, with the pot covered, for approximately 10 minutes. The resulting tea is then taken warm.

One herb notably does not rely on volatile oils to stimulate diaphoresis—*Ephedra sinensis (ma huang)*. It enhances circulation by stimulating the adrenal glands with its adrenaline-like alkaloids. It is the most effective herb for the treatment of asthma, but it is also very effective for all external-wind-cold conditions. Because it is so strongly stimulating, ephedra tea or one of its variants are generally not given to individuals who are weak and deficient. For them, cinnamon tea *(gui zhi tang)* or one of its variants is used.

Most of these herbs also dispel external wind, which represents the proliferation and penetration of pathogens throughout the surface of the body. Wind represents an element of sudden change, so symptoms that suddenly increase or lessen in intensity or otherwise change location are considered a manifestation of wind. The nervous system may be considered one aspect of wind. It is well recognized that there are at least two aspects to external disease: the irritating pathogenic factor and the body's reaction to it. This second aspect, the way our body reacts, can seem to be more severe than the actual cause, as in the case of some individuals' reactions to certain airborne pollens or dust particles. The histamine reactions of certain individuals to such particles is certainly more severe than the particles themselves, which cause little reaction for the majority of us. Severe histamine reactions are manifestations of wind in the traditional Chinese medicine (TCM) sense of the term. This makes antihistamines a class of drugs that help dispel external wind. From the herbalist's perspective, this alone is not enough. It is important to at least lessen if not eradicate the underlying immune weakness and/or toxicity that is the cause.

Another manifestation of wind is the tendency for bacteria to send forth a hyaluronidase enzyme that breaks down neighboring cell walls to enable them to penetrate further. The well-known Western herb echinacea, so effective for colds, influenza, and other infections, works by inhibiting the hyaluronidase enzyme. By confining bacteria—which would normally proliferate and penetrate as part of the manifestation of wind—to a local area, the hyaluronidase-inhibiting echinacea starves and chokes bacteria to extinction. In this way, the body's natural defenses are mobilized for its own protection and healing.

Diaphoretics, like all herbs in each of the categories, are chosen not only for their primary therapeutic properties but also for their secondary properties. For instance, many herbs in the surface-relieving categories have secondary properties that enable them to treat edema, cough, and such eruptive skin diseases as measles and to relieve pain.

Sweating therapy is a universal treatment for a variety of acute diseases in many cultures. If teas are used as part of this therapy, it is important to bundle up the patient afterward and have him or her lie still in a warm bed to allow diaphoresis to commence. Sweating must then continue for 10 to 20 minutes, and then the patient should be quickly sponged off with cool water to which a few tablespoons of apple-cider vinegar have been added. The patient is then returned to bed to rest under (and on) clean, fresh covers. To replenish energy after sweating, serve the patient a bowl of warm, lightly nourishing soup, like chicken soup or watery rice porridge. In fact, for those who are more deficient, cinnamon tea (gui zhi tang) is appropriate; following the tea with a bowl of thin rice porridge 20 minutes after sweating is absolutely essential. Excess sweating can exhaust yang qi and body fluids. Because of this, diaphoretic herbs are generally contraindicated for advanced stages of febrile diseases, in which the patient may have symptoms of severe fluid depletion, urinary problems, or anemia.

Warm-Pungent Herbs That Release the Exterior

External warm-pungent herbs are used to treat external wind-cold conditions. The most important indications include chills; fever; lack of sweating; headache; thin, white tongue coat; and a slow surface pulse. These herbs can also be used to treat upper-respiratory conditions, such as cough, asthma, and edema, and painful rheumatic conditions aggravated by wind and dampness.

Ephedra (MA HUANG)
Ephedra sinica; E. intermedia; E. equisetina
COMMON NAMES: Ephedra, *ma huang*

FAMILY: Ephedraceae

PART USED: Herb

ENERGY AND FLAVORS: Warm; bitter, acrid

ORGAN MERIDIANS AFFECTED: Lung, urinary bladder

PROPERTIES: Diaphoretic, bronchial dilator, diuretic

EFFECTS AND INDICATIONS: Induces perspiration, warms coldness, relieves wheezing, moves fluids. It is used for the common cold, wheezing, moves fluids. It is used for common cold, wheezing, bronchial asthma, bronchitis, and edema.

CONTRAINDICATIONS: Ephedra should not be used by those with external deficiency with symptoms of spontaneous sweating. Because the alkaloids have an effect similar to that of adrenaline, ephedra should not be used with symptoms of high blood pressure or insomnia.

DOSE: 3–9 grams

NOTES: While there are many species of ephedra that grow in diverse areas of the world, including the high desert of the North American Southwest, the one that originates in inner Mongolia has the greatest concentration of ephedrine and pseudoephedrine alkaloids. The greatest concentration of the active principle is in the portion of the stem between the joints. The best-quality ephedra has the joint removed. Interestingly, the root has exactly the opposite property and is used for excessive perspiration and diarrhea.

Cinnamon twig (GUI ZHI)

Ramulus cinnamomum cassiae

COMMON NAME: Cinnamon twig

FAMILY: Lauraceae

PART USED: Twigs and branches

ENERGY AND FLAVORS: Warm; sweet, acrid

ORGAN MERIDIANS AFFECTED: Lung, heart, urinary bladder

PROPERTIES: Diaphoretic, promotes circulation of blood

EFFECTS AND INDICATIONS: Induces perspiration, relieves muscle spasms, warms, promotes blood and *qi* circulation. It is indicated for the common cold and upper-respiratory congestion associated with external deficiency. It is also used for various circulatory disorders, including chest pains, palpitations, numbness, arthritic and rheumatic conditions, stopped menstruation, and abdominal cramps.

DOSE: 3–9 grams

CONTRAINDICATIONS: This herb should not be used for those with warm febrile diseases or those who are showing heat signs. It should be used with caution in women who are pregnant or are bleeding heavily.

NOTES: Cinnamon twig is one of the most important circulatory herbs in Chinese herbalism. It is in the same family as North American sassafras, and both herbs are good for circulation and promote urination.

Ginger (fresh) (SHENG JIANG)
Rhizoma zingiberis officinalis
COMMON NAME: Fresh ginger
FAMILY: Zingiberaceae
PART USED: Rhizome
ENERGY AND FLAVOR: Warm; acrid
ORGAN MERIDIANS AFFECTED: Lung, stomach, spleen
PROPERTIES: Diaphoretic, expectorant, antiemetic
INDICATIONS: Used for the common cold when there is thin white mucus and chills. Fresh ginger is also one of the best remedies for nausea associated with motion sickness and seafood poisoning.
CONTRAINDICATIONS: Ginger should not be used by those with heat signs in the lungs or stomach.
DOSE: 3–9 grams
NOTES: Perhaps the most versatile of all herbs, fresh ginger can be topically applied as a warm fomentation to relieve spasms pain and cramps. Simply cut several slices of the fresh root and place them in a pan of boiling water. Saturate a flannel cloth with the tea and apply it topically as warm as the body will bear. This is an ideal treatment for stiff neck and shoulders. The herb is cooked with meat to aid its assimilation and detoxify it. Fresh ginger tea is the most ideal herb to use for the first signs of mucus, cold, cough, and so on. To make it taste better, add honey. Drinking ginger tea with meals will greatly aid digestion and assimilation and is useful for those with weak, cold digestion.

Perilla leaf (ZI SU YE)
Folium perillae frutescentis
COMMON NAME: Perilla leaf
FAMILY: Labiatae
PART USED: Leaf

ENERGIES AND FLAVOR: Warm, aromatic; acrid

ORGAN MERIDIANS AFFECTED: Lung, spleen

PROPERTIES: Diaphoretic, carminative, antiemetic

EFFECTS AND INDICATIONS: Relieves wind cold, promotes sweating, circulates *qi*, relieves gastric congestion. It can be used for the common cold, cough, chest congestion, bloated stomach and abdomen, nausea, and vomiting. It is also used in cooking and as treatment to relieve symptoms related to seafood poisoning.

CONTRAINDICATIONS: Perilla leaf should not be used by those who have external diseases where there is already sweating or by those who have a damp-heat condition.

DOSE: 3–9 grams

NOTES: Perilla leaf, called *shiso* by the Japanese, is widely used as a condiment in much the same manner as sweet basil is used in Italian cooking.

Schizonepeta (JING JIE)

Herba seu flos schizonepetae tenuifolia

COMMON NAMES: Schizonepeta, Chinese catnip

FAMILY: Labiatae

PART USED: Leaves and flowers

ENERGIES AND FLAVOR: Slightly warm, aromatic; acrid

ORGAN MERIDIANS AFFECTED: Lung, liver

PROPERTIES: Diaphoretic, hemostatic (especially when charred), vents skin rashes, anti-inflammatory

EFFECTS AND INDICATIONS: Relieves wind cold, antispasmodic. It can be used for the onset of the common cold and influenza when they are accompanied by a headache and sore throat. It is also used for hastening the ripening and termination of eruptive skin diseases, such as measles and abscesses, as well as to alleviate itching. Finally, it can be used for blood in stools or uterine bleeding.

CONTRAINDICATIONS: Schizonepeta should not be taken by those with spontaneous sweating or with liver wind signs, such as headache, especially when there is a yin deficiency. It should not be used for full-blown skin diseases.

DOSE: 3–9 grams

Notopterygium (QIANG HUO)

Radix et rhizoma notopterygii incisum, Notopterygium forbesii

COMMON NAME: Notopterygium

FAMILY: Umbelliferae

PART USED: Root and rhizome

ENERGIES AND FLAVORS: Warm, aromatic; acrid, bitter

ORGAN MERIDIANS AFFECTED: Kidney, urinary bladder

PROPERTIES: Diaphoretic, antirheumatic

EFFECTS AND INDICATIONS: Relieves wind, cold, and damp conditions with associated pains. It is useful for the common cold and influenza, headache, soreness, and aching sensations throughout the body. It is especially effective for those with rheumatic, arthritic and other aches and pains in the upper back and shoulders.

CONTRAINDICATIONS: Notopterygium should not be used by those with weak or anemic conditions or arthritis caused by blood deficiency.

DOSE: 6–12 grams

Ledebouriella (FANG FENG)

Radix ledebouriellae divaricatae (formerly *siler divaricatum*)

COMMON NAME: Ledebouriella or siler

FAMILY: Umbelliferae

ENERGY AND FLAVORS: Warm; acrid, sweet

ORGAN MERIDIANS AFFECTED: Lung, liver, spleen, urinary bladder

PROPERTIES: Diaphoretic, antispasmodic, analgesic, antirheumatic, antimicrobial

EFFECTS AND INDICATIONS: Relieves coldness, wind, pain, spasms associated with coldness. It is used for the common cold or influenza when the symptoms include chills, headache, and body aches. It is also useful for rheumatic pains, especially when the pain seems to move from place to place (wind). This herb has also been used for intestinal spasms and for the treatment of trembling hands and feet. Finally, it is effective for itching skin and allergic rashes.

CONTRAINDICATIONS: This herb should not be used by those who are weak, those with anemia, or those with heat signs associated with yin deficiency.

DOSE: 3–9 grams

Scallion (CONG BAI)

Bulbus allii fistulosi

COMMON NAMES: Green onion, scallion

FAMILY: Liliaceae

PART USED: Bulb

ENERGY AND FLAVOR: Warm; acrid

ORGAN MERIDIANS AFFECTED: Lung, stomach

PROPERTIES: Diaphoretic, diuretic, antimicrobial, stomachic, expectorant

EFFECTS AND INDICATIONS: Dissipates coldness, induces perspiration, dispels dampness, relieves abdominal bloating. It is very effective in the initial stages of colds and influenza and for congestion of the lungs or sinuses. It can also be used when there is coldness or fullness in the stomach or chest area.

CONTRAINDICATIONS: Scallion should not be used when spontaneous sweating is occurring.

DOSE: 3–9 grams. It should be added near the end of making the decoction.

Coriander (HU SUI)

Coriandrum sativum

COMMON NAME: Coriander

FAMILY: Umbelliferae

PART USED: Herb

ENERGY AND FLAVOR: Warm; spicy

ORGAN MERIDIANS AFFECTED: Lungs, stomach

PROPERTIES: Diaphoretic, digestant, diuretic

EFFECTS AND INDICATIONS: Promotes sweating, brings rashes to the surface. Use with cicada (*chan tui*), schizonepeta (*jing jie*), and arctium (*niu bang zi*) for early stages of measles and other eruptive diseases. The tea can also be applied topically to help rashes erupt on the surface of the skin.

NOTES: Coriander herb, also known in Spanish as cilantro, is used as a condiment in both East Indian and Central American cuisine. Apart from its TCM classification as warm, the Chinese use it in cooking to counteract the heating effects of strongly spicy foods.

Cool-Pungent Herbs that Release the Exterior

Herbs in cool-pungent category can mildly stimulate diaphoresis. They are used to treat external wind-heat conditions with symptoms that include high fever, mild chills, sore throat, scanty or no sweating, thin yellow tongue coat, and rapid surface pulse. Some of these herbs are also useful for more quickly ripening and terminating measles and other eruptive diseases.

Burdock (NIU BANG ZI)

Fructus arctii lappae

COMMON NAMES: Burdock, arctium fruit

FAMILY: Compositae

PARTS USED: Seeds, root

ENERGY AND FLAVORS: Cold; bitter, acrid

ORGAN MERIDIANS AFFECTED: Lung, stomach

PROPERTIES: Antibiotic, antifungal, diaphoretic, diuretic, mild laxative, antipyretic

EFFECTS AND INDICATIONS: Burdock seed is very effective in venting rashes and other eruptive skin diseases, such as measles. It is also effective for hives, mumps, boils, carbuncles, and furuncles. While the seeds are especially effective for skin diseases as well as colds, influenza, fevers, and sore throats, the root is also effective as a general detoxifier of the blood and lymphatic system and as a treatment for cancer, especially lymphoma.

CONTRAINDICATIONS: Burdock should not be used by persons with diarrhea.

DOSE: 3–9 grams

Mint (BO HE)

Herba menthae haplocalycis

COMMON NAMES: Chinese mint

FAMILY: Labiatae

PART USED: Leaves

ENERGIES AND FLAVOR: Cool, aromatic; acrid

ORGAN MERIDIANS AFFECTED: Lung, liver

PROPERTIES: Diaphoretic, antipyretic, stomachic, carminative

EFFECTS AND INDICATIONS: Diaphoretic; clears wind-heat conditions associated with colds and influenza with fever, headache, sore throat, and red eyes (conjunctivitis). It can also be used for measles and rashes. Like peppermint, it is very good for stomach bloating and lifting the spirits. Finally, it can be used for mouth sores, toothache, allergic rashes, hives, and the early stages of measles.

CONTRAINDICATIONS: Mint, although not thought of as a strong herb by most people, should be used with caution by those with weakness and spontaneous sweating. This herb should not be used by nursing mothers, as it may slow lactation.

DOSE: 3–6 grams

Chrysanthemum flowers (JU HUA)

Flos chrysanthemum morifolium

COMMON NAME: Chrysanthemum flower

FAMILY: Compositae

PART USED: Flower

ENERGY AND FLAVORS: Slightly cold; bitter, sweet, acrid

ORGAN MERIDIANS AFFECTED: Lung, liver

PROPERTIES: Anti-inflammatory, antipyretic, antihypertensive

EFFECTS AND INDICATIONS: Clears heat, disperses wind, soothes the liver, improves vision. It can be used for the common cold, fevers, headaches, conjunctivitis, reddening of the eyes, and some cases of deafness. This herb is excellent for fevers with headache and for counteracting the effects of hot climate. While this is a surface-relieving herb, it also has some yin-nourishing properties.

CONTRAINDICATIONS: Those who are weak or have diarrhea should not use chrysanthemum flower.

DOSE: 5–12 grams

NOTES: The white chrysanthemum flower is used to relieve hypertension, pacify the liver, expel wind, and clear eyesight. The yellow chrysanthemum flower is more effective for wind-heat syndrome with symptoms of fever and sore throat.

White mulberry leaf (SANG YE)

Folium mori albae

COMMON NAME: White mulberry leaf

FAMILY: Moraceae

PART USED: Leaves

ENERGY AND FLAVORS: Cold; bitter, sweet

ORGAN MERIDIANS AFFECTED: Lung, liver

PROPERTIES: Diaphoretic, antibacterial, antihypertensive

EFFECTS AND INDICATIONS: Clears wind heat, soothes the liver, clears the eyes. It can be used for lung congestion with cough, sore throat, and yellow sputum. It brightens the eyes when they are red, painful, or dry and aching eyes. It can also be used when there is bleeding with heat signs.

CONTRAINDICATIONS: White mulberry leaf should not be used by those who have weakness with cold in the lungs.

DOSE: 5–12 grams

Black soybean (DAN DOU CHI)

Semen Sojae praeparatum

COMMON NAME: Fermented black soybean
FAMILY: Leguminosae
PART USED: Seed/bean
ENERGY AND FLAVORS: Cold; sweet, slightly bitter
ORGAN MERIDIANS AFFECTED: Lung, stomach
PROPERTIES: Weak diaphoretic, calmative
EFFECTS AND INDICATIONS: Prepared black soybean is subjected to a fermentive process. Prepared in this way, it has some nutritive properties and is also useful for treating the common cold accompanied by fever and headache. Because of its nourishing properties, it relieves irritability, restlessness, and insomnia especially, when the body has become exhausted from an acute feverish illness.
CONTRAINDICATIONS: Mothers who are nursing should not use black soybean, as it may inhibit lactation.
DOSE: 12–15 grams

Vitex fruit (MAN JING ZI)

Fructus viticis; Vitex rotundifolia, V. trifolia

COMMON NAMES: Vitex fruit, chaste berry
FAMILY: Verbenaceae
PART USED: Fruit
ENERGY AND FLAVORS: Cool; acrid, bitter
ORGAN MERIDIANS AFFECTED: Liver, stomach, urinary bladder
PROPERTIES: Diaphoretic, antipyretic, regulatory (of female hormones [*Vitex agnus castus*])
EFFECTS AND INDICATIONS: Relieves wind heat, clears heat from the liver channel. The Chinese variety is particularly useful for headache, dizziness, eye pain, and muscular aches and pains. The Western variety has a somewhat different usage—as a female hormonal regulator.
CONTRAINDICATIONS: Vitex should be used with caution by those who are weak or anemic.
DOSE: 5–12 grams (for external wind heat)

Pueraria (GE GEN)

Radix puerariae lobata

COMMON NAMES: Kudzu, Kuzu, Pueraria
FAMILY: Leguminosae

PARTS USED: Root, flowers

ENERGY AND FLAVORS: Cool; acrid, sweet

ORGAN MERIDIANS AFFECTED: Spleen, stomach, urinary bladder

PROPERTIES: Diaphoretic, antispasmodic, muscle relaxant, antipyretic

EFFECTS AND INDICATIONS: Clears wind heat; relieves muscular tension and spasms, especially of the neck and shoulders; vents eruptive skin diseases, such as measles. It is used for fevers caused by heat in colds and influenza and for stiff neck and shoulders. It has some demulcent properties, making it useful for thirst and dryness. It can also be used for many other diverse conditions, ranging from hypertension, dysentery, and colitis to sudden nerve deafness. The flowers have been shown to be effective in lessening the desire for alcohol and thus are used in the treatment of alcoholism.

CONTRAINDICATIONS: Pueraria should not be used by those with cold in the stomach and excessive sweating.

DOSE: 9–15 grams

Bupleurum (CHAI HU)

Radix bupleurum falcatum

COMMON NAME: Bupleurum, hare's ear

FAMILY: Umbelliferae

PART USED: Root

ENERGY AND FLAVORS: Cool; acrid, bitter

ORGAN MERIDIANS AFFECTED: Liver, gallbladder, pericardium, Triple Warmer

PROPERTIES: Diaphoretic, antipyretic, anti-inflammatory, antimalarial

EFFECTS AND INDICATIONS: Clears heat, regulates liver *qi,* raises the yang. It is used for treating the common cold that is accompanied by alternating symptoms of chills and fever; malaria; chest pain; prolapse of the anus, uterus, and other internal organs; and irregular menstruation. Though it is classified as a cool surface-relieving herb, it is commonly used in Chinese herbalism for stagnant liver *qi*, which refers to a pattern of symptoms including stifling feelings in the chest, flank pain, and emotional mood swings. For some, especially those with a tendency to yin deficiency, it can bring up unwarranted feelings of anger. This herb is also very well known for its sedative action, especially in the patented medicine *Xiao Yao Wan* (Bupleurum Sedative Pills). It is also effective for women with menstrual problems associated with premenstrual syndrome (PMS).

CONTRAINDICATIONS: Bupleurum should not be used by those with depleted fluids, those with liver yang rising, those with extreme headaches, or those with such eye diseases as conjunctivitis.

DOSE: 3–9 grams

NOTE: *Bupleurum longiradiatum* cannot be used because it is poisonous.

Cimicifuga (SHENG MA)

Rhizoma cimicifuga heracleifolia, Cimicfuga dahurica, C. foetida

COMMON NAMES: Chinese black cohosh, black cohosh, cimicifuga

FAMILY: Ranunculaceae

PART USED: Rhizome

ENERGY AND FLAVORS: Cool; sweet, acrid, slightly bitter

ORGAN MERIDIANS AFFECTED: Lung, spleen, stomach, large intestine

PROPERTIES: Diaphoretic, antipyretic, antifungal, antibacterial

EFFECTS AND INDICATIONS: Clears wind heat, regulates the circulation of *qi,* relieves pain. It can be used for headache caused by wind heat; gingivitis; hives; diarrhea; venting eruptive skin diseases, such as measles, in the early stages; and prolapsed internal organs, such as the anus and uterus. The Chinese say that this herb "lifts the sunken"; therefore, it is used to direct other herbs upward and is also indicated for prolapsed organs. North American cimicifuga may be similar though not identical to the Chinese variety.

CONTRAINDICATIONS: Black cohosh should not be used by those who have full-blown measles or those who are having trouble breathing. It should also not be used by those with excess in the upper regions and deficiency in the lower part of the body.

DOSE: 3–9 grams

Horsetail (MU ZEI)

Herba equiseti hiemalis

COMMON NAMES: Horsetail, shave grass, scouring rush

FAMILY: Equisetaceae

PART USED: Leaves (grass)

ENERGY AND FLAVORS: Neutral; sweet, bitter

ORGAN MERIDIANS AFFECTED: Lung, liver

PROPERTIES: Diaphoretic, diuretic, astringent

INDICATIONS: Although used in Western herbalism for urinary problems, horsetail is used in Chinese medicine for such ailments as bloodshot eyes and conjunctivitis. Because it is rich in trace minerals, it is excellent as a semiregular tonic, although it should not be used for extended periods of time.

CONTRAINDICATIONS: This herb should not be used by pregnant women, those who are weak, or those with excessive dryness or frequent urination.

DOSE: 3–9 grams

Herbs That Clear Heat

Herbs that clear internal heat are classified as alteratives in Western herbology. Heat belies the presence of toxic congestion. Any congestion in the body will eventually transform to heat from stagnation. As the body is overcome, it first tends to become cold and weak, but as it rallies to fight off the pathogenic evil, it changes to heat. In the process, this reversion from hot to cold to hot again, an essence or yin depletion occurs that requires yin tonics along with heat-clearing herbs to treat the disease. There are five subcategories of heat-clearing herbs:

- **Herbs that clear heat and purge fire:** When external pathogenic factors penetrate deeper, they are said to be at the *qi* level. At this stage, sweating therapy is no longer effective for relieving high fevers.
- **Herbs that clear heat and cool the blood:** When heat penetrates to the blood level, there may be symptoms of inflammation with bleeding.
- **Herbs that clear damp heat:** Damp heat includes pus, purulent discharges, and hepatitis. Herbs that clear damp heat may include cholagogues that increase liver filtering and the discharge of toxins through the bile.
- **Herbs that clear heat and remove toxins:** Some heat-clearing herbs clear various toxic conditions, such as toxic dysentery, boils, carbuncles, and epidemic infectious diseases.
- **Herbs that clear summer heat:** Summer heat refers to diseases associated with hot summer climates, such as heat stroke.

Because herbs that clear heat tend to have cold or cool properties, they may impair digestion as a result of injuring the spleen and stomach. In general, they should be used with caution for individuals with a tendency to low appetite, loose stools, and diarrhea.

HERBS THAT CLEAR HEAT AND PURGE FIRE

Herbs that clear heat and purge fire treat inflammation and heat at the *qi* level. This is a deeper layer of penetration than surface fevers, so external surface-relieving herbs are inappropriate. Symptoms to be treated include high fever, sweating (obviously, sweating therapy is contraindicated); thirst; delirium; irritability; scanty, dark urine; dry yellow tongue coat; and surging, forceful pulse. At this level, excess heat is centered in the lungs or stomach.

Gypsum (SHI GAO)
Gypsum fibrosum
COMMON NAME: Gypsum
CHEMICAL NAME: Calcium sulfate
CONDITION IN WHICH USED: Tea
ENERGY AND FLAVORS: Very cold; acrid, sweet
ORGAN MERIDIANS AFFECTED: Stomach, lung
PROPERTIES: Antipyretic, sedative
INDICATIONS: Gypsum is used for excess heat in the lungs or stomach manifesting as toothache, acute mouth sores, painful and bleeding gums, inflammation, or very high fever without chills. For inflammation, it can be used either externally or internally. It is used externally for wounds or burns.
CONTRAINDICATIONS: This substance should not be used by those with a weak stomach or without true heat.
DOSE: 10–50 grams

Gardenia fruit (ZHI ZI)
Fructus gardeniae jasminoidis
COMMON NAME: Gardenia, Cape Jasmine Fruit
FAMILY: Rubiaceae
PART USED: Fruit
ENERGY AND FLAVOR: Cold; bitter
ORGAN MERIDIANS AFFECTED: Heart, liver, gallbladder, lung, stomach, triple warmer
PROPERTIES: Cholagogue, anti-inflammatory, antipyretic, blood circulation promoter
EFFECTS AND INDICATIONS: Purges heat, disperses fire, dispels damp heat, cools blood, resolves bruises. Gardenia fruit is used for fever with

irritability or restlessness and urinary tract infections. It is effective for any bleeding in the mucous membranes, such as the nasal passages, the bowels, or the urinary tract. For bleeding, the ashes of the calcined herb are most effective; a teaspoon is taken internally at intervals or applied externally.

CONTRAINDICATIONS: Gardenia fruit should not be used by those who have diarrhea.

DOSE: 3–12 grams

Prunella (XIA KU CAO)

Spica prunellae vulgaris

COMMON NAME: Prunella, self heal, all heal

FAMILY: Labiatae

PART USED: Flower spike

ENERGY AND FLAVORS: Cold; sweet, acrid, bitter

ORGAN MERIDIANS AFFECTED: Liver, gallbladder, lung

PROPERTIES: Antipyretic, diuretic, anti-inflammatory antihypertensive vasodilator

INDICATIONS: Prunella, which grows both in the northwestern and northeastern parts of North America, is used for painful, red, and/or swollen eyes often associated with hypertension. It is also very effective for softening and resolving swollen lymph glands, goiter, breast lumps, cancer and tumors.

CONTRAINDICATIONS: Prunella should not be used by those with a weak stomach or spleen associated with coldness.

DOSE: 9–15 grams

Phragmites (LU GEN)

Phragmites communis

COMMON NAME: Phragmites, reed rhizome

FAMILY: Gramineae

PART USED: Rhizome

ENERGY AND FLAVOR: Cold; sweet

ORGAN MERIDIANS AFFECTED: Lung, stomach

PROPERTIES: Diuretic, antibiotic, antiemetic

INDICATIONS: Phragmites is effective for conditions of the lung involving thick yellow sputum, fever, and thirst. It can also be used for nausea and vomiting associated with stomach heat. For the Lower Warmer, it is used for damp heat with symptoms of urinary tract infections, such as dark urine, painful urination, and possibly blood in the urine. This is a common herb that resembles bamboo.

CONTRAINDICATIONS: This herb should not be used when there is weakness in the spleen and stomach caused by cold.

DOSE: 9–30 grams

Cassia seed (JUE MING ZI)

Semen cassiae tora

COMMON NAME: Cassia seed

FAMILY: Leguminosae

PART USED: Seed

ENERGY AND FLAVORS: Cool; sweet, bitter, salty

ORGAN MERIDIANS AFFECTED: Liver, kidney, large intestine, gallbladder

PROPERTIES: Antipyretic, antibiotic, antihypertensive, cholesterol reducing aid, mild laxative

INDICATIONS: This herb is especially good for conditions of the eyes. It will brighten them and relieve pain, congestion, itchiness, redness, or sensitivity to light when caused by wind-heat conditions. It can also be used when there is headache along with some of the above conditions in cases of liver yang rising. It is useful when there is either chronic or acute constipation accompanying liver yin deficiency. It has been shown to be effective in lowering cholesterol and reducing blood pressure.

CONTRAINDICATIONS: Cassia seeds should not be used by those with diarrhea or lethargy and should not be used with cannabis seed.

DOSE: 6–12 grams

NOTES: Toasted cassia seed has a coffeelike aroma and flavor. In China, it is a common household treatment item and the crushed toasted seeds are drunk as a warm beverage, instead of coffee, to lower high blood pressure.

Anemarrhena (ZHI MU)

Rhizoma anemarrhenae asphodeloides

COMMON NAME: Anemarrhena

FAMILY: Liliaceae

PART USED: Rhizome

ENERGY AND FLAVORS: Cold; sweet, bitter

ORGAN MERIDIANS AFFECTED: Stomach, lung, kidney

PROPERTIES: Anti-inflammatory, demulcent, antipyretic, antibacterial, nutritive

EFFECTS AND INDICATIONS: Purges heat, nurtures the yin, relaxes tension. It can be used for fevers accompanied with dryness (yin deficiency) in the lungs, stomach, or kidneys. This could manifest diversely with diseases such as tuberculosis, chronic bronchitis, chronic low-grade fever, irritability, nocturnal emissions, or abnormally high sex drive.

CONTRAINDICATIONS: Anemarrhena should not be used by those with diarrhea.

DOSE: 6–12 grams

Bamboo Leaf (DAN ZHU YE)
Herba lophatheri gracilis
COMMON NAME: Lophatherum
FAMILY: Gramineae
PART USED: Leaves
ENERGY AND FLAVORS: Cold; sweet, bland
ORGAN MERIDIANS AFFECTED: Heart, stomach, small intestine
PROPERTIES: Anti-inflammatory, antipyretic, diuretic
INDICATIONS: This herb is used for heat conditions associated with irritability and anxiety. It can also be used for swollen, painful gums and urinary tract infections with signs of irritability; because of its effect on the heart, which in Chinese theory corresponds to the mind.
CONTRAINDICATIONS: Bamboo leaf should not be used by pregnant women.
DOSE: 6–12 grams
NOTES: This is distinguished from black bamboo leaf, which similarly clears heat and relieves irritability but enters the heart, lung, and stomach.

Buddleia flower (MI MENG HUA)
Flos buddleiae officinalis
COMMON NAMES: Buddleia flower bud, butterfly bush
FAMILY: Loganiaceae
PART USED: Flower
ENERGY AND FLAVOR: Cool; sweet
ORGAN MERIDIAN AFFECTED: Liver
PROPERTIES: Antispasmodic, antipyretic, mild diuretic
INDICATIONS: This herb is used for conditions of the eyes, such as blood-

shot eyes, excessive tearing, excessive excretion, or sensitivity to light (photophobia). Because of its mild actions, it can be used for either excess or deficient conditions.

CONTRAINDICATIONS: None noted.

DOSE: 4–12 grams

NOTES: This herb is cultivated as an ornamental in the West.

HERBS THAT CLEAR HEAT AND COOL THE BLOOD

Herbs that cool the blood are used for inflammation and heat at the blood level. Symptoms include acute inflammatory conditions associated with various bleeding disorders, such as epistaxis, blood in the stool, blood in the urine, bleeding gums, coughing, vomiting, or spitting up of blood. We hear of many especially virulent and exotic viruses associated with bleeding that have this level of heat, and they are often deadly. These herbs are also used for severe high fevers with loss of consciousness, a deeply red tongue, and a rapid pulse. The herbs tend to have a cold energy with bitter, sweet, and salty flavors.

Rehmannia root (unprepared) (SHENG DI HUANG)
Radix rehmanniae glutinosae

COMMON NAMES: Raw rehmannia, Chinese foxglove

FAMILY: Scrophulariaceae

PART USED: Root

ENERGY AND FLAVORS: Cold; sweet, bitter

ORGAN MERIDIANS AFFECTED: Heart, liver, kidney

PROPERTIES: Antibacterial, antifungal, cardiotonic (dosage-sensitive), diuretic

INDICATIONS: Raw rehmannia is used in cases of heat caused by lack of fluids (yin deficiency) in the body. Its use therefore is well advised when there are heat signs with thirst. It is also recommended when there is bleeding in the stomach or uterus. Rehmannia is also effective when there is heart fire rising with sores in the mouth or on the tongue, irritability, insomnia, and/or chronic low-grade fever.

CONTRAINDICATIONS: Rehmannia root should not be used for spleen weakness with symptoms of diarrhea, lack of appetite, or excess phlegm. It should also be avoided by pregnant women.

DOSE: 9–30 grams

Scrophularia (XUAN SHEN)

Radix scrophulariae ningpoensis

COMMON NAMES: Chinese figwort, scrophularia

FAMILY: Scrophulariaceae

PART USED: Root

ENERGY AND FLAVORS: Cold; bitter, sweet, salty

ORGAN MERIDIANS AFFECTED: Lung, stomach, kidney

PROPERTIES: Anti-inflammatory, antihypertensive, antibacterial, antifungal, vasodilator

EFFECTS AND INDICATIONS: Nourishes the yin, relieves irritability and constipation. Chinese figwort is used when there are warm febrile diseases possibly associated with bleeding. It is especially helpful for swollen, inflamed lymph glands and severe sore throat. It is also useful for the treatment of cancers and tumors.

CONTRAINDICATIONS: Scrophularia should not be used by those with spleen or stomach weakness or dampness, especially when there is diarrhea. **Caution:** Scrophularia should not be used with *Radix veratri.*

DOSE: 9–30 grams

Cow bezoar (NIU HUANG)

Calculus bovis

COMMON NAME: Cow gallstone

FAMILY: Bovidae

PART USED: Gallstone or the bile of either an ox, water buffalo, or pig. It is dried and made into a powder for pills.

ENERGY AND FLAVORS: Cool; bitter, sweet

ORGAN MERIDIANS AFFECTED: Heart, liver

PROPERTIES: Anti-inflammatory, antipyretic, antibacterial

INDICATIONS: It is used for high fever with accompanying delirium and convulsion. It is also used for chronic sore throat or internal abscesses that have ruptured.

CONTRAINDICATIONS: Cow bezoar should not be used by pregnant women or those with spleen and stomach coldness and deficiency.

DOSE: 0.15–0.3 grams

NOTES: This substance is extremely expensive and primarily used in the Chinese patent called *Niu Huang Jie Du Pian,* which can be used for all of the above-mentioned conditions as well as mouth sores. The combination of *niu huang* with rhinoceros or water buffalo horn can be a lifesaver in the treatment of Legionnaire's disease, meningitis, and encephalitis.

Moutan peony (MU DAN PI)

Cortex moutan radicis, Paeonia suffruticosa
COMMON NAMES: Moutan peony, tree peony
FAMILY: Ranunculaceae
PART USED: Root bark
ENERGY AND FLAVORS: Slightly cold; acrid, bitter
ORGAN MERIDIANS AFFECTED: Heart, liver, kidney
PROPERTIES: Anti-inflammatory, antibacterial, antipyretic, analgesic
EFFECTS AND INDICATIONS: Invigorates the blood, clears blood stagnation. This herb has a wide variety of indications but is most effective in warm febrile diseases when there is blood in the sputum or nosebleeds, or when there is excessive menstrual bleeding. It is also used for amenorrhea, tumors, carbuncles, or blood stasis due to traumatic injury. It can be used topically for nondraining sores or abscesses.
CONTRAINDICATIONS: Moutan peony should not be used by women who are either pregnant or experiencing excessive menstrual flow. It should be avoided when there are cold signs or yin deficiency with excessive sweating.
DOSE: 3–9 grams

HERBS THAT CLEAR HEAT AND DRY DAMPNESS

Herbs that clear heat and dry dampness are generally bitter, cold, and drying in nature. North American goldenseal, barberry, Oregon grape root, and fringetree bark all would be in this category. Damp heat is characterized by fever, greasy tongue coat, scanty urine, jaundice, dysentery, diarrhea, purulent sores, eczema, psoriasis, abnormal discharges from the male or female reproductive organs, and cloudy urine. Because these herbs are bitter and drying, they can injure digestion and damage fluids. For this reason, demulcent, yin tonic herbs are sometimes added to formulas to offset any negative side effects.

Scutellaria (HUANG QIN)

Radix scutellariae baicalensis
COMMON NAMES: Scute, Chinese skullcap, scutellaria
FAMILY: Labiatae

PART USED: Root

ENERGY AND FLAVOR: Cold; bitter

ORGAN MERIDIANS AFFECTED: Liver, lung, heart, gallbladder, and large intestine

PROPERTIES: Anti-inflammatory, antibiotic, cholagogue, antihypertensive, calmative

INDICATIONS: A primary herb for damp heat conditions, especially of the upper body. It is indicated for symptoms of yellow phlegm, including phlegm with blood, diarrhea, dysentery, jaundice, urinary tract infections, and skin diseases. It can be used during pregnancy to help calm fetal restlessness. Scute, as it is commonly called, is excellent for liver yang rising (hypertension) with symptoms of irritability, red eyes, and flushed face.

CONTRAINDICATIONS: Scutellaria should not be used by those with deficiency heat in the lungs or with coldness in the Middle Warmer, such as diarrhea. It should not be used by those mothers with restless fetus due to cold conditions.

DOSAGE: 3–9 grams

NOTES: There are many varieties of scutellaria throughout the world. *Scutellaria lateriflora,* commonly used in Western herbalism, primarily uses the aerial portions for anxiety, restlessness, insomnia, or alcohol and drug addiction. It also relieves nervousness by clearing heat and toxins.

Coptis (*HUANG LIAN*)

Rhizoma coptidis, Coptis chinensis

COMMON NAME: Coptis

FAMILY: Ranunculaceae

PART USED: Rhizome

ENERGY AND FLAVOR: Cold; bitter

ORGAN MERIDIANS AFFECTED: Heart, liver, Stomach, large intestine

PROPERTIES: Anti-inflammatory, antibiotic, vasodilator, antipyretic, cholagogue

INDICATIONS: The anti-inflammatory property of coptis, because it enters the heart organ meridian, which governs the mind, makes it especially effective with heat conditions associated with nervousness, anxiety, and insomnia. Because it enters the liver organ meridian, it stimulates the flow of bile, relieving damp heat, making it effective for hepatitis, gallstones, cirrhosis, jaundice, and venereal diseases, including herpes simplex. It is also very effective for infections, fevers, conjunctivitis, inflammation, abscesses, and hemorrhage. It enters the stomach organ meridian, which governs the mouth, so it can be used for oral ulcers. In addition, it can be topically applied for scabies and external infections. It is impossible to overstate the wide scope of heat-clearing or alterative properties of such a valuable herb, but it is also useful for more serious diseases, from leukemia and cancer to tuberculosis and typhoid fever.

CONTRAINDICATIONS: Coptis should be used with caution because of its extreme bitterness. Large doses can injure the stomach.

DOSE: 1–9 grams

NOTES: Coptis contains berberine and is similar to North American goldenseal (*Hydrastis canadensis*), for which it can be substituted or used interchangeably.

Phellodendron (HUANG BAI)

Cortex phellodendron amurense

COMMON NAME: Philodendron bark

FAMILY: Rutaceae

PART USED: Bark

ENERGY AND FLAVOR: Cold; bitter

ORGAN MERIDIANS AFFECTED: Kidney, urinary bladder, large intestine

PROPERTIES: Anti-inflammatory, antipyretic, cholagogue, antibacterial, lowers blood sugar

EFFECTS AND INDICATIONS: Purges heat, detoxifies, clears damp heat. It is indicated for infections and inflammation with possible symptoms of discharge from the anus, vagina, or penis. It also is customarily used for symptoms of heat associated with kidney yin deficiency. These may include night sweats, afternoon fever, and nocturnal emissions. Phellodendron is an effective herb used topically for sores and damp heat conditions of the skin.

CONTRAINDICATIONS: Phellodendron should not be used by those with spleen or stomach deficiency with or without diarrhea.

DOSE: 3–9 grams

NOTE: Barberry leaves and rhizome, which also clear fever and heat associated with deficiency, can be used as an alternative to this herb.

Gentian root (LONG DAN CAO)

Radix gentianae longdancao

COMMON NAMES: Chinese gentian, gentian

FAMILY: Gentianaceae
PART USED: Root
ENERGY AND FLAVOR: Cold; bitter
ORGAN MERIDIANS AFFECTED: Liver, gallbladder, stomach
PROPERTIES: Cholagogue, antibacterial, anti-inflammatory, antispasmodic
INDICATIONS: This herb is used for inflammatory conditions associated
   with jaundice, itching, herpes virus, leukorrhea, venereal diseases,
   hepatitis, cholecystitis, and hypertension. Symptoms can include
   fever, headache, restlessness, abdominal pain, sore throat, bitter
   mouth taste, flank pain, and redness of the conjunctiva of the eyes.
CONTRAINDICATIONS: This herb should not be used by those with diarrhea caused by spleen/stomach deficiency or by persons without true
   damp heat symptoms.
DOSE: 3–9 grams

Sophora root (KU SHEN)

Radix sophorae flavescentis
COMMON NAME: Sophora
FAMILY: Leguminosae
PART USED: Root
ENERGY AND FLAVOR: Cold; bitter
ORGAN MERIDIANS AFFECTED: Heart, liver, stomach, large and small intes-
   tines, urinary bladder
PROPERTIES: Anti-inflammatory, diuretic, antibacterial, antifungal, anti-
   pruritic, parasiticide
INDICATIONS: Clears damp heat conditions, especially in the Lower
   Warmer, with symptoms such as acute urinary tract infections, vagi-
   nal or anal discharge with itching, or eczema. It also kills worms and
   is helpful in cases of ringworm. It can also be used topically to treat
   genital itching.
CONTRAINDICATIONS: Sophora root should not be used by those with
   weakness and cold in the spleen and stomach. **Caution:** Sophora
   root should not be used with *Radix veratri.*
DOSE: 3–12 grams

HERBS THAT CLEAR HEAT AND REMOVE TOXICITY

Toxic heat manifests as boils, carbuncles, erysipelas, sore throat, and
dysentery. Bites of venomous insects, snakes, and other animals are also

treated by these herbs. This presumably would include Lyme disease and Rocky Mountain fever.

Honeysuckle flowers (JIN YIN HUA)
Flos lonicerae japonicae
COMMON NAMES: Honeysuckle flower, lonicera
FAMILY: Caprifoliaceae
PARTS USED: Flowers
ENERGY AND FLAVOR: Cold; bitter, sweet
ORGAN MERIDIANS AFFECTED: Lung, heart, stomach, large intestine
PROPERTIES: Anti-inflammatory, antipyretic, antimicrobial
INDICATIONS: This herb has broad-spectrum antibiotic properties and can be used for all infections and inflammations. It is especially effective when the infection is in the Upper Warmer (respiratory tract) but is also effective for some Middle Warmer gastrointestinal tract inflammations. It is useful for the onset of wind-heat diseases associated with fevers, the common cold, sore throat, and influenza.
CONTRAINDICATIONS: This herb should not be used by those with weakness in the spleen/stomach system when there is cold or diarrhea. It should be used carefully when there are sores due to *qi* or yin deficiency.
DOSE: 6–15 grams; large doses (up to 60 grams) can be used effectively and safely in severe cases.
NOTE: The stems and leaves have more or less the same properties as the flowers but are more specific for arthritic and rheumatic conditions.

Dandelion (PU GONG YING)
Herba cum radix taraxaci mongolici
COMMON NAME: Dandelion
FAMILY: Compositae
PARTS USED: Herb, root
ENERGY AND FLAVORS: Cold; bitter, sweet
ORGAN MERIDIANS AFFECTED: Liver, stomach
PROPERTIES: Anti-inflammatory, cholagogue, diuretic, mild laxative, galactagogue, antimicrobial
INDICATIONS: A major herb in the West, dandelion is used whenever there is liver involvement with heat and toxins in the blood. This includes jaundice, hepatitis, red and swollen eyes, as well as urinary

tract infection, abscesses, or firm, hard sores in the breasts. It is also very effective to increase the production of mother's milk.

CONTRAINDICATIONS: This is a very safe herb, but overdoses could cause mild diarrhea.

DOSE: 10–30 grams

Isatis leaf (DA QING YE)

Folium isatidis tinctoria

COMMON NAME: Isatis leaf, indigo

FAMILY: Cruciferae

PART USED: Leaves

ENERGY AND FLAVOR: Cold; bitter

ORGAN MERIDIANS AFFECTED: Heart, lung, stomach

PROPERTIES: Antibacterial, antiviral, antipyretic

INDICATIONS: This herb is useful for febrile diseases and diseases associated with epidemics. Often, both the leaf and the root are used together for a variety of contagious diseases, including mumps. Despite the strength of this herb, it can be used by all, regardless of their constitution, for febrile epidemic diseases. Considering the fact that conventional Western medicine has little to offer for contagious viral diseases, this is one of a few herbs that deserve wider appreciation for their antiviral properties. It is especially effective when there is infection in the lungs and for skin conditions involving rashes or blotches.

CONTRAINDICATIONS: Isatis leaf should not be used long term by those with weak and cold spleen or stomach.

DOSE: 9–15 grams

Isatis root (BAN LAN GEN)

Radix isatidis

COMMON NAME: Isatis

FAMILY: Cruciferae

PART USED: Root

ENERGY AND FLAVOR: Cold; bitter

ORGAN MERIDIANS AFFECTED: Lung, heart, stomach

PROPERTIES: Antibacterial, antiviral, parasiticide

EFFECTS AND INDICATIONS: Isatis is one of the most effective antivirals. It is therefore useful for a wide range of infectious viral and bacterial conditions, including the common cold, influenza, sore throat, and epidemic diseases, such as mumps. It cools the blood and is effective for damp-heat conditions, such as jaundice.

CONTRAINDICATIONS: Isatis root should not be used by those who are weak or are without true fire toxicity.

DOSE: 10–30 grams

NOTE: Isatis and a relative, baptisia, are both presently cultivated in the West.

Forsythia fruit (LIAN QIAO)
Fructus forsythiae suspensae
COMMON NAME: Forsythia fruit
FAMILY: Oleaceae
PART USED: Fruit
ENERGY AND FLAVOR: Cool; bitter
ORGAN MERIDIANS AFFECTED: Heart, liver, lung, gallbladder
PROPERTIES: Antibacterial, antiemetic, parasiticide, antipyretic, anti-inflammatory
INDICATIONS: Forsythia, a major ingredient in the patented formula Honeysuckle and Forsythia Combination (*Yin Qiao San*), is commonly used for eliminating wind heat in the body, such as the common cold or influenza. It is also useful for toxic sores, carbuncles, swollen lymph nodes, Forsythia should be considered when there is high fever with thirst and delirium.
CONTRAINDICATIONS: Forsythia fruit should not be used by those with weak and cold spleen/stomach conditions or for sores that are already open or are caused by yin deficiency.
DOSE: 3–12 grams
NOTE: Forsythia fruit is commonly used for a variety of inflammatory conditions, including colds, sore throat, fevers, influenza, boils, carbuncles, and furuncles, and for the treatment of cancer (especially lung, throat, and breast cancer).

Violet (ZI HUA DI DING)
Herba cum radice violae
COMMON NAMES: Yedoens violet, viola
FAMILY: Violaceae
PART USED: Leaves and flowers
ENERGY AND FLAVORS: Cold; acrid, bitter
ORGAN MERIDIANS AFFECTED: Heart, liver

PROPERTIES: Anti-inflammatory, antibiotic, demulcent

INDICATIONS: This herb is used for inflammation, especially in the form of an abscess or boil, where it is topically applied as a poultice. The tea is useful for hot swellings of the throat, eyes, and ears, including such diseases as mumps and ulcers. It is also traditionally used in both Eastern and Western herbal traditions to soften and dissolve tumors.

CONTRAINDICATIONS: Violet should not be used by those who have a cold or deficiency condition.

DOSE: 9–15 grams

Houttuynia (YU XING CAO)

Herba cum radicis houttuyniae

COMMON NAME: Houttuynia

FAMILY: Saururaceae

PART USED: Leaves

ENERGY AND FLAVOR: Slightly cold; acrid

ORGAN MERIDIANS AFFECTED: Liver, lung, urinary bladder

PROPERTIES: Anti-inflammatory, antimicrobial, diuretic, expectorant

INDICATIONS: This herb is indicated for any toxic heat of the lungs in which there is thick yellow or green sputum. It can also be used for other hot swellings, either internally or externally, as it will help expel pus and cool the inflammation. It promotes urination for damp heat in the Lower Warmer.

CONTRAINDICATIONS: Houttuynia is contraindicated for those with cold deficiency symptoms.

DOSE: 15–40 grams, only lightly decocted

Portulaca (MA CHI XIAN)

Herba portulacae oleraceae

COMMON NAMES: Portulaca, purslane

FAMILY: Portulacaceae

PART USED: Leaves and stems

ENERGY AND FLAVOR: Cold; sour

ORGAN MERIDIANS AFFECTED: Liver, heart, large intestine

PROPERTIES: Anti-inflammatory, demulcent, antibiotic, antiparasitic, nutritive

EFFECTS AND INDICATIONS: Cools the blood. This herb is used internally for damp heat with symptoms of toxic dysentery, boils, sores, vaginal discharges, and urinary tract infections, as well as topically for venomous bites and stings.

CONTRAINDICATIONS: Pregnant women with digestive weakness should limit the use of portulaca because of its cold nature.

DOSE: 15–60 grams

HERBS THAT CLEAR SUMMER HEAT

Summer heat is a seasonal condition characterized by external heat caused by hot, humid weather and internal cold dampness caused by overeating cold, raw foods and ingesting cold drinks in hot weather. Because of the internal damp symptoms, the condition is associated with spleen dampness.

Mung bean (LU DOU)

Semen phaseoli radiati

COMMON NAME: Mung bean

FAMILY: Leguminosae

PART USED: Bean

ENERGY AND FLAVOR: Cool; sweet

ORGAN MERIDIANS AFFECTED: Heart, stomach

PROPERTIES: Antidote to toxic poisonings, antipyretic, antihypertensive, nutritive tonic

EFFECTS AND INDICATIONS: Mung bean is a nutritious protein food that can be used for all hot, inflammatory conditions, ranging from systemic infections to heat stroke to hypertension. It is also used for toxic poisoning, including aconite poisoning. It is very effective as a soup for heat stroke associated with thirst, irritability, and fever. Mung beans are commonly cooked with rice, ghee, coriander, turmeric, cumin, and salt in the justly famous therapeutic East Indian recipe called kichari, which can be eaten exclusively for 10 days to a month as a balanced general detoxification.

CONTRAINDICATIONS: Because of their cooling nature, mung beans should be avoided or cooked with warming spices for those with a weak digestion.

DOSE: 15–30 grams; 120 grams are cooked with 60 grams of licorice for aconite poisoning

Watermelon (XI GUA)

Fructus citrulli vulgaris

COMMON NAME: Watermelon

FAMILY: Cucurbitaceae
PART USED: Fruit, rind, seeds
ENERGY AND FLAVOR: Cold; sweet
ORGAN MERIDIANS AFFECTED: Heart, stomach, urinary bladder
PROPERTIES: Diuretic, antipyretic
INDICATIONS: Watermelon is useful for symptoms of overexposure to
   heat. For this, the rind should also be consumed. The ground seeds
   are an excellent diuretic and can also be used for urinary tract infec-
   tions.
CONTRAINDICATIONS: Watermelon should be avoided by those who have
   either too much dampness or too much coldness or a combination
   of both.
DOSE: 9–30 grams; 1 or 2 cups of the fresh juice is the best

Artemisia annua (QING HAO)
Herba artemisiae annuae
COMMON NAME: Sweet Annie
FAMILY: Compositae
PART USED: Leaves
ENERGY AND FLAVORS: Cold; acrid, bitter
ORGAN MERIDIANS AFFECTED: Liver, kidney, gallbladder
PROPERTIES: Antipyretic, antibacterial, antifungal, antimalarial
INDICATIONS: Artemisia annua can be used for heat stroke symptoms as
   well as a wide variety of inflammatory conditions, including all kinds
   of fevers. It is specific for both treating and preventing malaria. It can
   be used both topically and internally for bacterial and fungal infec-
   tions and is one of a few anti-inflammatory herbs that can be used
   with symptoms of wasting and yin deficiency.
CONTRAINDICATIONS: Artemisia annua should be avoided by those with
   diarrhea due to weak, cold spleen and stomach and by those without
   heat signs due to yin deficiency.
DOSE: 3–9 grams

Laxative and Purgative Herbs and Substances

Laxatives include herbs and other substances that stimulate evacuation of the bowels, as well as herbs that promote bowel movements by
helping to retain moisture and lubricating the large intestine. They are
mainly indicated for constipation. Herbalists believe that before any dis-

ease can be successfully treated, the bowels must be moving regularly, at least once daily if at all possible. Constipation and sluggishness of the bowels causes gradual accumulation of toxins in the body, which can lead to a myriad of serious diseases.

Down through time, purgatives and laxatives have been very popular. In the West, cascara and buckthorn bark are commonly used. In China, rhubarb is the most commonly used laxative. In India, the most effective of all bowel-regulating formulas is triphala, a common household item in that country. There are three subcategories of laxatives: purgatives, demulcent or lubricating laxatives, and strong cathartic purgatives that eliminate fluid accumulation.

A side discussion of triphala, an East Indian Ayurvedic formula, is important here because triphala can be easily integrated into the practice of TCM and is a great asset. Triphala is a mild bowel regulator that has digestive tonic properties and, unlike other laxatives, it causes no dependency. Triphala consists of three fruits, emblic myrobalan, beleric myrobalan, and chebulic myrobalan, the last of which is also used in TCM. Each of the three fruits regulates the three Ayurvedic humors of the body: the water humor is relieved by clearing high-lipid density in the circulatory system; the fire humor, residing in the liver, is cleared by stimulating the filtering of toxins from the blood and the discharge of bile; and the air humor is regulated through calming and toning the nervous system. Triphala eliminates all excesses without causing any deficiencies. In fact, the daily use of triphala will restore the proper intestinal chemistry so that the proper balance of favorable bacterial is naturally restored.

PURGATIVES

Purgatives are bitter and cold and can reduce fire and promote bowel movement. They are used for any condition associated with the retention of feces caused by excess heat in the stomach and intestines. They can be combined with herbs that clear heat whenever it seems advantageous to clear the accumulation of internal heat.

Rhubarb root (DA HUANG)
Radix et rhizoma rhei
COMMON NAME: Rhubarb root
FAMILY: Polygonaceae

PART USED: Root and rhizome

ENERGY AND FLAVOR: Cold; bitter

ORGAN MERIDIANS AFFECTED: Liver, spleen, large intestine, stomach, pericardium

PROPERTIES: Purgative, antibacterial, antitumor, antifungal, diuretic, hemostatic, cholagogue, antihypertensive, lowers serum cholesterol, anti-inflammatory

EFFECTS AND INDICATIONS: One of the more powerful herbs used in Chinese medicine, rhubarb is excellent for draining damp heat, especially when there is accompanying constipation. It moves the blood and is good for blood stagnation associated with acute stabbing pain and bruises, for which it can be taken both internally as well as externally in a liniment. Rhubarb is used for dysenteric conditions caused by damp heat with symptoms of bleeding in the stool. It can also be taken for vomiting of blood. It can be used both internally and topically for infections. It kills blood flukes. As an external remedy for inflammatory skin conditions such as boils and burns, rhubarb powder can be used alone or combined with other herbs with a little flour and water or honey to hold it together.

CONTRAINDICATIONS: Rhubarb root should only be used where there is excess heat and dampness. Nursing mothers should use it with extreme caution.

DOSE: 3–12 grams

Sodium sulfate (mirabilitum) (MANG XIAO)

COMMON NAME: Glauber's salt

ENERGY AND FLAVORS: Very cold; bitter, acrid, salty

ORGAN MERIDIANS AFFECTED: Stomach, large intestine

PROPERTIES: Purgative, anti-inflammatory, diuretic

EFFECTS AND INDICATIONS: This substance is used for constipation because of its softening properties, especially for stools that are dry and difficult to void. In addition, it is occasionally used to clear heat associated with sores in the mouth and on the breasts, for which it can be taken internally or applied externally.

CONTRAINDICATIONS: As this substance has a strong descending action, it should not be used during pregnancy, menstruation, or the postpartum period. It should also be avoided by those with spleen deficiency and by the elderly.

DOSE: 3–12 grams

Senna leaf *(FAN XIE YE)*

Folium sennae
COMMON NAME: Senna leaf
FAMILY: Leguminosae
PART USED: Leaf
ENERGY AND FLAVORS: Cold; sweet, bitter
ORGAN MERIDIAN AFFECTED: Large intestine
PROPERTIES: Antibacterial, purgative
INDICATIONS: Senna is used for accumulation of heat-causing stagnation in the intestines, with such symptoms as constipation and abdominal fullness.
CONTRAINDICATIONS: Senna leaf should not be overused by those with chronic constipation or by pregnant, menstruating, or postpartum women.
DOSE: 3–9 grams

Aloe *(LU HUI)*

Aloe vera
COMMON NAME: Aloe; aloe vera
FAMILY: Liliaceae
PARTS USED: Gel, leaves
ENERGY AND FLAVOR: Cold; bitter
ORGAN MERIDIANS AFFECTED: Liver, stomach, large intestine
PROPERTIES: Purgative, cholagogue, anthelmintic, antifungal
EFFECTS AND INDICATIONS: Aloe has become a common household plant and is widely known for its powerful effects on burns and wounds. When used externally on burns, aloe vera gel stops the burning sensation and promotes the healing process. Internally, the concentrated dried leaf is a powerful laxative and should be used with caution, as it is more potent than rhubarb. It is also effective against intestinal worms and parasites.
CONTRAINDICATIONS: This herb should not be used by pregnant or menstruating women or by those with cold, weak spleen and stomach.
DOSE: 0.5–2 grams

LUBRICATING LAXATIVES

A basic lubricating laxative is vegetable oil. For many, 1 tablespoon of olive oil or castor oil (which is stronger) makes a perfect demulcent laxative. Demulcent laxatives, such as psyllium seed husks, are commonly used to help the bowel retain moisture, which encourages regularity. The herbs in this category are often combined with angelica (*dang gui*) and other herbs that tonify blood, since from the TCM perspective, dryness can be a symptom of blood deficiency.

Cannabis seed (HUO MA REN)

Semen cannabis sativae
COMMON NAME: Cannabis seed, hemp seed
FAMILY: Moraceae
PART USED: Seed
ENERGY AND FLAVOR: Sweet and neutral
ORGAN MERIDIANS AFFECTED: Large intestine, spleen, stomach
PROPERTIES: Laxative, antihypertensive
INDICATIONS: Because they nourish the yin and lubricate the intestines, hemp seeds are used for constipation associated with dryness and yin deficiency. For external use, the seeds can be ground to a flour and applied as a poultice on sores and slow-healing wounds.
CONTRAINDICATIONS: Although cannabis seed is considered safe, it should not be taken for extended periods of time.
DOSE: 9–30 grams
NOTE: If cannabis seed is unavailable, flaxseed is often substituted.

STRONG CATHARTIC LAXATIVES

Cathartics and hydrogogues are strongly eliminating and are used only occasionally. Their main indications are severe abdominal swelling, ascites, edema, and bodily swelling. They can also be used for acute fluid retention in the chest associated with asthma.

Pharbitidis (QIAN NIU ZI)

Semen pharbitidis nil (Pharbitidis purpurea)
COMMON NAME: Morning glory seeds
FAMILY: Convolvulaceae
PART USED: Seed
ENERGIES AND FLAVORS: Cold, toxic; acrid, bitter
ORGAN MERIDIANS AFFECTED: Kidney, lung, large intestine
PROPERTIES: Laxative, diuretic, antiparasitic
EFFECTS AND INDICATIONS: This herb is a powerful laxative, driving out

stagnation of water, food, and damp heat conditions, as well as eliminating intestinal worms. It is also effective when there is stagnation of phlegm causing cough and wheezing.

CONTRAINDICATIONS: Pharbitidis should not be used by pregnant women and should be avoided by those with deficiency of the spleen or stomach.

DOSE: 3–9 grams in decoction; 1.5–3 grams used alone as a powder

Euphorbia kansui (GAN SUI)

Radix euphorbiae kansui

COMMON NAME: Kansui root

FAMILY: Euphorbiaceae

PART USED: Root

ENERGIES AND FLAVOR: Cold, toxic; bitter

ORGAN MERIDIANS AFFECTED: Lung, spleen, kidney, large intestine

PROPERTIES: Laxative, emetic, anthelmintic

EFFECTS AND INDICATIONS: Purges severe fluid accumulation, has a strong laxative action, eliminates intestinal worms. It is used for constipation with abdominal ascites in an excess pattern. It can be used for serious edema in the abdomen or for generalized edema but should be used with caution because of its violent nature. It might be considered for acute symptoms attendant to liver cirrhosis, hydrothorax, ascites, dysuria, pleurisy, constipation, and inflammation of the lymph glands.

CONTRAINDICATIONS: Euphorbia kansui should not be used by pregnant women or by those who are weak.

DOSE: 1–3 grams in decoction; 0.3–1 gram as a powder (when taken in this form, it should be roasted so as to reduce its toxicity—it can cause vomiting).

NOTE: This herb should not be used with *Radix glycyrrhizae uralensis* (gan cao).

Daphne genkwa (YUAN HUA)

Flos daphnes genkwa

COMMON NAME: Genkwa flower

FAMILY: Thymelaeceae

PART USED: Flower

ENERGIES AND FLAVOR: Warm, toxic; acrid

ORGAN MERIDIANS AFFECTED: Lung, kidney, large intestine

PROPERTIES: Laxative, diuretic, antibacterial, antifungal, antitussive, expectorant, antiparasitic

EFFECTS AND INDICATIONS: Drains dampness both through the intestines and bladder, soothes cough. Because of its toxicity, Daphne genkwa should be cautiously used for water stagnation in any of the Triple Burners. Externally, it is effective for eliminating parasites, such as ringworm and scabies. Because of its antitussive and expectorant properties, it is effective for chronic bronchitis, but owing to its potential toxicity, other herbs should be considered before trying this herb.

CONTRAINDICATIONS: Daphne genkwa should not be used by pregnant women or by those with weak constitutions.

DOSE: 1.5–3 grams used in a powder; it can be fried with vinegar to reduce its toxicity.

Phytolacca (SHANG LU)

Radix phytolacca esculenta, Phytolacca acinosa

COMMON NAME: Poke root

FAMILY: Phytolaccaceae

PART USED: Root

ENERGIES AND FLAVOR: Cold, toxic; bitter

ORGAN MERIDIANS AFFECTED: Spleen, kidney, large intestine, urinary bladder

PROPERTIES: Antibiotic, emetic, diuretic, antitussive, expectorant

EFFECTS AND INDICATIONS: Resolves lumps and tumors, is anticarcinogenic. It is used to treat lymphatic congestion, swollen lymph glands, edema, mastitis, abnormal congestion of all glands of the body, and severe ascites of the abdomen. The fresh herb is very strong and irritating to the gastrointestinal tract. Externally, it can be applied as a poultice to inflamed sores and infections.

CONTRAINDICATIONS: Phytolacca should be reserved for those with severe excess conditions and should not be used by pregnant women.

DOSE: 3–9 grams

Herbs That Drain Dampness: Diuretics

Diuretics are used to increase the secretion of bodily fluids through urination. One of the aspects of Chinese herbalism unique among all herbal traditions is its extensive use of mushrooms for this purpose, especially the polypores, such as poria cocos and *Polyporus umbellati*. These high-potassium substances are used to effect a balance of extra- and intracellular fluids. While sodium helps the body retain fluid within the cells, potassium promotes elimination of fluid. Of all plants in the botanical kingdom, mushrooms are the masters of water. When the right degree of rain and moisture arrives, they grow and swell, seem- ingly overnight, to their full size. The remainder of their life span is spent comfortably shedding any excess water. When taken internally, they help our body regulate fluid retention.

Most of the herbs in this category are very useful for both a lack of urination and frequent urination. Interestingly, the latter problem is treated by taking diuretics to ensure a more complete discharge of urine each time, which in turn causes the urge to urinate to become less frequent.

Generally, diuretics are classified as sweet or bland. The bland flavor (if you consider a mushroom's taste bland) is generally an indication of its diuretic properties. Some diuretics also clear heat and can be used for urinary tract infections. Diuretics are used for edema, jaundice, phlegm conditions, and weeping eczema. They should be used with caution for conditions of yin deficiency.

Poria cocos (FU LING)
Sclerotium poriae cocos
COMMON NAMES: Poria, hoelen
FAMILY: Polyporaceae
PARTS USED: Fruiting body
ENERGY AND FLAVORS: Neutral; sweet, bland
ORGAN MERIDIANS AFFECTED: Spleen, heart, lung, urinary bladder
PROPERTIES: Diuretic, sedative, lowers blood sugar, tonic
EFFECTS AND INDICATIONS: Clears dampness, tonifies the spleen functions, calms the mind. It is used for edema, mucus, urinary imbalances, diarrhea, palpitations, vertigo, restlessness, anxiety, and insomnia.
CONTRAINDICATIONS: Poria cocos should not be used when there is fre- quent, copious urination associated with deficiency and coldness.
DOSE: 6–15 grams
NOTE: Other parts of the poria mushroom that are used include the outer peel, called *fu ling pi*, which is the strongest part for clearing edema, and *fu shen*, which is the most effective part for calming the spirit.

Polyporus (ZHU LING)

Sclerotium polypori umbellati

COMMON NAMES: Polyporus, grifola

FAMILY: Polyporaceae

PART USED: Fruiting body

ENERGY AND FLAVORS: Neutral; sweet, bland

ORGAN MERIDIANS AFFECTED: Urinary bladder, kidney, spleen

PROPERTIES: Diuretic, lowers blood sugar, antibacterial, antitumor

EFFECTS AND INDICATIONS: Polyporus is similar to *fu ling*, but it is more
   diuretic and anti-inflammatory. It clears edema, heat, genitourinary
   infections, cystitis, urinary retention, diarrhea, and vaginal discharge.
   It has also recently been used in cancer treatment, as it has antitumor
   properties.

CONTRAINDICATIONS: Polyporus should not be used when there is an ab-
   sence of dampness.

DOSE: 6–15 grams

Talcum (HUA SHI)

COMMON NAME: Talcum

ENERGY AND FLAVOR: Cold; sweet

ORGAN MERIDIANS AFFECTED: Stomach, urinary bladder

PROPERTIES: Diuretic, antibacterial, antiemetic, antidiarrheal

EFFECTS AND INDICATIONS: Dispels dampness, clears heat, soothes irritation. It is used to treat difficult, scanty, or painful urination and to
   relieve damp heat and symptoms of summer heat, including diarrhea,
   fever, or thirt. This substance can also be used externally for damp
   heat conditions to both cool the heat and absorb the moisture. It can
   also be used when there is poisoning, both internally and externally,
   diluting and absorbing toxins and slowing the rate of poisoning. It
   can be applied to various skin rashes and/or used as a wash or
   douche for the mucous membranes. Finally, it can be taken internally
   to help stop diarrhea and vomiting.

CONTRAINDICATIONS: Talcum should not be used when there are no signs
   of damp heat, and it should be avoided during pregnancy.

DOSE: 9–12 grams in decoction; it should be placed in a cheesecloth to
   separate it from the rest of the herbs.

RECIPES: For the pain of urinary stones, combine 12 grams of talcum
   with 9 grams each of polyporus, poria, plantain seed, and alisma and
   4 grams of cinnamon twigs. For summer heat patterns with damp-

ness, thirst that is not satisfied with drinking, vomiting, and diarrhea, combine 12 grams of talcum and 6 grams of licorice.

Alisma (ZE XIE)

Rhizoma alismatis orientalis

COMMON NAME: Alisma, water plantain rhizome
FAMILY: Alismataceae
PART USED: Rhizome
ENERGY AND FLAVOR: Cold; sweet
ORGAN MERIDIANS AFFECTED: Kidney, urinary bladder
PROPERTIES: Diuretic, antihypertensive, lowers blood sugar, antibacterial
INDICATIONS: This herb is used for edema, damp heat of the Lower Warmer, urinary dysfunction, and diarrhea. It is also useful when there is kidney yin deficiency.
CONTRAINDICATIONS: Alisma should not be used when there are excretions caused by kidney yang deficiency or damp cold conditions, such as seminal emission or vaginal discharge.
DOSE: 6–12 grams

Coix (YI YI REN)

Semen coicis lachryma-jobi

COMMON NAMES: Job's tears, coix
FAMILY: Gramineae
PART USED: Seed
ENERGY AND FLAVORS: Slightly cold; sweet, bland
ORGAN MERIDIANS AFFECTED: Spleen, stomach, kidney, lung, large intestine
PROPERTIES: Diuretic, antirheumatic, antispasmodic, anti-inflammatory, antidiarrheal
EFFECTS AND INDICATIONS: Drains dampness, clears heat, eliminates pus, tonifies the spleen. This herb is valued because it can be used as a therapeutic food in rice porridge as well as added to medicinal formulas to regulate fluid retention and counteract inflammation. It is very good for all conditions and diseases associated with edema and inflammation, including pus, diarrhea, phlegm, edema or abscesses of either the lungs or the intestines, and rheumatic and arthritic conditions.
CONTRAINDICATIONS: Coix should not be used by pregnant women.
DOSE: 9–30 grams

RECIPES: For edema, blood in the urine, diarrhea, or dysentery, combine 20 grams of coix, 9 grams of alisma, 9 grams of poria, and 9 grams of atractylodes. For rheumatic and arthritic conditions, combine 30 grams of coix and cinnamon-twig tea cooked with rice to make a porridge.

Dianthus (QU MAI)

Herba dianthi

COMMON NAMES: Dianthus, Chinese pink flower

FAMILY: Caryophyllaceae

PART USED: Whole plant

ENERGY AND FLAVOR: Cold; bitter

ORGAN MERIDIANS AFFECTED: Heart, small intestine, urinary bladder

PROPERTIES: Diuretic, antibacterial, antiparasitic, stimulates peristalsis, lowers blood pressure

EFFECTS AND INDICATIONS: Drains dampness, clears heat, promotes urination. It is indicated for genitourinary tract infections associated with damp heat, with painful and difficult urination, and possibly with blood. It can be used for damp heat associated with constipation or cessation of menses due to blood stagnation.

CONTRAINDICATIONS: Dianthus should not be used by pregnant women or by those with deficiency of kidney or spleen *qi*.

DOSE: 6–12 grams

RECIPES: For urinary tract infections, combine 9 grams each of dianthus, plantain seeds, polyporus, and poria, 6 grams of cinnamon twigs, and 20 grams of talcum. For amenorrhea, combine 9 grams each of dianthus, peach seed, safflower, and leonurus.

Plantain seed (CHE QIAN ZI)

Semen plantaginis

COMMON NAME: Plantain seed

FAMILY: Plantaginaceae

PART USED: Seed

ENERGY AND FLAVOR: Slightly cold; sweet

ORGAN MERIDIANS AFFECTED: Kidney, lung, liver, urinary bladder, small intestine

PROPERTIES: Diuretic, antitussive, anti-inflammatory, expectorant, antidiarrheal, lowers blood pressure

EFFECTS AND INDICATIONS: Drains dampness, clears heat, brightens the eyes, resolves phlegm. It is used for urinary tract infections; scanty, painful, and/or frequent urination; dysentery; yellow phlegm in the lungs; conjunctivitis; blurred vision; photophobia; and cataracts caused by liver yin deficiency.

CONTRAINDICATIONS: Plantain seed should not be used in pregnancy, constipation, or deficiency of *qi* or without signs of damp heat.

DOSE: 3–9 grams

RECIPES: For urinary tract infections, combine 9 grams each of plantain seeds, alisma, and gardenia fruit and 30 grams of talcum. For diarrhea and dysentery caused by damp heat, combine 9 grams each of plantain seeds, poria, alisma, and atractylodes. For eyesight problems, blurred vision, photophobia, and cataracts, combine 9 grams of plantain seeds, 12 grams of unprepared rehmannia, 9 grams of lycii berries, and 9 grams of chrysanthemum. For cough with yellow mucus caused by heat in the lungs, combine 9 grams each of plantain seeds, trichosanthes, bamboo shavings, scutellaria, and fritillaria.

Akebia (MU TONG)

Caulis akebia trifoliata, Akebia quinata, vine of *Aristolochia manchuriensis*

COMMON NAMES: Akebia, clematis stem

FAMILY: Ranunculaceae (clematis)

PART USED: Stem

ENERGY AND FLAVOR: Cold; bitter

ORGAN MERIDIANS AFFECTED: Heart, small intestine, urinary bladder

PROPERTIES: Diuretic, antibiotic, antitumor, anti-inflammatory, analgesic, galactagogue

EFFECTS AND INDICATIONS: Drains dampness, clears heat, promotes urination, promotes menstruation and lactation, controls sleep apnea, calms irritability, and treats insomnia. It can be used for acute urinary tract infections, edema, and amenorrhea; to alleviate rheumatic conditions; to calm the mind; and to promote sleep. It has recently been used for tumors of the breast and digestive tract.

CONTRAINDICATIONS: Akebia should not be used during pregnancy and should be used with caution in patients with yin deficiency.

DOSE: 3–9 grams

RECIPE: For frequent or painful urination, urinary tract infections, or mouth and tongue ulcerations, combine 6 grams of akebia, 9 grams of bamboo leaf, and 10 grams of unprepared rehmannia.

Cornsilk (YU MI XU)

Stylus zeae mays
COMMON NAME: Cornsilk
FAMILY: Gramineae
PART USED: Silk
ENERGY AND FLAVOR: Neutral; sweet, bland
ORGAN MERIDIANS AFFECTED: Liver, gallbladder, urinary bladder, small intestine
PROPERTIES: Diuretic, lithotriptic (dissolves kidney stones), cholagogue, antihypertensive
INDICATIONS: This herb is used to treat edema, urinary dysfunction, urinary tract stones, jaundice, and hypertension. It is very effective for kidney stones and is a mild but effective diuretic. It is traditionally used both in Western and Chinese herbalism.
CONTRAINDICATIONS: There are no contraindications noted for cornsilk.
DOSE: 15–30 grams

Capillaris (YIN CHEN HAO)

Herba artemisiae capillaris
COMMON NAMES: Capillaris, Oriental wormwood
FAMILY: Compositae
PART USED: Whole plant
ENERGY AND FLAVORS: Cool; bitter, acrid
ORGAN MERIDIANS AFFECTED: Spleen, liver, gallbladder, stomach, urinary bladder
PROPERTIES: Diuretic, cholagogue, antipyretic, antimicrobial, lowers both cholesterol and blood pressure
INDICATIONS: Clears damp heat in the Lower Warmer, especially that caused by liver and/or gallbladder imbalances, with symptoms of hepatitis, jaundice, and gallbladder problems.
CONTRAINDICATIONS: Capillaris should not be used when there is jaundice caused by *qi* deficiency with no signs of damp heat.
DOSE: 9–15 grams
PRESCRIPTION: Capillaris Combination (*Yin Chen Hao Tang*)—10 grams of capillaris, 6 grams of gardenia fruit, and 6 grams of rhubarb. *Indications:* Clears internal damp heat with symptoms of hepatitis, jaundice, gallbladder inflammation, and gallstone attack. *Pulse:* Deep and rapid or slippery and rapid. *Tongue:* A yellow greasy coat.

Herbs That Dispel Wind and Dampness: Antirheumatics

Herbs that dispel wind damp are used to treat conditions of pain and obstructed circulation (called "Bi" pains) affecting the skin, muscles, tendons, and channels (acupuncture meridians), the joints, and bones. Primarily, they are used for arthritic and rheumatic aches, spasms, and pains, which are described as wind damp in TCM. These conditions can include fixed or migrating pains, numbness, spasms of the tendons or joints, lower-back and knee pains, and flaccidity of the limbs.

The herbs are selected based on the nature and location of the pain. If the cause is complicated by exterior factors of heat, cold, or wind, then the herbs for wind and damp conditions are combined with herbs from the exterior relieving category, such as ephedra or cinnamon twigs. If there is concomitant stagnation of *qi* or blood, then herbs that regulate *qi* and blood are added to the formula, such as angelica *dang gui*. If the condition is aggravated by excessive cold, then warming stimulants, such as prepared aconite or cinnamon bark, are added. If there is heat and inflammation as a result of prolonged stagnation, then anti-inflammatory herbs, such as honeysuckle stem, are used. Finally, for conditions of *qi*, blood, yin, or yang deficiency, appropriate tonics must be added.

Many of the herbs in this category are spicy, warm, and drying, and care should be taken when giving these to individuals with blood or yin deficiency.

Angelica *du huo* (DU HUO)

Radix angelicae pubescentis

COMMON NAME: Pubescent angelica

FAMILY: Umbelliferae

PART USED: Root

ENERGY AND FLAVORS: Warm; acrid, bitter

ORGAN MERIDIANS AFFECTED: Kidney, urinary bladder

PROPERTIES: Antibiotic, analgesic, sedative, antirheumatic, anti-inflammatory, antihypertensive

INDICATIONS: This is one of the best herbs for arthralgia symptoms caused by wind, cold, and dampness. It is especially useful for rheumatic pains of the lower body and for patients whose mobility is impaired as a result of pains in the waist, legs, and feet. It can also be used for external diseases caused by wind and internal dampness with symptoms of headaches, aching joints, and slight aversion to cold.

CONTRAINDICATIONS: Angelica *du huo* should not be used when there is yin deficiency, especially when there is heat.

DOSE: 3–9 grams

Stephania (FANG JI)

Radix stephaniae tetrandrae

COMMON NAME: Stephania root

FAMILY: Menispermaceae

PART USED: Root

ENERGY AND FLAVORS: Cold; acrid, bitter

ORGAN MERIDIANS AFFECTED: Spleen, kidney, lung, urinary bladder

PROPERTIES: Diuretic, analgesic, antipyretic, anti-inflammatory, antitumor, antibacterial, antihypertensive

INDICATIONS: This herb is used for arthritic and rheumatic conditions caused by wind, damp, and coldness; it can also be used for heat, depending on the other herbs with which it is combined. Its next most important uses are for generalized edema, ascites, lymphedema, and deficient mother's milk.

CONTRAINDICATIONS: Stephania should not be used by those with chronic dampness or those with yin deficiency.

DOSE: 3–9 grams

Large-leafed gentiana (QIN JIAO)

Radix gentianae qinjiao

COMMON NAME: Large-leafed gentian root

FAMILY: Gentianaceae

PART USED: Root

ENERGY AND FLAVOR: Cool; acrid, bitter

ORGAN MERIDIANS AFFECTED: Liver, gallbladder, stomach

PROPERTIES: Anti-inflammatory, antibiotic, antipyretic

INDICATIONS: This is an important herb for wind-damp-heat conditions associated with arthritic and rheumatic conditions that exhibit pain, swelling, and redness. It is also effective for muscular spasms. The second important use is for asthenic fever associated with wasting, such as infantile malnutrition, tuberculosis (TB) and acquired immunodeficiency syndrome (AIDS). For these conditions, it is combined with anemarrhena and lycii root bark. The third most important uses are as a diuretic and as a laxative. It is effective for relieving jaundice and dysuria.

DOSE: 3–9 grams

Acanthopanax (WU JIA PI)

Cortex acanthopanacis gracilistyliradicis

COMMON NAME: acanthopanax root bark

FAMILY: Araliaceae

PART USED: Root bark

ENERGY AND FLAVOR: Warm; acrid

ORGAN MERIDIANS AFFECTED: Liver, kidney

PROPERTIES: Antirheumatic, diuretic, circulatory stimulant

EFFECTS AND INDICATIONS: Promotes the circulation of *qi* and blood and will relieve fluid stagnation. This herb therefore can be especially helpful for the elderly and for underdeveloped or slow-to-develop children. It is effective for chronic rheumatic and arthritic conditions caused by cold, wind, and dampness and for weakness of the bones and sinews.

CONTRAINDICATIONS: This herb should not be used when there is yin deficiency with heat signs.

DOSE: 3–12 grams

RECIPE: Soak 30 grams of the herb in a ½ quart of strong spirits, such as vodka or gin. Take a teaspoon 3 times daily.

NOTE: This herb is very closely related to Siberian ginseng (*Eleutherococcus senticosus*) and probably shares many of its antistress attributes.

Mulberry twig (SANG ZHI)

Mori albae, Ramulus

COMMON NAME: Mulberry twig

FAMILY: Moraceae

PART USED: Twig

ENERGY AND FLAVOR: Neutral; bitter

ORGAN MERIDIAN AFFECTED: Liver

PROPERTIES: Antirheumatic, diuretic, antispasmodic

INDICATIONS: The twigs of the white mulberry tree are used to promote circulation, dispel dampness, relieve wind and spasms, and treat arthritic and rheumatic pains of the extremities. The herb has also been used for high blood pressure and edema.

CONTRAINDICATIONS: No contraindications for mulberry twig have been noted.

DOSE: 9–15 grams

Clematis root (WEI LING XIAN)
Radix clematidis chinensis
COMMON NAME: Clematis root
FAMILY: Ranunculaceae
PART USED: Root
ENERGY AND FLAVORS: Warm; acrid, salty
ORGAN MERIDIAN AFFECTED: Urinary bladder
PROPERTIES: Antirheumatic, analgesic, antidiuretic, antibacterial, lowers blood sugar
EFFECTS AND INDICATIONS: Relieves rheumatic aches and pains, numbness, and motor impairment; opens the circulation of *qi* through the channels and acupuncture meridians. Its properties make it specific for helping to remove fish bones stuck in the throat.
CONTRAINDICATIONS: Clematis root should not be used by those with deficiency of either *qi* or blood.
DOSE: 3–12 grams

Chinese quince (MU GUA)
Fructus chaenomelis speciosa
COMMON NAMES: Chinese quince, chaenomeles fruit
FAMILY: Rosaceae
PART USED: Fruit
ENERGY AND FLAVOR: Warm; sour
ORGAN MERIDIANS AFFECTED: Liver, spleen
PROPERTIES: Antirheumatic, anti-inflammatory, antispasmodic, digestive, antiemetic
EFFECTS AND INDICATIONS: Promotes circulation, moves blood and *qi*, relaxes the muscles and tendons, dispels dampness, harmonizes the stomach. It is used for arthritic and rheumatic conditions, especially of the legs, and to relieve food stagnation in the stomach.
CONTRAINDICATIONS: Chinese quince should not be used by those with a yin deficiency. It should also be avoided in exterior conditions.
DOSE: 3–9 grams

Xanthium (CANG ER ZI)
Fructus xanthii sibirici
COMMON NAMES: Xanthium, cocklebur fruit

FAMILY: Compositae
ENERGIES AND FLAVORS: Warm, slightly toxic; sweet, bitter, pungent
ORGAN MERIDIAN AFFECTED: Lung
PROPERTIES: Decongestant, antirheumatic, analgesic, antifungal
INDICATIONS: One of the most important herbs for sinus congestion, chronic nasal discharge, respiratory allergies, and loss of smell. It is also used to relieve aches and pains caused by wind-damp-cold conditions.
CONTRAINDICATIONS: Xanthium should not be used by those with blood deficiency (anemia). **Caution:** Overdose can result in vomiting, abdominal pain, and diarrhea.
DOSE: 3–9 grams

Herbs That Transform Phlegm and Stop Cough

Herbs that transform phlegm and stop cough are used for conditions with cough and asthma and conditions related to phlegm accumulation, such as swollen glands (scrofula), goiter, epilepsy, convulsions, and yin carbuncles (the type that swell up and lack the strength to properly discharge).

Herbs are selected and formulated according to the underlying cause and symptomology. If there are symptoms of heat, cold, or deficiency, herbs that clear heat, warm coldness, and tonify *qi,* blood, yin, or yang are added accordingly. If there are symptoms of epilepsy or convulsions as a result of internal liver wind, then herbs that subdue and extinguish liver wind as well as herbs that calm the spirit are added. For yin carbuncles, herbs that warm and eliminate stagnation are added. Finally, for hard swellings, such as goiter and scrofula, herbs that soften hardness are added.

The herbs and substances in this category are subdivided into cool items that transform hot phlegm and warm herbs that transform cold Phlegm.

COOL HERBS AND SUBSTANCES THAT TRANSFORM HOT PHLEGM

Fritillaria (*CHUAN BEI MU*)
Bulbus fritillariae cirrhosae
COMMON NAME: Fritillaria

FAMILY: Liliaceae

PART USED: Bulb

ENERGY AND FLAVORS: Slightly cold; sweet, bitter

ORGAN MERIDIANS AFFECTED: Heart, lung

PROPERTIES: Expectorant, antitussive, demulcent, alternative

EFFECTS AND INDICATIONS: Clears phlegm heat; good for many kinds of coughs, especially chronic cough and those caused by yin deficiency, in which there may be difficulty expectorating or unproductive coughs with patterns of constrained *qi*. This herb can be used internally and externally for swollen glands and other nodular swellings and abscesses in the lungs or breasts.

CONTRAINDICATIONS: Fritillaria is ineffective for coughs caused by cold dampness. The raw unprocessed herb is toxic and should not be taken internally.

DOSE: 3–9 grams; 1–2 grams when taken as a powder.

NOTE: There are two varieties of Fritillaria. *Chuan bei mu* has more lung-nourishing properties, while another variety, called *zhe bei mu,* clears heat from the lungs more effectively.

Trichosanthes fruit (*GUA LOU*)

Fructus trichosanthes

COMMON NAME: Trichosanthes fruit

FAMILY: Cucurbitaceae

PARTS USED: Various parts of this herb are used for different purposes. The fruit and seed are very similar, except the seed has more strength for lubricating the intestines, transforming phlegm, and dissolving nodules. The peel of the fruit is more effective in treating the stomach and aiding the circulation of *qi*.

ENERGY AND FLAVOR: Cold; sweet

ORGAN MERIDIANS AFFECTED: Lung, stomach, large intestine

PROPERTIES: Expectorant, anti-inflammatory, demulcent, antibiotic, anticancer

EFFECTS AND INDICATIONS: Helps circulate the lung *qi* for tight or painful chest obstruction, promotes bowel movement by relaxing and lubricating the intestines. For hot, difficult-to-expectorate phlegm, possibly accompanied with a stifling sensation in the chest (Stagnant lung *qi*). It is also used for swollen glands, boils and carbuncles, and lung and breast abscesses. More recently, it has been successfully used for high blood lipid levels and hypertension.

CONTRAINDICATIONS: Trichosanthes fruit should not be used by those with coldness and dampness, especially when there is spleen deficiency.

DOSE: 6–18 grams

Trichosanthes seed (GUA LOU REN)

Semen trichosanthes kirilowii

COMMON NAME: Trichosanthes seed

FAMILY: Cucurbitaceae

PART USED: Seed

ENERGY AND FLAVOR: Cold; sweet

ORGAN MERIDIANS AFFECTED: Lung, stomach, large intestine

PROPERTIES: Expectorant, emollient, mild laxative

INDICATIONS: This herb can be used similarly to *gua lou,* except it is more useful for dry stool or mild constipation with the ailments for which *gua lou* is used. It can also be used either internally or externally to help wounds heal.

CONTRAINDICATIONS: Trichosanthes seed should not be used when there is diarrhea or when there is no heat.

DOSE: 9–15 grams

Trichosanthes root (TIAN HUA FEN)

Radix trichosanthes kirilowii

COMMON NAME: Trichosanthes root

FAMILY: Cucurbitaceae

PART USED: Roots

ENERGY AND FLAVOR: Cold; bitter, slightly sweet, sour

ORGAN MERIDIANS AFFECTED: Lung, stomach

PROPERTIES: Anti-inflammatory

INDICATIONS: This herb is used for lung heat conditions when there is both phlegm and dryness. It helps generate fluids evaporated from heat conditions, and aids expectoration. It is helpful for toxicity manifested by inflammation, pus, sores, carbuncles, and especially breast abscesses. It can be used either externally or internally as needed.

CONTRAINDICATIONS: Trichosanthes root should not be used by pregnant women, those without heat, or those with diarrhea.

DOSE: 9–15 grams

Dried bamboo sap (ZHU LI)

Succus bambusae

COMMON NAME: Dried bamboo sap

FAMILY: Gramineae

ENERGY AND FLAVOR: Very cold; sweet

ORGAN MERIDIANS AFFECTED: Heart, lung, stomach

PROPERTIES: Expectorant, antipyretic

INDICATIONS: This herb is very cold and is therefore used for upper-respiratory infections where there is heat, which includes symptoms of yellow phlegm. It is very effective for cough with yellow phlegm that is difficult to expectorate. It is also used for mental imbalances described as invisible phlegm obstructing the heart.

CONTRAINDICATIONS: Dried bamboo sap should not be used for coughs that are associated with cold or by those with spleen deficiency with symptoms such as diarrhea.

DOSAGE: 30–60 grams; 9–15 grams for coughs. The herb is often taken with ginger juice to help offset its extreme coldness.

Bamboo shavings (ZHU RU)

Caulis bambusae in taeniis

COMMON NAME: Bamboo shavings

FAMILY: Gramineae

PART USED: Shavings of the stem

ENERGY AND FLAVOR: Slightly cold; sweet

ORGAN MERIDIANS AFFECTED: Stomach, gallbladder, and lung

PROPERTIES: Expectorant, antipyretic, antiemetic, hemostatic

INDICATIONS: This herb is used for thick, yellow, hard-to-expectorate phlegm when there is respiratory infection. A second use is for vomiting caused by heat in the stomach, for which it can be combined with pinellia and coptis. It can also be used for morning sickness and a restless fetus when combined with scutellaria and pinellia. A third use is to cool blood heat for various symptoms of bleeding, such as hemoptysis (spitting up of blood and phlegm), hematemesis (vomiting blood), epistaxis (bloody nose), and metrorrhagia (menstrual flooding).

CONTRAINDICATIONS: Bamboo shavings should not be used in cases of spleen deficiency or cough caused by cold.

DOSE: 4.5–9 grams

Pumice (FU HAI SHI)

COMMON NAME: Pumice

ENERGY AND FLAVOR: Cold; salty

ORGAN MERIDIAN AFFECTED: Lung

PROPERTIES: Expectorant, antipyretic, diuretic

INDICATIONS: This herb is used when there is heat present with yellow, difficult-to-expectorate phlegm. It is used to soften hard lymph glands and nodules caused by stagnant phlegm heat. It is also used for urinary stones and infections.

CONTRAINDICATIONS: Pumice should not be used for a cough caused by cold and weakness.

DOSE: 6–15 grams

Sargassum (HAI ZAO)

Herba sargassii

COMMON NAME: Sargassum, seaweed

FAMILY: Sargassum

PART USED: Whole plant

ENERGY AND FLAVOR: Cold; bitter, salty

ORGAN MERIDIANS AFFECTED: Lung, kidney, liver, spleen, stomach

PROPERTIES: Expectorant, diuretic, regulates the thyroid, antifungal, antiparasitic, antihypertensive, lowers cholesterol levels

INDICATIONS: Although an expectorant, this herb is mostly used to reduce swollen lymph glands, various lumps, and nodules, especially in the neck, associated with goiter, scrofula, or tuberculosis. It is also used in formulas for fluid retention. Traditionally, it has been used for hernia pain and pain in the testes.

CONTRAINDICATIONS: Sargassum should not be used by those with coldness due to spleen and stomach deficiency.

DOSE: 6–15 grams

WARM HERBS THAT TRANSFORM COLD PHLEGM

Pinellia (BAN XIA)

Rhizoma pinelliae ternatae

COMMON NAME: Pinellia

FAMILY: Araceae

PART USED: Rhizome

ENERGIES AND FLAVOR: Warm, toxic; acrid

ORGAN MERIDIANS AFFECTED: Lung, spleen, stomach

PROPERTIES: Antitussive, expectorant, antiemetic, antitoxin, anodyne

EFFECTS AND INDICATIONS: Draws out cold and damp, directs *qi* downward. It is the most important herb for cold phlegm and dampness, especially when the root of the problem is a cold, damp spleen. Its ability to direct *qi* downward makes it useful for cough, phlegm, nausea, and vomiting; for this, it is commonly combined with citrus peel and ginger. It is also used for swollen glands, nodules, and goiter caused by stagnation of cold phlegm.

CONTRAINDICATIONS: Pinellia should not be used by pregnant women or those with any blood disorders, especially bleeding. It should be used with caution by those with heat conditions. Ancient texts describe pinellia as incompatible with aconite.

DOSE: 5–12 grams

Inula flower (XUAN FU HUA)

Flos inula japonica

COMMON NAME: Inula flower, elecampane flower

FAMILY: Compositae

PART USED: Flower

ENERGY AND FLAVOR: Warm; acrid, bitter

ORGAN MERIDIANS AFFECTED: Lung, spleen, stomach, liver, large intestine

PROPERTIES: Expectorant, antinausea

INDICATIONS: This herb is used for stagnant phlegm conditions where the spleen and stomach are deficient, causing rebellious movement of fluids manifesting as coughing and wheezing. It is also used for vomiting and hiccups due to spleen deficiency.

CONTRAINDICATIONS: Inula flower should be avoided by those with tuberculosis or cough due to wind heat.

DOSE: 3–9 grams

Arisaema rhizome (TIAN NAN XING)

Rhizoma arisaema consanguineum

COMMON NAMES: Jack-in-the-pulpit, arisaema rhizome

FAMILY: Araceae

PART USED: Rhizome

ENERGIES AND FLAVORS: Warm, toxic; bitter, acrid

ORGAN MERIDIANS AFFECTED: Lung, liver, spleen

PROPERTIES: Expectorant, analgesic, anticonvulsive, sedative, antitumor

INDICATIONS: This herb is used for cold, stubborn phlegm with a full distended feeling in the chest and difficult expectoration. It is also used for wind conditions that cause convulsions, paralysis, spasms, stroke, dizziness, or epilepsy. It has been used with success in some kinds of cancers and can be used externally for suppurating sores and abscesses. When used externally, the unprepared root is indicated; otherwise it is used in its prepared form or with fresh ginger to counteract its toxic properties.

CONTRAINDICATIONS: Arisaema rhizome should not be used during pregnancy or by those with yin-deficient cough with dry phlegm.

DOSE: 4–9 grams

Platycodon (JIE GENG)
Radix platycodi grandiflori

COMMON NAME: Platycodon, Balloon Flower Root
FAMILY: Campanulaceae
PART USED: Root
ENERGY AND FLAVOR: Neutral; acrid, bitter
ORGAN MERIDIAN AFFECTED: Lung
PROPERTIES: Expectorant, demulcent, anti-inflammatory
INDICATIONS: This herb can be used for both hot and cold phlegm. It assists the lung *qi* to expectorate phlegm and stop cough. It is also used for pulmonary abscesses, throat inflammations, and loss of voice. It also eliminates pus, reducing inflammation and promoting healing. Finally, this is one of the herbs with a rising *qi*, meaning that it is used in formulas to direct the activity of other herbs to the upper part of the body. It can be used to quell cough, clear phlegm, and treat the common cold, influenza, bronchitis, and pulmonary tuberculosis.

CONTRAINDICATIONS: Because of its ascending energy, platycodon is generally contraindicated for hemoptysis (blood in the sputum).

DOSE: 3–9 grams

HERBS THAT RELIEVE COUGH AND WHEEZING

Herbs that relieve cough and wheezing have properties similar to those of the previous category but they more specifically lessen the cough reflex, ease breathing, and treat emphysema and asthma.

Apricot seed (XING REN)
Semen pruni armeniaceae

COMMON NAME: Apricot seed

FAMILY: Rosaceae

PART USED: Seed

ENERGIES AND FLAVOR: Slightly warm, slightly toxic; bitter

ORGAN MERIDIANS AFFECTED: Lung, large intestine

PROPERTIES: Antitussive, antiasthmatic, demulcent

INDICATIONS: Apricot seed is one of the finest herbs for acute cough and bronchitis. It can be used for either hot or cold conditions when combined with the appropriate herbs and is especially good for dry coughs because of its moistening nature. It has a secondary action of moistening the intestines; therefore, it is good to use when there is constipation associated with the aforementioned conditions.

CONTRAINDICATIONS: Apricot seed herb should be used with caution for diarrhea caused by yin deficiency.

DOSE: 3–9 grams

Coltsfoot flower (KUAN DONG HUA)

Flos tussilago farfara

COMMON NAME: Coltsfoot flower

FAMILY: Compositae

PART USED: Flower

ENERGY AND FLAVOR: Warm; acrid

ORGAN MERIDIAN AFFECTED: Lung

PROPERTIES: Antitussive, expectorant, antiasthmatic

INDICATIONS: In small doses, coltsfoot flower dilates the bronchial passages and can be used for asthmatic and other chronic upper-respiratory conditions that are of a cold nature.

CONTRAINDICATIONS: Coltsfoot flower should not be used for conditions that are of a hot nature.

DOSE: 3–9 grams

NOTES: Coltsfoot is a common herb used throughout history for coughs and wheezing. It is the Chinese, however, who primarily emphasize the use of the flowers for this purpose. Interestingly, while the leaves used in the West are primarily used as an anti-inflammatory, the flowers are mostly used by the Chinese for coughs that are due to cold.

Loquat leaf (PI PA YE)

Folium eriobotryae japonicae

COMMON NAME: Loquat leaf

FAMILY: Rosaceae

ENERGY AND FLAVOR: Cool; bitter

ORGAN MERIDIANS AFFECTED: Lung, stomach

PROPERTIES: Antitussive, expectorant, antiemetic

EFFECTS AND INDICATIONS: Directs the *qi* of the lung and stomach downward so as to alleviate coughing, nausea, and belching; dissolves phlegm. The expectorant properties of loquat leaf makes it useful for eliminating phlegm that causes lung heat coughs. It is most effective when the condition is one of phlegm and heat, as it dissolves phlegm and is an expectorant.

CONTRAINDICATIONS: Loquat leaf should not be used for cough caused by cold.

DOSE: 6–15 grams

Perilla seed (ZI SU ZI)

Fructus perillae frutescentis

COMMON NAME: Perilla seed

FAMILY: Labiatae

PART USED: Seed

ENERGY AND FLAVOR: Warm; acrid

ORGAN MERIDIANS AFFECTED: Lung, large intestine

PROPERTIES: Antitussive, expectorant, emollient, antiasthmatic, mild laxative

INDICATIONS: Perilla seed is used for cold phlegm conditions associated with copious phlegm and wheezing. It is most useful when there is a stuffy feeling in the chest causing a more labored exhalation rather than inhalation. Perilla seed is also useful when there is constipation due to dryness in the intestines.

CONTRAINDICATIONS: Perilla seed should not be used when there is diarrhea or cough due to weakness and deficiency.

DOSE: 3–9 grams

Stemona root (BAI BU)

Radix stemonae

COMMON NAME: Stemona root

FAMILY: Stemonaceae

ENERGY AND FLAVORS: Slightly warm; sweet, bitter, acrid

ORGAN MERIDIAN AFFECTED: Lung

PROPERTIES: Demulcent, antitussive, antifungal, antiparasitic

INDICATIONS: Because of its lubricating and nutritive properties, stemona root is useful for acute or chronic coughs, especially those caused by yin deficiency. This herb can also be employed to expel parasites.

CONTRAINDICATIONS: Stemona root should not be used when there is spleen and stomach deficiency with diarrhea.

DOSE: 3–9 grams

Aristolochia fruit (MA DOU LING)

Fructus aristolochiae

COMMON NAME: Aristolochia fruit, birthwort fruit

FAMILY: Aristolochiaceae

PART USED: Fruit

ENERGY AND FLAVORS: Cold; bitter, slightly acrid

ORGAN MERIDIANS AFFECTED: Lung, large intestine

PROPERTIES: Expectorant, antitussive, anti-inflammatory, antibacterial, antifungal

INDICATIONS: This herb is useful when there is lung heat and inflammation, with or without deficiency, but with the presence of phlegm. For these conditions, it stops coughing and wheezing. It is also used internally to treat bleeding hemorrhoids.

CONTRAINDICATIONS: Aristolochia fruit should not be used in cases of spleen deficiency with diarrhea or conditions of cold and deficiency with cough and wheezing.

DOSE: 3–9 grams

Aromatic Herbs that Transform Dampness

The aromatic herbs that transform dampness are warm, dry, mostly spicy, and pungent. They help circulate *qi*, relieve dampness, and strengthen the spleen and stomach, thereby benefiting digestion. The primary indication of dampness in this category is a sense of fullness and congestion in the epigastric and abdominal areas. As a result, there may also be symptoms of poor appetite, nausea, vomiting, acid regurgitation, lassitude, diarrhea, a cloyingly sweet taste in the mouth, and a greasy tongue coat. These herbs can also be used to treat summer heat and damp heat conditions.

Aromatic herbs can be combined with herbs from other categories as appropriate. For damp heat, aromatic herbs are combined with herbs that clear heat and dry dampness. If there is damp cold, they can also be used in combination with herbs that warm the interior. Dampness is a by-product of digestive weakness with spleen and stomach deficiency, so herbs in this category are often combined with herbs that tonify spleen *qi*. In general, because of their warm, drying nature, they should be used with caution for conditions of yin deficiency.

Agastache (*HUO XIANG*)

Herba agastaches seu pogostemi
COMMON NAME: Agastache, patchouli, pogostemon, wrinkled giant hyssop
FAMILY: Labiatae
PART USED: Whole plant
ENERGY AND FLAVOR: Slightly warm; acrid
ORGAN MERIDIANS AFFECTED: Lung, spleen, stomach
PROPERTIES: Stomachic, diaphoretic
INDICATIONS: Agastache has a multitude of uses, the most important being to relieve internal dampness, aid digestion, and relieve nausea. When internal dampness obstructs the spleen, it loses its ability to transform fluids, resulting in digestive disorders, including nausea, abdominal distension, and vomiting. In many cases, this makes it also appropriate for the treatment of morning sickness. Additionally, it can be used for externally contracted diseases, such as the common cold and influenza. Specifically, agastache alone or taken in formula is good for diseases associated with so-called summer heat, characterized by internal dampness, nausea, thirst with no satisfaction by drinking, and summer colds. I have found that the common Western herb sweet basil has similar characteristics and can be used in tea for similar imbalances.
CONTRAINDICATIONS: Agastache should not be used for conditions of yin deficiency or heat.
DOSE: 3–9 grams

Magnolia bark (*HOU PO*)

Cortex magnolia officinalis
COMMON NAME: Magnolia bark
FAMILY: Magnoliaceae
ENERGY AND FLAVORS: Warm; acrid, bitter, aromatic
ORGAN MERIDIANS AFFECTED: Spleen, lung, stomach, large intestine
PROPERTIES: Digestant, carminative
EFFECTS AND INDICATIONS: Regulates stomach *qi*, relieves food stagnation,

dries the dampness that impairs digestion and assimilation (spleen *qi*). As such, it is generally good to use for a stifling chest sensation, abdominal and chest fullness, bloating, gas, and nausea, as well as upward-rising *qi* of the lungs with symptoms of wheezing, phlegm, and asthma.

CONTRAINDICATIONS: Magnolia bark should not be used by pregnant women or by those with stomach or spleen deficiency.

DOSE: 3–9 grams

Black atractylodes (*CANG ZHU*)

Rhizoma atractylodes lancea

COMMON NAME: Black atractylodes

FAMILY: Compositae

PART USED: Rhizome

ENERGY AND FLAVORS: Warm; aromatic, bitter, acrid

ORGAN MERIDIANS AFFECTED: Spleen, stomach

PROPERTIES: Carminative, diuretic, antispasmodic

INDICATIONS: This herb's strong drying properties help relieve spleen dampness and congestion of the stomach and spleen; therefore, it promotes gastric circulation, improving appetite and relieving abdominal fullness, bloating, nausea, and vomiting. Its second major property is to counter cold-damp-wind symptoms associated with arthritic and rheumatic conditions, such as aching soreness of the joints. Depending on the other herbs with which it is combined, it can be used for either wind-cold-dampness or wind-damp-heat conditions. It also has diaphoretic properties and can be used for external disorders, such as initial stages of colds, headaches, lack of sweating, and suppurating sores and ulcers. Finally, this herb seems to improve night vision and a sensation of sand in the eyes.

CONTRAINDICATIONS: As for many herbs that promote sweating and are drying, there is a tendency that inappropriate use or overuse of black atractylodes can exhaust the *qi* and blood. This herb therefore should not be used by those with *qi* deficiency or yin deficiency with heat signs.

DOSE: 3–9 grams

Cardamom (*SHA REN*)

Fructus amomi

COMMON NAME: Cardamon, amomi

FAMILY: Zingiberaceae
PART USED: Fruit
ENERGIES AND FLAVOR: Warm, aromatic; acrid
ORGAN MERIDIANS AFFECTED: Spleen, stomach
PROPERTIES: Carminative, stomachic, expectorant, tonic
EFFECTS AND INDICATIONS: Transforms dampness, counteracts nausea and
  vomiting, relieves abdominal fullness and diarrhea; calms a restless
  fetus, helps prevent miscarriage, relieves morning sickness. It is used
  as a carminative to relieve stomach stagnation and aid digestion. It is
  commonly added to tonic formulas to prevent stagnation.
CONTRAINDICATIONS: Cardamom should not be used by those with yin
  deficiency when there are heat signs.
DOSE: 2–6 grams

Herbs That Relieve Food Stagnation

Herbs that relieve food stagnation are used to promote digestion.
They are indicated for symptoms of abnormal distension, belching, acid
regurgitation, nausea, vomiting, or abnormal bowel movement as a result of spleen and stomach deficiency. These can be used alone, such as
medicated leaven, but they are often combined with herbs that warm
the spleen and stomach if there is coldness or with bitter herbs that
clear heat if heat is present. The symptoms are very similar to those
described under Aromatic Herbs That Transform Dampness (pages
209–12), but in this category, it is food stagnation rather than dampness
that is at issue. It is very possible, however, to have both conditions
simultaneously, so it is not uncommon to have herbs from both categories, as well as *qi* regulators and *qi* tonics, in the same formula. In this
group, hawthorn berries are specific for aiding the digestion of fats and
protein, while barley sprouts and chicken gizzards relieve stagnation of
carbohydrates and grains.

Hawthorn berry (SHAN ZHA)

Fructus crataegi
COMMON NAMES: hawthorn berry, crataegus
FAMILY: Rosaceae
PART USED: Berry (fruit)
ENERGY AND FLAVORS: Slightly warm; sour, sweet
ORGAN MERIDIANS AFFECTED: Liver, spleen, stomach

PROPERTIES: Relieves food congestion, counteracts fatty foods, promotes circulation, regulates blood pressure, lowers cholesterol

INDICATIONS: Chinese food therapy teaches that sour taste counteracts oils and fat. For this purpose, vinegar and lemon are often used. Hawthorn, with its sour flavor, is specifically used to help digest animal protein and greasy, fatty foods. It also promotes blood circulation. These two attributes make it very appropriate as a heart tonic for the treatment of certain types of hypertension, arteriosclerosis, and high cholesterol and blood lipid levels. Burned and charred, the powder (1 teaspoon) can be taken with warm water to treat diarrhea and dysentery. Finally, hawthorn is useful for relieving hernial pain.

CONTRAINDICATIONS: Hawthorn berry should be avoided by those with spleen and stomach deficiency or acid stomach.

DOSE: 9–15 grams

Barley sprouts (MAI YA)

Fructus hordei vulgaris germinatus

COMMON NAMES: Barley sprouts, germinated barley, malt

FAMILY: Gramineae

PART USED: Sprout

ENERGY AND FLAVOR: Neutral; sweet

ORGAN MERIDIANS AFFECTED: Liver, spleen, stomach

PROPERTIES: Carminative (when raw), galactagogue, increases appetite and digestive (when stir-baked)

INDICATIONS: Barley sprouts, fresh or dry, are specifically useful for stagnation of starchy foods, such as bread and cereal, when the accumulation of foods has caused dyspepsia and other abdominal symptoms. For infants who have problems digesting milk, a tea of barley sprouts can be mixed with the milk. They can also be used for women who wish to reduce or stop the flow of breast milk or to relieve engorgement. They are also used for stagnation of *qi* with abdominal swelling, gas, and loss of appetite. To make barley sprouts, soak barley seeds for a day, then place it in an open jar with a cloth over the top. Once or twice a day, rinse the sprouts with water and immediately strain them. When the seeds develop small "tails," they are ready to use. They may be dried for storage.

CONTRAINDICATIONS: Barley sprouts should not be used by nursing mothers who don't want to decrease milk flow or by those without food stagnation.

DOSE: 9–15 grams; a dose of up to 60 grams can be used to stop lactation

Rice sprouts (GU YA)

Fructus oryzae sativae germinatus
COMMON NAME: Rice sprouts, germinated rice
FAMILY: Graminae
PART USED: Fruit
ENERGY AND FLAVOR: Neutral; sweet
ORGAN MERIDIANS AFFECTED: Spleen, stomach
PROPERTIES: Digestive
EFFECTS AND INDICATIONS: Sprouted rice has properties similar to those of sprouted barley except that it is milder. Dry-fried, it is more strengthening to the spleen, while in its unprepared form, it is stronger in relieving food stagnation. Because these sprouted grains depend a lot on their enzyme activity, the most effective way is to grind the dried sprout to a fine powder and simply take as a pill or powder mixed with water.
CONTRAINDICATIONS: Sprouted rice should not be used by nursing mothers, because it can reduce milk flow, or by those without symptoms of food stagnation.
DOSE: 9–15 grams

Medicated leaven (SHEN QU)

Massa fermentata
COMMON NAME: Medicated leaven
ENERGY AND FLAVORS: Warm; sweet, acrid
ORGAN MERIDIANS AFFECTED: Spleen, stomach
PROPERTIES: Digestive, appetite stimulant
INDICATIONS: *Shen qu* is composed of a group of herbs, including artemisia annua, xanthium, polygonum hydropiper, and other herbs that are mixed with a fermented mixture of wheat flour and bran. This is sometimes called "Chinese yogurt" because its intention is to supplement favorable bacteria and enzymes for the digestive tract. It is used for a variety of digestive problems, including stomach distension, poor appetite, and stagnation of food.
CONTRAINDICATIONS: Medicated leaven should not be used by pregnant women or by those with stomach fire.
DOSE: 9–15 grams

Radish seed (LAI FU ZI)

Semen raphani sativi

COMMON NAME: Radish seed

FAMILY: Cruciferae

ENERGY AND FLAVORS: Neutral; acrid, sweet

ORGAN MERIDIAN AFFECTED: Spleen, stomach, lung

PROPERTIES: Digestive, carminative, expectorant

EFFECTS AND INDICATIONS: Radish seed reduces food stagnation and helps the qi to descend to treat symptoms of belching, regurgitation, and abdominal distension and pain. It is also used for chronic cough to help dissolve phlegm and redirect lung qi downward for such conditions as chronic bronchitis and other upper-respiratory conditions.

CONTRAINDICATIONS: Radish seed should not be used by those who are weak and have deficient qi.

DOSE: 6–12 grams

Chicken gizzard (JI NEI JIN)

FAMILY: Phasianidae

PART USED: The lining of the chicken gizzard

ENERGY AND FLAVOR: Neutral; sweet

ORGAN MERIDIANS AFFECTED: Small intestine, bladder, spleen, stomach

EFFECTS AND INDICATIONS: Strongly unblocks food stagnation, dissolves stones in either the biliary or urinary tract. For all kinds of food stagnation, this substance improves the spleen's transportive function. It is also used for frequent and nighttime urination and bed-wetting, gallstones and urinary stones, and for childhood malnutrition.

CONTRAINDICATIONS: No contraindications are noted for chicken gizzard.

DOSE: 1.5–3 grams 2 or 3 times daily, taken as a powder (considered more effective than a decoction)

NOTES: Combine chicken gizzard with any of the herbs in this category for food stagnation. If there is accompanying spleen qi deficiency with diarrhea, add atractylodes (bai zhu), codonopsis (dang shen), and dioscorea (shan yao). For childhood malnutrition, combine with atractylodes (bai zhu), codonopsis (dang shen), poria (fu ling), and dioscorea (shan yao). For biliary and urinary tract stones, combine with lysimachia (jin qian cao).

HERBS THAT REGULATE *QI*

Qi stagnation is generally manifested with feelings of stagnation and pain, belching, nausea, vomiting, cough, and asthma. The herbs that regulate *qi* are aromatic, pungent, and bitter.

Qi stagnation is one of the five stagnations, the others being blood, cold, food, and phlegm stagnations. *Qi* stagnation especially relates to conditions associated with the stomach, liver, and, to a lesser extent, the lungs. Stagnation of the stomach calls for herbal carminatives with a spicy flavor that promote the circulation of *qi* in the stomach.

Because the liver is responsible for the smooth flow of *qi*, stagnant liver *qi* can indicate an impairment of the liver's ability to store and release glycogen to help maintain a steady level of energy and the transformation of stress hormones. Stagnant liver *qi* is also associated with various psychological symptoms, such as depression and severe mood swings. Since these can be hormonally influenced, stagnant liver *qi* is one of the causes of PMS, menopausal symptoms, the development of breast and lower-pelvis fibroid cysts and swellings, as well as symptoms of inappropriate or inordinate anger, irritability, and hypertension.

When stagnant liver *qi* symptoms coexist with digestive disorders, they give rise to a variety of food-related disorders, such as food allergies. These are described as liver and stomach *qi* stagnation or liver attacking the spleen. Because of their drying, spicy, and bitter flavors, which are dispersing by nature, *qi*-regulating herbs are contraindicated or should be used cautiously for conditions of deficient *qi*, blood, or yin.

Citrus peel *(CHEN PI)*

Pericarpium citri reticulatae

COMMON NAMES: Tangerine peel, citrus peel

FAMILY: Rutaceae

PART USED: Peel of fruit

ENERGIES AND FLAVORS: Warm, aromatic; acrid, bitter

ORGAN MERIDIANS AFFECTED: Spleen, lung

PROPERTIES: Carminative, expectorant, stomachic

INDICATIONS: Citrus peel has a drying, carminative action that makes it one of the best substances to use to assist the spleen's transforming and transporting functions. It is effective for conditions of phlegm and dampness as well as other symptoms of stagnant spleen and lung *qi,* such as indigestion, food stagnation, hiccups, belching, nausea, vomiting, and cough. It is often used in conjunction with tonifying herbs to help reduce their cloying effect.

CONTRAINDICATIONS: Citrus peel should not be used when there is cough with yin deficiency; this could manifest as a dry cough or coughing blood. It should also be avoided when there is sticky yellow phlegm.

DOSE: 3–9 grams

Green tangerine peel (QING PI)

Pericarpium citri reticulatae viride

COMMON NAMES: Green tangerine peel, blue citrus peel

FAMILY: Rutaceae

PART USED: Fruit peel

ENERGY AND FLAVORS: Warm; bitter, acrid

ORGAN MERIDIANS AFFECTED: Liver, gallbladder, stomach

PROPERTIES: Carminative, stomachic, cholagogue, mild laxative, analgesic for abdominal pains

EFFECTS AND INDICATIONS: While citrus peel regulates spleen *qi,* green tangerine peel, with its cholagoguic and mild laxative properties, has a downward energy that regulates the action of the liver and gallbladder. As such, it regulates liver *qi* stagnation and is effective for epigastric pains as well as for food stagnation. It is also used to dissolve masses and hard nodules, especially in the breasts, which are symptoms of irregular liver *qi.*

CONTRAINDICATIONS: Green tangerine peel should be used with caution by those who are weak and have low energy because of *qi* deficiency.

DOSE: 3–9 grams

Immature bitter orange (ZHI SHI)

Fructus immaturus citri aurantii

COMMON NAME: Bitter orange, *zhi shi, chih-shih*

FAMILY: Rutaceae

PART USED: Fruit peel

ENERGY AND FLAVORS: Slightly cold; bitter, sour, acrid

ORGAN MERIDIANS AFFECTED: Spleen, stomach, large intestine

PROPERTIES: Tonic, increases blood pressure, carminative; small doses relax the intestines and large doses increase peristalsis

INDICATIONS: This herb is used similarly to the other citrus herbs as a carminative and to break up food stagnation, as well as to help disperse stagnant *qi*. It is also used as a tonic for the uterus and for prolapse of the uterus, anus, or stomach.

CONTRAINDICATIONS: Immature bitter orange should be used with caution during pregnancy, when there is *qi* deficiency, or when there is cold in the stomach.

DOSE: 3–9 grams

Areca peel (DA FU PI)

Pericarpium arecae catechu

COMMON NAME: Areca peel, betel husk

FAMILY: Palmae

ENERGY AND FLAVOR: Warm; acrid

ORGAN MERIDIANS AFFECTED: Spleen, stomach, large and small intestines

PROPERTIES: Carminative, laxative (by increasing peristalsis), diuretic

INDICATIONS: This herb is excellent in cases of stagnation of foods and fluids when there is constipation, edema, and abdominal distension. It can be used for many digestive problems but is most often used for constipation or edema.

CONTRAINDICATIONS: Areca peel should not be used by those who are weak from *qi* deficiency.

DOSE: 3–9 grams

Cyperus (XIANG FU)

Rhizoma cyperi rotundi

COMMON NAME: Cyperus, nutgrass

FAMILY: Cyperaceae

PART USED: Rhizome

ENERGY AND FLAVORS: Neutral; acrid, bitter, sweet

ORGAN MERIDIANS AFFECTED: Liver, Triple Burner, stomach

PROPERTIES: Carminative, antispasmodic, analgesic, estrogenic

INDICATIONS: Cyperus is especially effective for regulating menstrual and digestive discomfort caused by disharmony between the liver and the spleen. Because of its neutral properties, it is widely used for either cold or hot conditions.

CONTRAINDICATIONS: Cyperus is quite drying and may not be appropriate for conditions of yin or *qi* deficiency.

DOSE: 4–12 grams

NOTES: There are many different species growing on all continents and most have been traditionally used for similar purposes. A species growing in the Peruvian rain forest is used by local tribes to prevent conception. This may be because of its estrogenic properties, but it may also be as a result of an ergot oxytoxic fungus that grows on its roots. Northern California Native Americans ate the small tubers as food.

Saussurea (MU XIANG)
Radix aucklandiae lappae

COMMON NAME: Saussurea, costus root, aucklandia
FAMILY: Compositae
PART USED: Root
ENERGY AND FLAVORS: Warm; acrid, bitter
ORGAN MERIDIANS AFFECTED: Spleen, liver, lung, gallbladder, large intestine, stomach
PROPERTIES: Carminative, digestant, antispasmodic
EFFECTS AND INDICATIONS: Promotes the circulation of spleen and stomach *qi* and thereby relieves abdominal pain, lack of appetite, nausea, and vomiting. It also regulates and circulates liver and gallbladder *qi* and is effective for jaundice. It can be used for stagnation of *qi* in the intestines and is useful for dysenteric disorders and tenesmus.
CONTRAINDICATIONS: Saussurea should not be used by those with dehydration, anemia, or yin deficiency.
DOSE: 3–9 grams
NOTE: Saussurea should not be boiled but should be steeped at the end of making the decoction.

Lindera root (WU YAO)
Radix linderae Strychnifoliae

COMMON NAME: Lindera root
FAMILY: Lauraceae
PART USED: Root
ENERGY AND FLAVOR: Warm; acrid
ORGAN MERIDIANS AFFECTED: Spleen, lung, kidney, urinary bladder, stomach
PROPERTIES: Carminative, anodyne, antispasmodic, diaphoretic, mild laxative, vasodilator (increases blood pressure by increasing blood flow)
INDICATIONS: Lindera is primarily used for stagnation of *qi* due to cold with symptoms of pain in the abdominal region, including menstrual

pain. It is also useful when the stagnation of *qi* affects the urinary bladder, causing frequent urination and/or inability to hold urine. These symptoms must be caused by cold in order for this herb to be effective.

CONTRAINDICATIONS: Lindera root should not be used by those who are weak from *qi* deficiency or those with interior heat.

DOSE: 3–9 grams

Persimmon calyx (SHI DI)

Diospyri kaki

COMMON NAMES: Persimmon calyx, Kaki calyx

FAMILY: Ebenaceae

PART USED: Calyx

ENERGY AND FLAVOR: Neutral; bitter

ORGAN MERIDIANS AFFECTED: Lung, stomach

PROPERTIES: Carminative, astringent

INDICATIONS: This commonly grown tree yields a fine medicine that is very effective for redirecting *qi* that is flowing upward, with symptoms such as hiccups and belching. Because of its neutral energy, it can be used for both hot and cold conditions, according to the other herbs used in the formula.

CONTRAINDICATIONS: Persimmon calyx should be used with caution by those with prolapsed organs due to deficient *qi,* as it has an energy that directs the *qi* downward.

DOSE: 3–9 grams

NOTE: The dried calyx is ground to a powder and 3 grams at a time is taken internally with warm water.

Aquilaria (CHEN XIANG)

Lignum aquilariae

COMMON NAMES: Aquilaria, aloe wood, eagle wood

FAMILY: Thymelaeceae

PART USED: Wood

ENERGIES AND FLAVORS: Warm, aromatic; acrid, bitter

ORGAN MERIDIANS AFFECTED: Spleen, kidney, lung, stomach

PROPERTIES: Carminative, anodyne

EFFECTS AND INDICATIONS: Relieves abdominal and epigastric pain caused by cold and *qi* stagnation, directs the *qi* downward. It is used for relieving hiccups, belching, nausea, or vomiting, as well as for such lung symptoms as wheezing and asthma. It is especially effective for lung *qi* imbalances when the underlying cause is kidney–adrenal deficiency. This herb can be used for *qi* stagnation caused either by excess or deficiency.

CONTRAINDICATIONS: Aquilaria should not be used by those with prolapsed organs caused by *qi* deficiency or by those with yin deficiency and heat signs.

DOSE: 1–3 grams

Herbs That Regulate the Blood

Herbs that regulate blood are further subdivided into those that stop bleeding and those that promote blood circulation. Interestingly, some herbs that promote or regulate blood circulation can actually be used to stop bleeding because hemorrhage, being a concentration of blood in a specific area, is a form of blood stagnation. For this reason, Western herbalists use cayenne pepper, either taken internally or applied topically, for bleeding and hemorrhage. *Tian qi* ginseng (*Radix notoginseng*), one of the most powerful trauma herbs, is used for both internal and external injuries with associated bruising, clots, and hemorrhage. It is also one of the most effective herbs for dissolving blood clots. For trauma and first aid, one of the best forms of ginseng to use, *Tian qi* ginseng, is in the Chinese patented formula *Yunnan Paiyao*.

For severe hemorrhage, hemostatic herbs and substances are indicated. While nowadays it is best to refer such emergency cases to a physician, it is useful to know how to deal with them if a physician is unavailable. Certainly, one should try to directly stanch the flow of blood either directly over the area or through the use of a tourniquet. Generally, the carbonized ashes of astringent and hemostatic herbs and substances, including mugwort (*ai ye*), agrimony (*xian he cao*), and human hair (*xue yu tan*), are most effective to stop bleeding. Internally, 1 or 2 teaspoons of the ashes can be taken with a little water, but they are also effective when applied externally. Mugwort ashes, the residue of moxibustion, are saved by acupuncturists in the highly unlikely event that any abnormal bleeding occurs after treatment. Mugwort ashes are also very effective for diabetics with bleeding sores on their feet.

Herbs that invigorate blood are classified as emmenagogues in Western herbalism. In TCM, they have many important uses, including to warm and promote circulation of blood in cardiovascular conditions or menstrual irregularities; treat sharp, acute pains caused by blood stagnation; and break blood stasis in certain tumors, cysts, hardened clots, and scar tissue.

HERBS THAT STOP BLEEDING

Tian qi or *san qi* ginseng
Radix notoginseng
COMMON NAMES: Notoginseng, panax pseudoginseng
FAMILY: Araliaceae
PART USED: Root
ENERGY AND FLAVORS: Warm; sweet, slightly bitter
ORGAN MERIDIANS AFFECTED: Liver, stomach
PROPERTIES: Hemostatic, anti-inflammatory, tonic, diuretic, antifungal, antiviral, lowers blood sugar
EFFECTS AND INDICATIONS: This trauma herb par excellence combines hemostatic, blood-moving, and tonic properties. It can be taken for internal wounds and bleeding and applied externally for the same purpose. It dissolves blood clots, relieves all kinds of bleeding and painful menstruation, and alleviates swelling and pain. Recently, it has been found to be effective for coronary heart disease, angina pectoris, and hyperlipidemia. Finally, it can be used to treat chronic infectious hepatitis and other inflammatory diseases.
CONTRAINDICATIONS: *Tian qi* should not be used during pregnancy. It should be used with caution by those with anemia, blood deficiency, or yin deficiency or those without stagnation of blood. Its strong blood-moving or *qi*-moving effects can further deplete and exhaust the *qi* if taken with these conditions.
DOSE: 1–9 grams; 1–3 grams when taken as a powder; can be used topically

Bletilla *(BAI JI)*
Rhizoma bletillae striatae
COMMON NAME: Bletilla rhizome
FAMILY: Orchidaceae
PART USED: Rhizome
ENERGY AND FLAVORS: Slightly cold; bitter, sweet
ORGAN MERIDIANS AFFECTED: Liver, lung, stomach

PROPERTIES: Hemostatic, astringent, anti-inflammatory, antibacterial, vulnerary

EFFECTS AND INDICATIONS: Besides stopping bleeding, this herb also nourishes blood and yin. It is used for different kinds of bleeding from the stomach or lungs, with symptoms of vomiting blood, coughing blood, or nosebleeds. It is also very good used externally for bleeding from traumatic injury. It can be used externally to help heal wounds of all kinds, including burns, as it helps the flesh to grow and promotes healing. Its antibacterial and anti-inflammatory effects help to heal the acute symptoms of the burn or wound.

CONTRAINDICATIONS: Bletilla is contraindicated for acute bleeding caused by externally contracted or excess conditions involving bleeding from the lungs or stomach. It should also not be used with aconite.

DOSE: 3–12 grams

Mugwort (AI YE)

Folium artemisiae argyi

COMMON NAME: Mugwort, Chinese mugwort

FAMILY: Compositae

PART USED: Leaves

ENERGY AND FLAVORS: Warm; bitter, acrid

ORGAN MERIDIANS AFFECTED: Liver, spleen, kidney

PROPERTIES: Antibacterial, antifungal, expectorant, antiasthmatic, cholagogue, antipyretic, emmenagogue, hemostatic, antispasmodic

EFFECTS AND INDICATIONS: The Chinese mugwort is used to warm all the meridians and expel coldness, especially in the uterus, and helps with cramping and pain associated with menstruation, PMS, and other abdominal pains. It is used when there is danger of miscarriage due to a cold womb or bleeding. It is also used for cold lung conditions with phlegm and asthma.

CONTRAINDICATIONS: Mugwort should not be used when there is heat in the blood due to yin deficiency and should be used with caution during pregnancy.

DOSE: 3–9 grams

Sanguisorba (DI YU)

Radix sanguisorbae officinalis

COMMON NAMES: Sanguisorba, burnet-bloodwort root

FAMILY: Rosaceae

PART USED: Root

ENERGY AND FLAVORS: Slightly cold; bitter, sour

ORGAN MERIDIANS AFFECTED: Liver, large intestine, stomach

PROPERTIES: Hemostatic, astringent, antibacterial, vulnerary, antiemetic

EFFECTS AND INDICATIONS: This herb is used for cooling the blood (bleeding can be a sign of excess heat or inflammation) when there is bleeding in the Lower Burner, bleeding from the bowels or the uterus, or bleeding hemorrhoids. It can also help stop diarrhea because of its astringent action. It is excellent used externally, especially for burns; it helps guard against infection and promotes the healing of the skin.

CONTRAINDICATIONS: Sanguisorba should not be used when there is coldness or weakness, especially when there is deficient *qi* causing uterine bleeding.

DOSE: 6–12 grams

Cattail pollen (PU HUANG)

Pollen typhae

COMMON NAME: Cattail pollen

FAMILY: Typhaceae

ENERGY AND FLAVOR: Neutral; sweet

ORGAN MERIDIANS AFFECTED: Heart, liver, spleen, pericardium

PROPERTIES: Hemostatic, astringent, lowers blood pressure, mild laxative, diuretic

INDICATIONS: This herb has a powerful effect on the blood, increasing the platelet count. Because of its astringent action, it is very effective in stopping bleeding anywhere in the body. By invigorating blood and breaking blood stasis, it relieves pain associated with such a condition. It has a quite powerful action on the uterus; it is more powerful in a normal uterus than in a pregnant one. Nonetheless, it may cause strong contractions.

CONTRAINDICATIONS: Cattail pollen should not be used during pregnancy.

DOSE: 5–10 grams

Agrimony (XIAN HE CAO)

Herba agrimoniae pilosae

COMMON NAME: Agrimony

FAMILY: Rosaceae

PART USED: Whole plant

ENERGY AND FLAVOR: Neutral; bitter

ORGAN MERIDIANS AFFECTED: Lung, liver, spleen

PROPERTIES: Hemostatic, astringent, antiparasitic, anti-inflammatory, antibacterial, increases blood pressure, tonic, analgesic

INDICATIONS: This herb is used for most all types of bleeding anywhere in the body. When used for different types of bleeding, it should be combined with the appropriate herbs for the condition, whether deficiency, excess, hot, or cold. Because of its astringent action, it is useful for diarrhea. It can also be used for parasites in the intestines.

CONTRAINDICATIONS: Agrimony is generally very safe but should be used with caution in cases of extreme heat or fire symptoms.

DOSAGE: 6–15 grams; it can be used externally as a wash

Biota leaves (CE BAI YE)

Cacumen biotae orientalis

COMMON NAME: Biota leaves

FAMILY: Cupressaceae

PART USED: Leaves

ENERGIES AND FLAVOR: Slightly cold, astringent; bitter

ORGAN MERIDIANS AFFECTED: Liver, lung, heart, large intestine

PROPERTIES: Hemostatic, astringent, antitussive, sedative, anti-inflammatory, antibacterial, antiviral, expectorant, antispasmodic, promotes the growth of hair

INDICATIONS: Biota is used for any kind of bleeding when it is associated with heat. It can also be used for bleeding with cold conditions when it is combined with the right herbs. It is also used for coughs when there is heat in the lungs, difficulty expectorating, and blood in the sputum. Biota is also useful externally for early stages of burns, but only when they are relatively minor.

CONTRAINDICATIONS: Biota leaves should not be used when there are no signs of heat or dampness or over long periods of time.

DOSE: 6–12 grams

Charred human hair (XUE YU TAN)

Crinis carbonisatus hominis

COMMON NAME: Charred human hair

FAMILY: Hominidae

ENERGY AND FLAVOR: Neutral; bitter

ORGAN MERIDIANS AFFECTED: Liver, kidney, heart

PROPERTIES: Hemostatic, diuretic

INDICATIONS: This is one of the best agents to stop bleeding of all kinds; because of its availability, it can be very useful in situations in which nothing else is at hand. It can also be used for difficulty in urination.

CONTRAINDICATIONS: No contraindications for charred human hair are noted.

DOSE: 3–9 grams; the powder can be applied directly to a wound as needed

Lotus rhizome node (OU JIE)
Nodus nelumbinis nuciferae rhizomatis

COMMON NAME: Lotus rhizome node

FAMILY: Nymphaeaceae

PART USED: Rhizome node

ENERGIES AND FLAVOR: Astringent, neutral; sweet

ORGAN MERIDIANS AFFECTED: Lung, liver, stomach

PROPERTIES: Hemostatic, astringent

INDICATIONS: This herb can be used for many kinds of bleeding, but it is most often used for bleeding of the lung or stomach when there is coughing of blood or vomiting of blood. This herb works not only by its astringent activity but also by breaking up blood stasis.

CONTRAINDICATIONS: No contraindications for lotus rhizome node are noted.

DOSE: 6–15 grams; the fresh juice is often used and is best in that form in doses of 30–60 grams

Imperata (BAI MAO GEN)
Rhizoma imperatae cylindricae

COMMON NAMES: Imperata, woolly grass, white grass

FAMILY: Gramineae

PART USED: Leaves (grass)

ENERGY AND FLAVOR: Cold; sweet

ORGAN MERIDIANS AFFECTED: Lung, stomach, urinary bladder

PROPERTIES: Hemostatic, antibacterial, diuretic, lowers blood pressure

INDICATIONS: Imperata is used when there is hot blood that is leaving its pathways, as in blood in the urine, vomiting up of blood, coughing up of blood, or nosebleed. It is especially useful to regulate the flow of urine and for the treatment of cystitis.

CONTRAINDICATIONS: Imperata should not be used where there is cold associated with spleen deficiency.

DOSE: 10–30 grams; more is often used when the herb is used alone (without any other herb) or if used fresh

HERBS THAT INVIGORATE THE BLOOD

Ligusticum (CHUAN XIONG)
Radix ligustici chuanxiong
COMMON NAMES: Ligusticum, Szechuan lovage root, cnidium
FAMILY: Umbelliferae
PART USED: Root
ENERGY AND FLAVOR: Warm; acrid
ORGAN MERIDIANS AFFECTED: Liver, gallbladder, pericardium
PROPERTIES: Emmenagogue, antibacterial, antihypertensive, sedative, anticonvulsive
EFFECTS AND INDICATIONS: Ligusticum is one of the primary herbs used for moving blood and *qi*. It can be used in any case of blood stasis with pain and stagnation, including amenorrhea (painful menstruation) or dysmenorrhea. This herb can also be used for wind conditions in which there is painful obstruction or in any externally contracted wind condition; it is also used for skin conditions having to do with wind. Ligusticum is one of the finest herbs for many kinds of headaches, depending on the herbs with which it is used in conjunction.
CONTRAINDICATIONS: Ligusticum should not be used for headaches that occur because of yin deficiency or from rising liver yang. It should not be used where there is abnormal bleeding or during pregnancy.
DOSE: 3–9 grams

Red sage root (DAN SHEN)
Radix salviae miltiorrhizae
COMMON NAMES: Red sage, Salvia root
FAMILY: Labiatae
PART USED: Root
ENERGY AND FLAVOR: Slightly cold; bitter
ORGAN MERIDIANS AFFECTED: Heart, liver, pericardium
PROPERTIES: Vasodilator, anticoagulant, lowers cholesterol, antibacterial, sedative, lowers blood sugar
EFFECTS AND INDICATIONS: This is a very important herb because it combines strong blood-moving properties but with a cooling, so it can be

used for patterns of heat with blood stasis without overstimulating the system and aggravating an inflammatory condition. In fact, it is calming and mildly sedating. It is one of the premier herbs for most heart conditions, relieving angina (heart pains) and powerfully reducing blood levels of cholesterol and other lipids. It is also used for blood stagnancy in the lower abdomen, mostly associated with menstrual difficulties, when there is pain. It can also be used when there is blood stasis associated with stagnant liver *qi*.

CONTRAINDICATIONS: Red sage root should not be used if there is no blood stasis. It should not be used in conjunction with *Rhizoma et radix veratri* (Chinese Hellebore)

DOSE: 3–15 grams

Corydalis (YAN HU SUO)
Rhizoma corydalis yanhusuo
COMMON NAME: Corydalis
FAMILY: Papaveraceae
PART USED: Rhizome
ENERGY AND FLAVORS: Warm; acrid, bitter
ORGAN MERIDIANS AFFECTED: Liver, lung, spleen, heart
PROPERTIES: Circulatory stimulant, analgesic, sedative, antispasmodic
EFFECTS AND INDICATIONS: Corydalis is an excellent agent to allay pain. It invigorates the blood, breaks blood stasis, and circulates the *qi*, and it can be used for traumatic injuries, dysmenorrhea, pain in the chest, or any other pain in the epigastric region caused by blood stasis. It can also be used for insomnia.
CONTRAINDICATIONS: Corydalis should not be used during pregnancy.
DOSE: 3–9 grams

Turmeric tuber (YU JIN)
Tuber curcumae
COMMON NAMES: Turmeric tuber, curcuma
FAMILY: Zingiberaceae
PART USED: Tuber
ENERGY AND FLAVORS: Cool; acrid, bitter
ORGAN MERIDIANS AFFECTED: Liver, lung, heart, gallbladder
PROPERTIES: Promotes blood and *qi* circulation, analgesic, cholagogue, antibacterial, antifungal
EFFECTS AND INDICATIONS: This is not the same turmeric that is used in

cooking, which is the next herb in this section, *jiang huang*. Another important difference is that *yu jin* is cooler than *jiang huang*, which is warm and more circulating. Yu jin is also used for moving both stagnant blood and *qi*, however. It is used for traumatic injuries because it breaks up blood stasis. It is also very useful for conditions of stagnant liver *qi* because it regulates the *qi* and promotes the movement of both *qi* and blood for conditions such as pain in the chest, flanks, or abdominal pains. It cools the blood and removes phlegm from the heart when there are symptoms such as delirium and mania. It is specific for jaundice.

CONTRAINDICATIONS: Turmeric tuber should not be used during pregnancy or by those without signs of stagnant blood or *qi*. It should also be used with caution by those with yin deficiency from blood loss. Turmeric tuber should not be used with *Flos caryophylli* (cloves).

DOSE: 3–9 grams

Turmeric (*JIANG HUANG*)

Rhizoma curcumae longae

COMMON NAME: Turmeric rhizome

FAMILY: Zingiberaceae

PART USED: Rhizome

ENERGY AND FLAVORS: Warm; acrid, bitter

ORGAN MERIDIANS AFFECTED: Liver, spleen

PROPERTIES: Promotes blood and *qi* circulation, cholagogue, emmenagogue, analgesic, antibacterial, antifungal, anti-inflammatory

EFFECTS AND INDICATIONS: This is the turmeric that imparts a yellow color to curry powder. Unlike the previous herb, *yu jin*, this herb is warming in nature and thus has different indications. It is used for stagnation of both blood and *qi* and is effective for such conditions as amenorrhea, dysmenorrhea, and other pains in the abdominal region caused by stagnation of blood or *qi*. It is excellent for traumatic injuries when there is pain and swelling from stagnation. It should be considered when there are rheumatic conditions of wind-cold dampness. It is also an effective herb for traumatic injuries.

CONTRAINDICATIONS: Turmeric should be avoided during pregnancy. It should not be used when there is anemia (blood deficiency) with signs of stagnation of blood or *qi*.

DOSE: 3–9 grams

NOTES: Turmeric, also called *haldi*, is extensively used in Ayurvedic medicine for a wide variety of conditions ranging from arthritis to ulcers, flatulence, blood in the urine, bruises, colic, respiratory diseases, chest pains, jaundice, hepatitis, diabetes, menstrual irregularities, hemorrhage, and toothache. As a single herb, it is a medicinal treasure chest. One family tradition in India is to take ¼–½ teaspoon of turmeric root powder daily with triphala. Triphala is used to help maintain intestinal regularity, while turmeric is an antibiotic and antiviral for the prevention of infectious diseases. Actually called goldenseal in India, it has many similar liver acting, antibiotic properties as *Hydrastis canadensis*. It is also effective both as a treatment and preventive for intestinal worms and parasites. Externally, turmeric powder has been commonly used as a wash to clear the skin and treat acne. Turmeric, coriander, and cumin seeds make a potent digestive combination. These are also the three basic herbs of Indian curry powder. This same combination—1 teaspoon mixed with honey—is also one of the most effective treatments for all respiratory diseases, from bronchitis to asthma. Curcumin, the compound responsible for turmeric's yellow color, is considered its primary anti-inflammatory component. Even in high doses, turmeric has not been shown to have any toxicity. The major points to consider about turmeric are that it promotes circulation and digestion because of its warming energy and mildly pungent flavor and that it is an anti-inflammatory, indicated by its bitter taste. It is also highly respected for its antioxidant properties, being regarded as more potent than either vitamin C or E. Because of this, it is useful for the treatment of all stages of cancers. One estimate based on statistical research is that as little as ½ teaspoon of turmeric daily can prevent the DNA (deoxyribonucleic acid) damage associated with all cancers. Its antioxidant properties also account for its use as a food preservative and an inhibitor of rancidity of fats and oils. Obviously, turmeric has a wide range of uses, beginning with all diseases and symptoms associated with inflammation, such as arthritic and rheumatic diseases, gout and joint degeneration. It is used to increase ligament flexibility for the practice of yoga and other exercises requiring stretching. It is also a blood-detoxifying herb with a chemical action similar to that of NDGA (nordihydroquaiaretic acid), found in the North American desert herb chaparral (*Laurrea tridentata*). Dimethylbenzyl alcohol, another component of turmeric, benefits the cardiovascular system by normalizing cholesterol, first by reducing it in the blood and then by removing its accumulation in the liver. It removes arterial plaque, effectively treats anemia, and is a potent hemostatic used to reduce bleeding. Because of its blood-moving properties, turmeric is a very effective herb for regulating menstruation. Turmeric is perhaps the best herb for all liver and gallbladder diseases because of its ability to lower liver enzymes. Because it can increase bile output by up to 100%, it is one of the most effective treatments for gallstones.

Motherwort (YI MU CAO)
Herba leonuri heterophylli
COMMON NAME: Chinese motherwort
FAMILY: Labiatae
PART USED: Aerial portion, leaves
ENERGY AND FLAVOR: Slightly cold; acrid, bitter
ORGAN MERIDIANS AFFECTED: Heart, liver, urinary bladder
PROPERTIES: Emmenagogue, antihypertensive, antispasmodic, diuretic, antibacterial, antifungal
INDICATIONS: A slightly different species from Western motherwort (Leonurus cardiaca), Chinese motherwort is used in many of the same ways; its usage in the West extends back to Greek and Roman times and probably earlier. It is used to regulate menstruation, invigorate the blood, and break up blood stasis when there is pain and swelling in the abdominal region. It can be used to expel the placenta as well as to decrease postpartum pain. It is widely used in infertility when caused by blood stasis or immobile masses (tumors or cysts that are hard and cannot be moved). It is also used to promote urination for systemic edema, especially when there is blood in the urine.
CONTRAINDICATIONS: Motherwort should not be used during pregnancy or by those with anemia (blood deficiency) or yin deficiency.
DOSE: 9–30 grams

Bugleweed (ZE LAN)
Herba lycopi lucidi
COMMON NAME: Bugleweed
FAMILY: Labiatae
PART USED: Whole plant
ENERGY AND FLAVOR: Warm; acrid, bitter
ORGAN MERIDIANS AFFECTED: Liver, spleen, urinary bladder
PROPERTIES: Circulatory stimulant, cardiac tonic, diuretic

EFFECTS AND INDICATIONS: Bugleweed is used for invigorating the blood when there are menstrual difficulties associated with stagnant blood. It can be used for trauma where there is blood stasis and swelling. It can also be used for edema.

CONTRAINDICATIONS: Bugleweed should be used with caution during pregnancy and should not be used when there is no blood stasis.

DOSE: 3–9 grams

Red peony root (CHI SHAO)

Radix paeoniae rubrae
COMMON NAME: Red peony root
FAMILY: Ranunculaceae
PART USED: Root
ENERGY AND FLAVORS: Slightly cold; sour, bitter
ORGAN MERIDIANS AFFECTED: Liver, spleen
PROPERTIES: Circulatory stimulant, emmenagogue, analgesic, antispasmodic, anti-inflammatory, antibacterial, diuretic, sedative, antipyretic
EFFECTS AND INDICATIONS: Red peony root is used when there is heat in the blood and blood stasis associated with such conditions as amenorrhea, abdominal pain, menorrhagia, and other gynecological difficulties. It is also used for injuries, either internal or external, where there are symptoms of heat in the blood, blood stasis, or swelling. It also clears rising liver fire, which causes red, swollen, and painful eyes.
CONTRAINDICATIONS: Red peony root should not be used by those with blood deficiency (anemia).
DOSE: 6–12 grams

Peach seed (TAO REN)

Semen persicae
COMMON NAMES: Peach seed, peach kernel, persica
FAMILY: Rosaceae
PART USED: Kernel/seed (within pit)
ENERGY AND FLAVORS: Neutral; sweet, bitter
ORGAN MERIDIANS AFFECTED: Liver, heart, lung, large intestine
PROPERTIES: Circulatory stimulant, emmenagogue, anticoagulant, analgesic, antitussive, antiasthmatic, demulcent, aperient
EFFECTS AND INDICATIONS: This is a very important herb for breaking up blood stasis and invigorating the blood. It is used in most cases of

blood stagnation, including menstrual difficulties, traumatic injury, and immobile masses. It also has a mild action of lubricating the intestines for constipation caused by dryness.

CONTRAINDICATIONS: Peach seed should not be used by pregnant women.

DOSE: 5–10 grams

Safflower (HONG HUA)
Flos carthami tinctorii

COMMON NAME: Safflower, carthamus

FAMILY: Compositae

PART USED: Flower

ENERGY AND FLAVORS: Warm; acrid, bitter

ORGAN MERIDIANS AFFECTED: Heart, liver

PROPERTIES: Circulatory stimulant, emmenagogue, lowers blood pressure, lowers cholesterol, analgesic

INDICATIONS: Safflower is commonly used to alleviate pain caused by blood stagnation. It is therefore useful for menstrual disorders, abdominal pains caused by blood stasis, and most other kinds of pain caused by blood stasis. It is also effective for traumatic injury when there is pain and swelling; for this, it can be used both internally or externally.

CONTRAINDICATIONS: Safflower should not be used by pregnant women.

DOSE: 3–9 grams

Myrrh (MO YAO)
Resina myrrhae

COMMON NAME: Myrrh

FAMILY: Burseraceae

ENERGY AND FLAVOR: Neutral; bitter

ORGAN MERIDIANS AFFECTED: Heart, liver, spleen

PROPERTIES: Circulatory stimulant, emmenagogue, analgesic, promotes healing, antibacterial, antifungal, lowers cholesterol

INDICATIONS: Myrrh resin works excellently when used for blood stasis and swelling when there is pain caused by traumatic injury as well as for menstrual irregularities. It is indicated externally for pain and swelling caused by blood stasis with inflammation. It is also very good for wounds and sores that are not healing. Its antibacterial and antifungal properties are very appropriate in these cases, as is its ability to stimulate flesh growth. Myrrh also is an important addition to mouthwashes.

CONTRAINDICATIONS: Myrrh should not be used by pregnant women or taken internally for extended periods of time.

DOSE: 3–9 grams

Frankincense (RU XIANG)
Resina olibani

COMMON NAME: Frankincense, mastic, olibanum

FAMILY: Burseraceae

ENERGY AND FLAVORS: Warm; acrid, bitter

ORGAN MERIDIANS AFFECTED: Heart, liver, spleen

PROPERTIES: Circulatory stimulant, emmenagogue, analgesic, vulnerary, promotes wound healing

INDICATIONS: Frankincense is used for breaking blood stasis and alleviating pain caused by stagnant blood and *qi* caused by traumatic injuries and epigastric pain. It is also used for cases of wind-cold dampness (arthritic and rheumatic) conditions where there is obstruction of blood and *qi* causing pain and spasm. It can be used externally to promote wound healing and alleviate pain. Like myrrh resin, with which it is commonly combined, it is effective as a mouthwash for the treatment of gum disease.

CONTRAINDICATIONS: Frankincense should not be used by pregnant women. It should be used with caution by those with spleen deficiency.

DOSE: 3–9 grams

Achyranthes root (NIU XI)
Radix achyranthis bidentatae

COMMON NAME: Achyranthes root

FAMILY: Amaranthaceae

PART USED: Root

ENERGY AND FLAVORS: Neutral; bitter, sour

ORGAN MERIDIANS AFFECTED: Liver, kidney

PROPERTIES: Emmenagogue, analgesic, diuretic, tonic

EFFECTS AND INDICATIONS: This herb is used for pain caused by blood stasis and is especially useful when the blood stagnation is in the upper body, as it promotes the movement of blood and *qi* downward. Despite this, it is also used both as a circulatory herb and as a tonic for the liver and kidneys and is specific for soreness and pain in the lower back, knees, and the joints. Having anti-inflammatory properties, it can be used for clearing damp heat in the Lower Burner. Finally, achyranthes is effective for other symptoms, such as toothache, bleeding gums, and vomiting of blood.

CONTRAINDICATIONS: Achyranthes root should not be used by pregnant women. It should be used with caution by those with weak digestion and spleen deficiency.

DOSE: 6–9 grams

Herbs that Warm the Interior and Expel Cold

Herbs that warm the interior and expel cold are used for internal coldness with *qi* and yang deficiencies. Coldness often indicates yang *qi* deficiency, so these herbs are also added to formulas that tonify yang. For cases of yang collapse with convulsions or coma, these herbs are particularly indicated. In Western herbalism, cayenne pepper is often used in such cases; in Ayurvedic herbalism, a formula called *trikatu,* consisting of equal parts black pepper, pippali (long pepper), and ginger, is used.

The herbs in this category are all spicy-hot and treat conditions of deficient yang or *qi* of the spleen and kidney as well as of other organs, including the heart and lungs. Because of their spicy-hot nature, they are contraindicated for conditions of excess heat or yin deficiency.

Prepared aconite *(FU ZI)*
Radix lateralis aconiti, Aconitum carmichaeli
COMMON NAME: Prepared aconite
FAMILY: Ranunculaceae
PART USED: Root
ENERGIES AND FLAVOR: Very hot, toxic; acrid
ORGAN MERIDIANS AFFECTED: Heart, kidney, spleen
PROPERTIES: Metabolic warming stimulant, cardiotonic, analgesic, anti-inflammatory
EFFECTS AND INDICATIONS: Being the most yang of all herbs, prepared aconite is a very important metabolic stimulant. In its raw form, it is quite toxic, but in the prepared form described here, the poisonous alkaloids have been mostly neutralized and it is considered quite safe. Nevertheless, to further reduce toxicity, aconite root should be

cooked for at least 1 hour. It strongly dispels cold and raises the yang when it has undergone incredible strain and is separating from the yin. It helps unblock the heart, assisting in circulation, and tonifies kidney yang to help prevent the separation of yin and yang, which will result in death. It can be used for yang deficiency throughout the body, including the yang of the kidney, heart, or spleen, when there is interior cold associated with the condition. Because of its hot nature, it is used to dispel cold from the channels (acupuncture meridians) and alleviate pain from obstruction.

CONTRAINDICATIONS: Prepared aconite should not be used by those with yin deficiency, with true heat, with false chills, or during pregnancy.

DOSE: 3–9 grams; it should be decocted for 30–60 minutes before adding the rest of the herbs.

Dry ginger (GAN JIANG)

Rhizoma zingiberis officinalis

COMMON NAME: Dry ginger

FAMILY: Zingiberaceae

PART USED: Rhizome

ENERGY AND FLAVOR: Hot; acrid

ORGAN MERIDIANS AFFECTED: Heart, lung, spleen, stomach

PROPERTIES: Warming stimulant, carminative, emmenagogue, expectorant, antispasmodic

INDICATIONS: Unlike fresh ginger, which is used for external diseases and including perspiration, dry ginger is hotter and is used to warm the interior and benefit the yang when it has been injured by cold or deficiency. It can be used for either internally or externally contracted cold and is especially useful in warming the spleen and stomach and raising the yang *qi*. It can also be used for a wide variety of digestive problems with symptoms such as vomiting, abdominal pain, and nausea. It is very good for motion sickness. It is also useful when there is thin, white, watery mucus in the lungs; it warms and dries excess mucus from the lungs and assists expectoration.

CONTRAINDICATIONS: Dry ginger should not be used by those with yin deficiency and heat signs or bleeding associated with hot blood. This herb should be used with extreme caution during pregnancy.

DOSE: 3–9 grams

Cinnamon bark (ROU GUI)

Cortex cinnamomi cassiae

COMMON NAME: Cinnamon bark

FAMILY: Lauraceae

PARTS USED: Bark, twigs

ENERGY AND FLAVOR: Very hot; acrid, sweet

ORGAN MERIDIANS AFFECTED: Spleen, liver, kidney, heart, urinary bladder

PROPERTIES: Warming, metabolic stimulant, stomachic, antihypertensive, yang tonic

EFFECTS AND INDICATIONS: Cinnamon bark is considered to be one of the hottest herbs in the Chinese materia medica. It is used to assist the yang of the kidneys and bring the fire back to its origin, which is the kidneys–adrenals, when it has been moved out by cold. It tonifies spleen yang to treat weak digestive metabolism. It is also used for asthma and symptoms associated with wheezing caused by the kidneys' inability to grasp and circulate the *qi* from the lungs. It breaks up blood stasis and moves *qi* when there is painful obstruction associated with cold. For this, cinnamon twigs are more often used. Cinnamon twigs are also used as a milder alternative to cinnamon bark. Cinnamon is commonly used with tonifying herbs, as it helps in the generation of *qi* and blood.

CONTRAINDICATIONS: Cinnamon bark should not be used by those with yin deficiency with heat signs or when there is interior heat; it should be used with extreme caution during pregnancy.

DOSE: 1–6 grams

Evodia (WU ZHU YU)

Fructus evodiae rutaecarpae

COMMON NAME: Evodia

FAMILY: Rutaceae

PART USED: Fruit

ENERGIES AND FLAVORS: Hot, slightly toxic; acrid, bitter

ORGAN MERIDIANS AFFECTED: Liver, spleen, kidney, stomach

PROPERTIES: Warming stimulant, analgesic, emmenagogue, antibacterial, antiparasitic, antihypertensive

EFFECTS AND INDICATIONS: Evodia warms the spleen and stomach and helps when there are digestive problems associated with cold. It relieves pain caused by liver *qi* stagnation and is effective when there is a disharmony between the liver and the spleen with *qi* moving upward, causing vomiting, nausea, or headaches. It is effective when there is dampness and cold in the spleen causing diarrhea, especially in the morning.

CONTRAINDICATIONS: Evodia should not be used by those with yin deficiency, especially if dryness is an issue, as this herb is very drying and therefore should not be used for extended periods of time because it may injure the yin. It should not be used with red sage root (*Radix salviae miltiorrhizae [dan shen]*).

DOSE: 3–6 grams

Fennel seed (*XIAO HUI XIANG*)

Fructus foeniculi vulgaris
COMMON NAME: Fennel
FAMILY: Umbelliferae
ENERGY AND FLAVOR: Warm; acrid
ORGAN MERIDIANS AFFECTED: Liver, kidney, spleen, stomach
PROPERTIES: Carminative, stomachic, analgesic
EFFECTS AND INDICATIONS: Fennel is used to move constrained liver *qi* and warm the spleen and stomach. It is especially helpful when there are such digestive problems as vomiting, nausea, cramping, or pain in the abdomen caused by coldness. It is also used to alleviate pain in the testes caused by cold and deficiency.
CONTRAINDICATIONS: Fennel seed should not be used by those with yin deficiency with heat signs or by those with excess heat.
DOSE: 3–9 grams

Long pepper fruit (*BI BA*)

Fructus piperis longi
COMMON NAME: Long pepper fruit, pippali
FAMILY: Piperaceae
PART USED: Fruit
ENERGY AND FLAVOR: Hot; acrid
ORGAN MERIDIANS AFFECTED: Spleen, lung, kidney, stomach, large intestine
PROPERTIES: Stimulant, analgesic, digestive, decongestant
INDICATIONS: Long pepper fruit is used to expel cold in the stomach and intestines when there is pain and cramping with symptoms of nausea

and vomiting. It can be applied topically to disperse stagnation and is especially effective for toothache.

CONTRAINDICATIONS: Long pepper fruit should not be used by those with heat signs from either excess or deficiency.

DOSE: 1–3 grams

Galangal (GAO LIANG JIANG)

Rhizoma alpiniae officinari

COMMON NAME: Galangal, lesser galangal

FAMILY: Zingiberaceae

PART USED: Rhizome

ENERGY AND FLAVOR: Hot; acrid

ORGAN MERIDIANS AFFECTED: Spleen, stomach

PROPERTIES: Antibacterial, stomachic

INDICATIONS: Galangal is used for pain in the epigastric region caused by cold, with such symptoms as vomiting, pain, or diarrhea. It is also indicated when there are immobile masses associated with cold.

CONTRAINDICATIONS: Galangal should not be used by those with deficiency with heat signs or by those with true heat signs.

DOSE: 3–6 grams

Tonic Herbs

Tonics are used for patterns of deficiency. They are further subdivided into four subcategories: deficient *qi*, deficient blood, deficient yin, and deficient yang. Called the Four Treasures, the herbs in each of the four categories are not necessarily exclusive of each other and may be combined or used singly as appropriate for each individual. As one example, ginseng *ren shen,* the most well known of all tonic herbs, is regarded as useful for all deficiencies, even though it is classified according to its primary use as a *qi* tonic.

Yin tonics have a heavy, moist nature. They can be divided into two types, those that nourish the kidneys and liver and those that moisten the lungs and stomach. The kidneys and liver are the deepest aspects of the body, so that the deepest levels of yin deficiency always affect these organs. Stomach and lung yin deficiency are conditions that can evolve over time or result from the prolonged presence of a high fever or an acute viral disease.

Tonics should not be taken when there are patterns of excess stagnation, because they may aggravate the excess symptoms. This is also true of the use of rich foods, such as sugar, dairy, eggs, and fatty meat. One strategy to consider before taking tonics is to follow a light vegetarian diet or take detoxifying herbs for 1 to 3 days before administering tonic herbs and formulas. Another more common method is to include smaller amounts of *qi* and/or blood-moving herbs, such as ligusticum (*Radix ligustici chuanxiong*) and citrus peel, as assistants to *qi* or blood tonics.

Individuals with weak digestion may find it difficult to digest tonics and may even develop symptomatic heat reactions, such as dry mouth, irritability, insomnia, abdominal bloating, indigestion, nausea, and loss of appetite. Food is considered the best tonic; therefore, after a brief period of detoxification, the combination of tonic foods and herbs is superior and will often prevent adverse reactions to tonics. Even when taken with food, however, tonics may be better assimilated if they are combined with *qi* and/or blood-regulating herbs such as cardamon, ginger, and/or ligusticum, for instance.

Most tonic herbs have a mild energy and can be cooked with rice or other cereals to make congee or can be used in various soups and stews. According to the Five Elements system, salt goes to the kidneys, so when tonifying the kidneys, it is always helpful to take the appropriate herbs with a pinch of salt. Sweet flavors go to earth spleen; thus, for spleen tonification, a small amount of honey, barley, or rice syrup or raw, unrefined sugar can serve as a carrier to the spleen stomach.

The deepest levels of tonification will be more satisfactorily achieved if tonic herbs are taken with animal protein. In Ayurvedic medicine, and for the general Hindu lactovegetarian diet, tonic herbs are usually combined with warm milk. In fact, Ayurveda predates Indian vegetarianism, so its original texts describe the use of various flesh foods and animal parts to be used with herbs for deficiency conditions. The Chinese Five Elements assign pork to the kidneys and the cow, or beef, to the spleen, so that taking a minimum (2 to 4 ounces daily, for example) of these corresponding flesh foods with the appropriate herbs will allow them to be more powerfully assimilated and better used. Many of the symptoms of spleen deficiency correspond in Western physiology to thyroid and pancreas weakness, which may be subclinical and thus not indicated by results of standard blood tests. It is a good idea to combine the use of spleen tonics with glandular extracts of thyroid and pancreas. For kidney deficiency, one should use adrenal extracts—the adrenal cortex extract for yin deficiency and the adrenal medulla extract for yang deficiency, if they are available in this way. Similarly, combining organ extracts of liver and heart with corresponding tonic herbs will be more effective.

For yang tonification, exercise is extremely important, while for yin tonification, rest and sleep are best. Since yin tonification cannot replace sleep, prescribing calming and sedative herbs is another method to indirectly tonify yin. While tonics constitute the most renowned aspect of Chinese medicine, from a holistic perspective it is always a good idea to attempt to determine the underlying cause of a deficiency. In most cases, deficiencies are caused by stress, for which the best remedy is rest and good food.

QI TONICS

Qi tonics are generally sweet and slightly warm. They enter the spleen and lungs. Symptoms of spleen qi deficiency include fatigue, weakness, edema, poor appetite, loose stool, abdominal distension, and prolapse of the anus and/or other internal organs. Lung qi deficiency will have many of the characteristic qi deficiency symptoms along with shortness of breath and spontaneous perspiration.

Qi deficiency can occur simultaneously with blood, yang, or yin deficiency, and herbs are combined accordingly. Qi is also responsible for the generation and circulation of blood, so that qi tonics are used after acute blood loss.

Qi tonic herbs such as astragalus, the most characteristic herb for the deep immune system (wei qi), can be used to tonify all four deficiencies. Qi tonics may be used alone or in combination with qi-regulating herbs, such as saussurea (mu xiang) or citrus peel (chen pi) to aid their assimilation.

Ginseng (REN SHEN)

Radix ginseng, or Panax ginseng
COMMON NAMES: Ginseng, Chinese or Korean ginseng
FAMILY: Araliaceae
PART USED: Root
ENERGY AND FLAVORS: Warm; sweet, slightly bitter
ORGAN MERIDIANS AFFECTED: Spleen, lung, heart
PROPERTIES: Qi tonic, stomachic, stimulant, nutritive, rejuvenative, demulcent

INDICATIONS: Ginseng is used as a *qi* tonic mainly for the spleen and lungs. It is used when there has been a loss of *qi* caused by any one of many factors, such as loss of blood or chronic deficiency. It is used for such symptoms as spontaneous sweating, difficulty breathing, extreme fatigue, and weak digestion, which may manifest as lack of appetite, chronic diarrhea, or prolapse of internal organs. It can be used when there is thirst that is insatiable and heart *qi* deficiency with symptoms such as fatigue, insomnia, palpitations, or forgetfulness. It is generally indicated for mild usage by individuals over 45 or 50 years old and is not recommended during youth unless there are clear symptoms of *qi* deficiency, since it can increase sexual libido. Ginseng is generally not used as a stimulant; an overly high dose can cause symptoms of uneasiness, irritability, headache, and palpitations.

CONTRAINDICATIONS: Ginseng should not be used by those with yin deficiency with heat signs or by those with heat because of excess. It should also not be used when there are acute pathogenic conditions. It should be avoided by those with very high blood pressure.

DOSE: 3–9 grams; higher dosages are sometimes used for shock because of blood loss.

NOTES: Codonopsis is considered to have similar *qi* tonic effects as ginseng *ren shen* but at approximately half the potency. American ginseng is cooler and is more of a yin tonic, making it more suitable for stressed individuals who have a great deal of nervous energy and wish to support their essence.

Codonopsis (DANG SHEN)

Radix codonopsis pilosulae

COMMON NAME: Codonopsis

FAMILY: Campanulaceae

PART USED: Root

ENERGY AND FLAVOR: Neutral; sweet

ORGAN MERIDIANS AFFECTED: Spleen, lung

PROPERTIES: *Qi* tonic, lowers blood pressure, regulates (raises or lowers) blood sugar, increases numbers of white and red blood cells

INDICATIONS: This herb is often and routinely used in all formulas in place of ginseng when the stronger herb is not required. It is used for spleen *qi* deficiency that causes lack of appetite or prolapse of internal organs. It is useful for fatigue and weakness of the limbs and is effective for deficiency of lung *qi* that causes shortness of breath or chronic cough. It can be used in small doses when there is an acute illness with an underlying deficiency as long as the acute attack is addressed in the formula used.

CONTRAINDICATIONS: Codonopsis should be used with caution when there is acute illness.

DOSE: 9–30 grams

Astragalus *(HUANG QI)*

Radix astragali membranaceus

COMMON NAME: Astragalus

FAMILY: Leguminosae

PART USED: Root

ENERGY AND FLAVOR: Slightly warm; sweet

ORGAN MERIDIANS AFFECTED: Lung, spleen

PROPERTIES: *Qi* tonic, immune tonic, diuretic, lowers blood pressure

EFFECTS AND INDICATIONS: Astragalus is the primary herb used in Chinese medicine to tonify the immune system, or *wei qi,* of the lungs. It is useful for conditions of immune deficiency that lead to spontaneous sweating. It is also used for spleen *qi* deficiency with symptoms of weak, low metabolism; edema; and prolapse of internal organs, as it raises the spleen yang and *qi*. It can be used for *qi* and blood deficiency caused by loss of blood or after childbirth.

CONTRAINDICATIONS: Astragalus should not be used for cases of excess or when there is deficiency of yin with heat signs, and it should not be used when there is stagnation of *qi* or dampness, especially when there is painful obstruction.

DOSE: 9–30 grams; more can be used when indicated

Dioscorea *(SHAN YAO)*

Radix dioscoreae oppositae

COMMON NAME: Dioscorea, Chinese yam, mountain potato

FAMILY: Dioscoreaceae

PART USED: Root, tuber

ENERGY AND FLAVOR: Neutral; sweet

ORGAN MERIDIANS AFFECTED: Spleen, lung, kidney, stomach

PROPERTIES: *Qi* tonic, nutrient, demulcent

INDICATIONS: Tonifies spleen and lung *qi* and also tonifies both the yin and the yang of the kidneys and the lungs. It is used for spleen deficiency when there is chronic diarrhea, stagnation of food, and fatigue. It is also useful when there is lung *qi* deficiency with symptoms such as spontaneous sweating, chronic cough, and difficulty breathing. It can also be used for such symptoms as frequent urination, incontinence of seminal fluid, and vaginal discharge.

CONTRAINDICATIONS: Dioscorea should be used with caution when there is excess heat or dampness.

DOSE: 9–30 grams; a very large dosage can be used in special cases of wasting diseases

NOTES: This herb is eaten as a vegetable in both China and Japan. Only recently has it begun to be cultivated in the West. Perhaps because of the hormone precursors the herb contains, there are few reports of adverse symptoms associated with menopause in countries where it is included as part of the diet.

Atractylodes (BAI ZHU)
Rhizoma atractylodes macrocephalae

COMMON NAMES: Atractylodes *bai zhu,* white atractylodes
FAMILY: Compositae
PART USED: Rhizome
ENERGY AND FLAVOR: Warm; sweet, bitter
ORGAN MERIDIANS AFFECTED: Spleen, stomach
PROPERTIES: *Qi* tonic, carminative, diuretic
EFFECTS AND INDICATIONS: Atractylodes combines *qi*-tonifying, dampness dispelling, and carminative properties, making it perfect for strengthening the spleen and digestive metabolism. It is useful for both deficiency of *qi* or yang, with such symptoms as diarrhea, lack of appetite, and edema, and for other dampness conditions, including damp painful obstruction. It can also be used for spontaneous sweating and restless fetus when associated with spleen deficiency.

CONTRAINDICATIONS: Atractylodes should not be used by those with yin deficiency with heat signs or with extreme thirst.

DOSE: 3–9 grams

Pseudostellaria (TAI ZI SHEN)
Radix pseudostellariae heterophyllae

COMMON NAME: Pseudostellaria
FAMILY: Caryophyllaceae
PART USED: Root

ENERGY AND FLAVORS: Neutral; sweet, slightly bitter

ORGAN MERIDIANS AFFECTED: Spleen, lung

PROPERTIES: Qi tonic, nutritive, demulcent

EFFECTS AND INDICATIONS: Pseudostellaria is used to tonify the qi of the spleen and lung and is used for such ailments as chronic cough, lack of appetite, and weakness. It is also used when there are insufficient fluids from febrile diseases.

CONTRAINDICATIONS: Pseudostellaria should not be used with Rhizoma et radix veratri (Chinese Hellebore).

DOSE: 9–30 grams

Jujube date (DA ZAO)

Fructus zizyphi jujubae

COMMON NAME: Jujube date

FAMILY: Rhamnaceae

PART USED: Dates

ENERGY AND FLAVOR: Neutral; sweet

ORGAN MERIDIANS AFFECTED: Spleen, stomach

PROPERTIES: Qi tonic, sedative, nutritive, antihepatotoxin

EFFECTS AND INDICATIONS: This herb is used for deficiency of the spleen and stomach with such symptoms as fatigue, loose stools, and lack of appetite. It nourishes the blood and can be used when there are such symptoms as restlessness, insomnia, and emotional instability associated with blood deficiency. It is also used in formulas to harmonize the actions of the other herbs.

CONTRAINDICATIONS: Jujube date should not be used when there are conditions of dampness or food stagnation, intestinal parasites, or dental diseases.

DOSE: 10–30 grams; this roughly calculates to 2–10 dates, since the size varies.

Licorice (GAN CAO)

Radix glycyrrhiza uralensis

COMMON NAME: Chinese licorice

FAMILY: Leguminosae

PART USED: Roots

ENERGY AND FLAVOR: Neutral; sweet

ORGAN MERIDIANS AFFECTED: All twelve meridians

PROPERTIES: *Qi* tonic, anti-inflammatory, cholagogue, antitussive, anti-histamine, detoxicant

EFFECTS AND INDICATIONS: Licorice is probably the most used herb in the Chinese materia medica; because of its harmonizing effects on other herbs, it can be found in many formulas. It is used as a tonic for spleen *qi* deficiency, for the heart when there are symptoms of palpitations and irregular pulses, and to lubricate the lungs when there is a deficient dry cough. Because of its neutral energy, licorice can be used in formulas to treat either hot or cold conditions. It should be considered when there has been poisoning of any part of the body either internally or externally. Licorice has an excellent anti-inflammatory action similar to that of cortisone; in fact, excessive prolonged use can intensify and prolong the effects of cortisone.

CONTRAINDICATIONS: Licorice should not be used when there is excess dampness, nausea, or vomiting and generally should be used with caution by those who tend to retain water.

DOSE: 2–9 grams

NOTE: Prepared licorice is made by stir-frying the dried licorice root in a wok with honey. This makes it warmer and more of a *qi* tonic.

BLOOD TONICS

Blood tonics tend to be bitter and sweet with either a warm or neutral nature. They are primarily used for treating blood deficiency, including anemia and symptoms of pale complexion, lips, and nails; dizziness; blurred vision; palpitations; anxiety; and scanty, light red menses or stopped menstruation. The Chinese describe blood as the mother of *qi* and *qi* as the mother of blood. Because of this, *qi* and blood tonics are often combined to treat symptoms of blood deficiency. Often, blood-regulating herbs, such as ligusticum (*chuan xiong*) and red peony root are added to assist circulation. Blood's being a part of yin is reflected in the fact that certain blood tonics, such as prepared rehmannia, are used to tonify blood and yin. Both blood and yin tonics are indicated for dryness, with the difference being that yin deficiency is associated with symptoms of heat as well as dryness. As with all tonics, individuals with weak digestion may have trouble assimilating these herbs, so herbs that strengthen and regulate spleen *qi* are often added to blood tonic formulas.

Prepared rehmannia (SHU DI HUANG)

Radix rehmanniae glutinosae

COMMON NAME: Prepared rehmannia

FAMILY: Scrophulariaceae

PART USED: Root

ENERGY AND FLAVOR: Slightly warm; sweet

ORGAN MERIDIANS AFFECTED: Heart, liver, kidney

PROPERTIES: Blood tonic, yin nutritive tonic, cardiotonic, diuretic, nutritive, demulcent, lowers blood sugar, lowers blood pressure

EFFECTS AND INDICATIONS: This herb is the primary blood and yin tonic and is used for deficient liver and kidney yin with symptoms including night sweats, nocturnal emissions, and wasting disorders. It is used as a blood tonic for such conditions as irregular menses, pale complexion, and dizziness. It can also be used to tonify the blood and augment the essence for lower back pain, weakness in the lower extremities, premature graying of the hair, and general exhaustion.

CONTRAINDICATIONS: Prepared rehmannia should be used with caution by those with weak digestion and spleen *qi;* it should be avoided by those with stagnation of *qi* or phlegm.

DOSE: 9–30 grams

NOTES: The distinction between unprepared and prepared rehmannia (which is cured nine times in alcohol) is that prepared rehmannia is slightly warm and more of a blood tonic, while unprepared rehmannia is cool and anti-inflammatory with milder tonic properties.

Fleeceflower (HE SHOU WU)

Radix polygoni multiflori

COMMON NAME: Fleeceflower, *he shou wu*

FAMILY: Polygonaceae

PART USED: Root

ENERGIES AND FLAVORS: Astringent, slightly warm; sweet, bitter

ORGAN MERIDIANS AFFECTED: Liver, kidney

PROPERTIES: Blood tonic, lowers cholesterol, laxative, antibacterial

EFFECTS AND INDICATIONS: *He shou wu* is a liver and kidney blood and yin tonic. It helps to retain the essence and treats such symptoms as premature graying of the hair, anemia, dizziness, weak lower back and knees, nocturnal emissions, and vaginal discharge. This herb is excellent as a tonic because, unlike most tonics, it is not cloying in nature and therefore does not tend to stagnate. It is good for constipation in the elderly because it tonifies while having a mild laxative effect.

CONTRAINDICATIONS: Fleeceflower should not be used by those with diarrhea or when there are phlegm conditions associated with spleen deficiency.

DOSE: 9–30 grams

NOTES: Fleeceflower is now being cultivated throughout many Western countries. While the roots are a blood tonic, it is useful to know that the stems are used as a sedative for nervousness and insomnia. Fleeceflower is prepared by cooking the root in black soybean soup and then drying it for use.

Chinese angelica (DANG GUI)

Radix angelicae sinensis

COMMON NAME: *Dong quai, dang gui,* Chinese angelica

FAMILY: Umbelliferae

PART USED: Root

ENERGY AND FLAVOR: Warm; sweet, acrid, bitter

ORGAN MERIDIANS AFFECTED: Heart, liver, spleen

PROPERTIES: Blood tonic, emmenagogue, sedative, analgesic, mild laxative, antibacterial, anti-inflammatory

INDICATIONS: *Dang gui* is the premier herb for blood deficiency, just as ginseng is for *qi* deficiency. Because of this, it is sometimes called women's ginseng, because women's health is as closely related to blood as men's is to *qi*. Therefore, it is widely used for all gynecological conditions, including irregular menstruation, infertility, postpartum weakness, menopause imbalances, and anemia. It is also indicated for blurred vision, dizziness, or palpitations when these symptoms are caused by blood deficiency. It invigorates the blood and can be used for conditions of blood stagnation causing painful obstruction or abdominal or menstrual pains. It can also be used for wind-damp painful obstruction associated with blood deficiency. It unblocks the intestines, having a mild laxative effect when there is constipation due to blood deficiency.

CONTRAINDICATIONS: Chinese angelica should not be used by those with diarrhea or abdominal distension due to dampness or by those with yin deficiency with heat signs.

DOSE: 3–9 grams

NOTES: There are several species of angelica that are used as the herb *dang gui.* One species used is *angelica acutiloba,* the Japanese regard this herb as having blood tonic properties equal to or even superior to those of *angelica sinensis. Dang gui* is finely sliced and soaked in wine to make it warmer and more bioavailable. The body of the root is used more for tonifying blood, while the tails are considered to be more for the *qi* of the blood, meaning blood circulation. *Dang gui* is now being cultivated in North America.

White peony *(BAI SHAO)*
Radix paeoniae lactiflorae
COMMON NAME: White peony
FAMILY: Ranunculaceae
PART USED: Root
ENERGY AND FLAVOR: Slightly cold; bitter, sour
ORGAN MERIDIANS AFFECTED: Liver, spleen
PROPERTIES: Blood tonic, antispasmodic, analgesic, sedative, anti-inflammatory, diuretic, antibacterial
EFFECTS AND INDICATIONS: This herb is used to nourish the blood and nourish the ying nutritive energy. It is effective for helping to astringe the yin to restrain uprising of yang. It is used to help regulate menstrual disorders, such as dysmenorrhea, vaginal discharge, and uterine bleeding. It is used when the liver yang is in excess and when there is stagnant liver *qi.* It opens and softens the liver and can be used for spasms of the abdomen and pain in the abdominal region.
CONTRAINDICATIONS: White peony should not be used by those with diarrhea and spleen and stomach deficiency. It should be avoided when there is an exterior condition. Avoid using white peony with rhubarb root *(Radix et rhizoma rhei [da huang]).*
DOSE: 3–12 grams
NOTES: White peony is more nourishing and blood tonifying, while red peony is more blood moving. In older times, however, no distinction was made between the two. Today, we recognize wild peony as the source for red peony root and cultivated peony as the source for white peony root.

Lycii berries *(GOU QI ZI)*
Fructus lycii
COMMON NAME: Lycii berries, Chinese wolfberries
FAMILY: Solanaceae

PART USED: Fruit

ENERGY AND FLAVOR: Neutral; sweet

ORGAN MERIDIANS AFFECTED: Liver, kidney, lung

PROPERTIES: Blood and yin tonic, lowers cholesterol and blood sugar, antihepatotoxin

EFFECTS AND INDICATIONS: This herb is used for deficiency of both blood and yin and is especially useful when these deficiencies occur in the liver and kidneys, causing such symptoms as weak lower back and knees, nocturnal emissions, impotence, and wasting disorders. It nourishes the liver and benefits the essence. It is commonly combined with chrysanthemum flower for blurred vision and poor night vision. It is also used for yin deficiency of the lungs when there is consumptive cough.

CONTRAINDICATIONS: Lycii berries should not be used by those with patterns of heat and excess or when there is spleen deficiency with dampness or loose stools.

DOSE: 6–18 grams

Mulberry fruit (SANG SHEN)

Fructus mori albae

COMMON NAME: Mulberry

FAMILY: Moraceae

PART USED: Fruit

ENERGY AND FLAVOR: Cold; sweet

ORGAN MERIDIANS AFFECTED: Liver, heart, kidney

PROPERTIES: Blood and yin tonic, nutritive, sedative, mild laxative

EFFECTS AND INDICATIONS: This herb is used to tonify the blood and yin for such symptoms as dizziness, tinnitus, and anemia. It has also been used for premature graying of hair, diabetes, and insomnia due to blood deficiency. Having mild demulcent laxative properties, it is good for constipation in the elderly.

CONTRAINDICATIONS: Mulberry fruit should not be used by those with diarrhea due to spleen deficiency.

DOSE: 9–30 grams

Longan berries (LONG YEN ROU)

Arillus euphoriae longanae

COMMON NAMES: Longan berries, dragon's eyes

PART USED: Fruit

FAMILY: Sapindaceae
ENERGY AND FLAVORS: Warm; sweet
ORGAN MERIDIANS AFFECTED: Heart, spleen
PROPERTIES: Nourishes the blood, calms the spirit, relieves fatigue (especially mental fatigue)
INDICATIONS: This herb can be used for anxiety, neurosis, insomnia, and forgetfulness; heart palpitations caused by heart blood deficiency; exhaustion and fatigue caused by spleen deficiency; and exhaustion caused by worry, overthinking, or overwork.
CONTRAINDICATIONS: Longan berries should not be used for conditions of dampness and heat.
DOSE: 6–15 grams.
NOTE: Longan berries are also eaten as a confection or food.

Donkey-hide gelatin (E JIAO)

Gelatinum corii asini (equus asinus)
COMMON NAMES: Ass's-hide gelatin, black donkey-skin gelatin
FAMILY: Equidae
ENERGY AND FLAVORS: Neutral; sweet
ORGAN MERIDIANS AFFECTED: Kidney, liver, lungs
PROPERTIES: blood tonic and nourishment, hemastatic, yin lubricant and moistener
INDICATIONS: It is used for dizziness, pale complexion, and palpitations; for bleeding with coughing of blood, blood in the stool, metrorrhagia, and uterine bleeding; for yin deficiency with symptoms of irritability, insomnia, and yin deficient heat; and for coughs caused by lung yin deficiency.
CONTRAINDICATIONS: Donkey-hide gelatin should not be used for external conditions or conditions associated with dampness caused by spleen deficiency.
DOSE: 3–15 grams
NOTE: Donkey-hide gelatin should be dissolved in a strained decoction, dissolved in red wine, or taken in pills.

YANG TONICS

Yang tonics are generally used to treat spleen and kidney yang deficiency. Yang deficiency exhibits symptoms of dislike of cold; cold extremities; aching soreness of the lower back, knees, and joints;

impotence; frigidity; infertility; enuresis; clear leukorrhea; loose stool; wheezing; white tongue coat; and deep pulse. Yang tonics are generally warm and drying. If inappropriately taken for conditions of yin deficiency, they can further injure yin and cause yin fire to arise. Commonly, yang tonics are taken with prepared rehmannia to protect kidney yin and actually enhance the body's ability to use yang tonics. Finally, two of the most common herbs added to formulas to tonify yang are prepared aconite and cinnamon bark. Neither of these are directly included in this category; they are actually in the category of internal warming herbs.

Eucommia bark (DU ZHONG)
Cortex eucommiae ulmoidis
COMMON NAME: Eucommia bark
FAMILY: Eucommiaceae
ENERGY AND FLAVORS: Warm; sweet, slightly acrid
ORGAN MERIDIANS AFFECTED: Kidney, liver
PROPERTIES: Yang tonic, lowers blood pressure, diuretic, sedative
EFFECTS AND INDICATIONS: This herb is used to nourish the liver and tonify kidney yang and is specific for the bones and sinews. It treats such symptoms as weak lower back and knees, fatigue, impotence, and frequent urination. It is especially useful when there is threatened miscarriage or bleeding during pregnancy due to deficiency and coldness with back pain. It is a major herb for the treatment of both hypertension and lower back pain.
CONTRAINDICATIONS: Eucommia bark should not be used by those with heat signs associated with either hyperactivity or yin deficiency; it should not be used in conjunction with scrophularia (*Radix scrophulariae ningpoensis [xuan shen]*).
DOSE: 6–12 grams

Dipsacus root (XU DUAN)
Radix dipsaci asperi
COMMON NAMES: Dipsacus, teasel
FAMILY: Dipsacaceae
PART USED: Root
ENERGY AND FLAVOR: Warm; bitter, acrid
ORGAN MERIDIANS AFFECTED: Kidney, liver
PROPERTIES: Yang tonic, bone healing, antirheumatic, hemostatic

EFFECTS AND INDICATIONS: For symptoms of kidney yang deficiency with poor circulation. It is used to strengthen the bones and tendons and promote circulation. It stops bleeding during pregnancy when it is caused by deficiency and threatened miscarriage. It can also be used either internally or externally for trauma when there is stagnation of blood causing pain. Because of its blood-moving properties its power to promote growth of flesh, dipsacus is excellent for healing of bones and sores; in fact, the translation of the Chinese name is "bone-healing herb." It is commonly found in many areas of the Western world.

CONTRAINDICATIONS: Dipsacus should not be used by those with yin deficiency with signs of heat.

DOSE: 6–18 grams

Psoralea (BU GU ZHI)

Fructus psoraleae corylifoliae

COMMON NAME: Psoralea

FAMILY: Leguminosae

PART USED: Fruit

ENERGY AND FLAVORS: Warm; acrid, bitter

ORGAN MERIDIANS AFFECTED: Kidney, spleen

PROPERTIES: Yang tonic, astringent

EFFECTS AND INDICATIONS: Psoralea seed tonifies both kidney and spleen yang. It is useful for a variety of yang-deficiency symptoms, including impotence, premature ejaculation, weak lower back, diarrhea, urine incontinence, and frequent urination. Psoralea is also useful when there is wheezing and asthma caused by weak kidneys unable to pull down the *qi* of the lungs. It has been used to treat vitiligo, alopecia, and psoriasis. For vitiligo, a paste is made of the powdered seeds and topically applied to affected areas.

CONTRAINDICATIONS: Psoralea should not be used by those with yin deficiency when there are heat signs. It may be hard on the stomach.

DOSE: 3–9 grams

Walnuts (HU TAO REN)

Semen juglandis regiae

COMMON NAME: Walnuts

FAMILY: Juglandaceae

ENERGY AND FLAVOR: Warm; sweet

ORGAN MERIDIANS AFFECTED: Lung, kidney, large intestine

PROPERTIES: Yang tonic, nutrient, dissolves stones, mild laxative, emollient

EFFECTS AND INDICATIONS: Walnuts are used for the kidney yang deficiency signs of lower back pain and urinary incontinence. They are an agent that astringes essence and therefore can be used when there is premature ejaculation or other similar reproductive issues. Another use is for chronic cough caused by lung and kidney deficiency. Walnuts are also effective when there is constipation due to yang deficiency or there has been loss of fluids due to a febrile disease. Finally, because of their high oil content, walnuts are helpful for constipation in the elderly.

CONTRAINDICATIONS: Walnuts should not be used by those with yin deficiency when there are heat signs present or in those with heated phlegm and a hot cough.

DOSE: 9–30 grams

Morinda root (BA JI TIAN)
Radix morindae officinalis
COMMON NAME: Morinda
FAMILY: Rubiaceae
PART USED: Root
ENERGY AND FLAVOR: Warm; acrid, sweet
ORGAN MERIDIANS AFFECTED: Liver, kidney
PROPERTIES: Yang tonic, diuretic, antirheumatic
EFFECTS AND INDICATIONS: This herb is used for the kidney-yang Deficiency signs of premature ejaculation, male and female infertility, and irregular menstruation. It strengthens the bones and tendons and is useful for weakness in the extremities and back. It is also useful for painful obstruction caused by dampness and coldness.

CONTRAINDICATIONS: Morinda root should not be used by those with heat signs caused by yin deficiency, those with damp heat patterns, or those who are having difficulty urinating. It should not be combined with red sage root (*Radix salviae miltiorrhizae [dan shen]*).

DOSE: 3–12 grams

Epimedium leaf (YIN YANG HUO)
Herba epimedii
COMMON NAME: Epimedium, horny goat herb

FAMILY: Berberidaceae

PART USED: Leaf

ENERGY AND FLAVOR: Warm; sweet, acrid

ORGAN MERIDIANS AFFECTED: Kidney, liver

PROPERTIES: Yang tonic, aphrodisiac, antirheumatic

INDICATIONS: This herb is used for kidney-yang deficiency with such symptoms as impotence, urinary incontinence, forgetfulness, and weakness in the lower back and knees. It is also used for wind-damp cold painful obstruction of the joints and extremities. Epimedium tonifies both the yin and the yang and is useful when there is liver and kidney deficiency in which the liver yang is rising, causing such symptoms as hypertension, headaches, dizziness, and irregular menstruation.

CONTRAINDICATIONS: Epimedium leaf should not be used by those with yin deficiency with heat signs; nor should it be used alone for extended periods of time, since overuse may result in dizziness, dry mouth, thirst, vomiting, or nosebleed.

DOSE: 6–12 grams

NOTE: Epimedium is grown as an ornamental in Western herb gardens.

Cordyceps (DONG CHONG XIA CAO)

Cordyceps sinensis

COMMON NAMES: Cordyceps, winterworm, caterpillar fungus

FAMILY: Clavicipitaceae

PART USED: The caterpillar larvae fungus

ENERGY AND FLAVOR: Warm; sweet

ORGAN MERIDIANS AFFECTED: Lung, kidney

PROPERTIES: Tonic, astringent, expectorant, antiasthmatic

EFFECTS AND INDICATIONS: Cordyceps tonifies the kidney yang and is useful for weak back and knees, impotence, and most of the other common kidney yang deficiency symptoms. It is also good for lung yin deficiency when accompanied with kidney yang deficiency, when there are symptoms of chronic cough and cough with blood in the sputum. This is a very safe herb and can be taken for extended periods of time. Cordyceps has been found to be very effective for increasing stamina, making it useful for competitive sports.

CONTRAINDICATIONS: Cordyceps should be used with caution when there is an exterior condition.

DOSE: 6–12 grams

NOTE: The potency of cordyceps is increased when it is cooked with duck.

Cistanche (ROU CONG RONG)

Herba cistanches deserticolae
COMMON NAME: Cistanche
FAMILY: Orobanchaceae
PART USED: Whole plant
ENERGY AND FLAVOR: Warm; sweet, salty
ORGAN MERIDIANS AFFECTED: Kidney, large intestine
PROPERTIES: Yang tonic, sialagogue (increases the secretion of saliva), mild laxative
INDICATIONS: Tonifies kidney yang for symptoms of premature ejaculation, impotence, weak and cold lower back and knees, and female frigidity and infertility. It can be used when there is abnormal bleeding or vaginal discharge in women with kidney yang deficiency symptoms of a cold womb. This herb is excellent for the elderly and severely weak individuals with *qi* and blood deficiency and constipation, as it moistens the intestines and helps the movement of the feces while gently tonifying.
CONTRAINDICATIONS: Cistanche should not be used when there is yin deficiency with heat signs or when there is diarrhea from either deficient spleen or stomach or pathogenic heat.
DOSE: 6–12 grams

Human placenta (ZI HE CHE)

Placenta hominis
COMMON NAME: Human placenta
FAMILY: Hominidae
ENERGY AND FLAVOR: Warm; sweet, salty
ORGAN MERIDIANS AFFECTED: Lung, kidney, heart, liver
PROPERTIES: Yang tonic, nutritive, immune tonic, galactagogue
EFFECTS AND INDICATIONS: The human placenta is used for deficiency of yang, *qi*, and blood. It tonifies kidney yang and *qi*, liver blood, and the heart and lung *qi*. It also benefits the essence, which is stored in the kidney. It can be used in any of these deficiencies but is especially indicated for yang deficiency. It is indicated for infertility, impotence, pain in the lower back and knees, insufficient lactation, anemia, general weakness, and chronic cough.

CONTRAINDICATIONS: Human placenta is very safe, but it should be used with caution when there is heat from yin deficiency and should not be used for prolonged periods.

DOSE: 1.5–4.5 grams

Deer antler (LU RONG)

Cornu cervi parvum (cervus nippon)

COMMON NAME: Deer antler

FAMILY: Cervidae

PART USED: The antler

ENERGY AND FLAVORS: Warm; sweet, salty

ORGAN MERIDIANS AFFECTED: Kidneys, liver

PROPERTIES: Kidney yang tonic, governor vessel (spine meridian) tonic, *qi* and blood tonic

EFFECTS AND INDICATIONS: Augments essence and growth, strengthens sinews and bones, treats infertility and impotence. This herb is used for kidney yang deficiency patterns, including impotence, fatigue, coldness, dizziness, tinnitus, weakness of the lower back and extremities, and frequent, clear urination. It is considered effective in the treatment of maldevelopment of children, including rickets, learning disabilities, mental retardation, and failure to thrive. It strengthens the bones (for healing fractures and osteoporosis) and ligaments. It is also used to treat female infertility, uterine coldness, cold deficient uterine bleeding and vaginal discharge, and sores that do not heal.

CONTRAINDICATIONS: Deer antler is a powerful yang tonic, so one should begin with a low dose and gradually increase it. Too much can cause hyperactive yang symptoms, including hypertension with dizziness and conjunctivitis. It can also injure the yin and cause hemorrhage. It is therefore strongly contraindicated in patients with yin deficiency with patterns of heat.

DOSAGE: 3–9 grams as a powder divided into 2 or 3 daily doses; it can also be boiled into a tea or soaked in rice wine

Curculigo (XIAN MAO)

Rhizoma curculiginis orchioidis

COMMON NAME: Curculigo orchioides, circuliginis

FAMILY: Amaryllidaceae

PART USED: Rhizome

ENERGY AND FLAVORS: Hot, toxic; acrid

ORGAN MERIDIANS AFFECTED: Kidney, liver

PROPERTIES: Kidney yang tonic

EFFECTS AND INDICATIONS: Strengthens bones and sinews, clears cold and dampness. This herb is used to treat impotence, urinary incontinence, cold intolerance, aching soreness of the lower back and knees, lower back pain, and hypertension associated with menopause.

DOSE: 3–9 grams

CONTRAINDICATIONS: Curculigo should not be used for symptoms of hyper–yang fire.

Cibotium (GOU JI)

Rhizoma cibotii barometz

COMMON NAME: Cibotium barometz

FAMILY: Dicksoniaceae

PART USED: Rhizome

ENERGY AND FLAVORS: Warm; bitter, sweet

ORGAN MERIDIANS AFFECTED: Kidneys, liver

PROPERTIES: Kidney yang tonic

EFFECTS AND INDICATIONS: Treats kidney yang deficiency patterns, strengthens the bones and sinews, treats cold wind-dampness conditions with stiffness and aching soreness of the lower back and knees, treats urinary incontinence and chronic vaginal discharge. This herb is used to promote healing of the bones and ligaments from injuries. It is also used to treat lower back and knee weakness and reduce edema of the legs. In addition, it is used for urinary incontinence and chronic vaginal discharge.

DOSE: 5–9 grams

CONTRAINDICATIONS: Cibotium should not be used for difficult urination caused by yin deficiency. It is also considered to be antagonistic to *Herba cum radice patriniae (bai jiang cao)*.

Drynaria (GU SUI BU)

Rhizoma drynariae fortunei

COMMON NAME: Drynaria fortunei

FAMILY: Polypodiaceae

PART USED: Rhizome

ENERGY AND FLAVORS: Warm; bitter

ORGAN MERIDIANS AFFECTED: Kidneys, liver

PROPERTIES: Kidney yang tonic, blood circulation stimulator

EFFECTS AND INDICATIONS: Heals bones and ligaments from injuries, stimulates hair growth, treats kidney yang deficiency patterns. The herb is used to treat lower back and knee weakness, diarrhea, tinnitus, failing hearing, and bleeding gums from kidney deficiency. It heals broken bones and torn ligaments from injuries and can be applied topically as a tincture for alopecia.

DOSE: 6–18 grams

CONTRAINDICATIONS: Drynaria should not be used for symptoms of yin deficiency or when there is no blood stagnation.

YIN TONICS

The yin of the body represents its material and fluid substance. It becomes exhausted and wasted as a result of hyperactivity of yang or an overstimulation of the sympathetic nervous system. Yin is an all-inclusive representation of a number of complex physiological substances, including blood, lubricating material, muscles, organic material, and physical hormones. It is these yin substances that nourish and contain the very material essence of our being and create a receptable for life energy, called *qi*, to flow.

From one Chinese perspective, the yin of the body is of paramount importance, because without it, the yang, in the form of life energy, cannot be received and contained. Some of us seem to inherit a body with a strong yin substance. Such a body seems able to withstand higher levels of internal stress from bad food, negative emotions, and external stress as a result of injury and excessive physical activity than others. Still others may have a yin bodily substance that ages faster. Thus, the yin of the body is absolutely involved with longevity, so that the longer we can preserve our yin, the longer and better quality our lives will be.

We experience yin deficiency in many ways. When we think or work beyond our capacity, we experience burnout, which is the West's way of understanding the Chinese concept of yin deficiency. For Western athletes who seem always in quest of more yang, the concept of yin deficiency seems strange, yet it is not uncommon for them to experience total collapse, exhaustion, and burnout, from which no amount of yang or *qi* tonics, such as panax ginseng or Siberian ginseng (*Eleutherococcus senticosus*), can rescue them. In fact, any type of further stimulation, whether from physical or emotional exertion or food and herbs, will further contribute to their exhaustive yin deficiency.

The unique quality of yin tonics is that they nourish and refresh the system and repair the vehicle for the proper reception and experience of vital *qi*. As such, their quality is usually moist, heavy, and otherwise nutritive and demulcent. Being dense and concentrated, they may be difficult to digest, indicating that there may be a simultaneous yang and *qi* deficiency as well. Oils have a concentrated yin quality. In Ayurveda, oils like ghee (clarified butter), sesame, and olive oils are used to nourish the nerve energy, known as *vata*. An excess of *vata*, from an Ayurvedic perspective, is synonymous with Chinese yin deficiency.

The understanding of yin deficiency represents the most fundamental key to the understanding of traditional Chinese medical theory. Somehow, it is not within most Americans' way of life and thinking to understand how a lack of yin can cause us to experience an apparent excess of yang. We think of ebullient enthusiasm and energy as always positive; however, without being grounded in yin, these result in scattered and unfocused energy.

We experience ungrounded yin deficiency when we are sleep-deprived and suddenly feel wide awake and energized. It is at this time that we are desperately running on empty and we are in danger of seriously depleting our yin reserves. The most fundamental yin tonic is sleep, just as physical exercise becomes a yang tonic. It is during sleep that the body naturally refreshes and renews itself. In the West, hard-driving aerobic exercise is strongly recommended by many as a cure-all for all physical deficiencies. What many do not realize, however, is that there is never a lack of potential energy, only the capacity to receive and use it. Eastern exercises, such as yoga and *tai chi*, for instance, endeavor to circulate and move the physical yang energy without depleting or injuring the yin. This is an important distinction. Besides employing slow movements, *tai chai* uses thought—subtle yin energy—to direct and circulate physical energy.

True yin deficiency means that there are signs of burnout in the form of heat or inflammation. This may take the form of infectious and inflammatory diseases that are unresponsive to the usual anti-inflammatory drugs and antibiotics. This is so little understood in the practice of conventional Western medicine that often, the result is further injury of the body's yin reserves through prescribing more and stronger drugs. To treat such yin deficient inflammations, it is necessary to prescribe heat-clearing drugs and/or herbs along with yin and other tonics so that the body is given the strength to use the more active anti-inflammatories.

There are many characteristic yin deficiency diseases: multiple sclerosis, diabetes, osteoporosis, AIDS, TB, and all other autoconsumptive diseases, to name only a few. Aging, while not a disease, is an essential degeneration or weakening of yin that sets the stage for the body's decay. As a result, our skin tends to become drier as we age—our skin wrinkles, we become stiff, and we have more aches and pains. Our reproductive secretions decrease, our memory wanes, and we become more irritable and sensitive to strong lights, sounds, and other sensory experiences. All of this is aggravated by the fact that with incipient yin deficiency, we tend to sleep shorter hours.

Yin-nourishing tonics make up for the waning of natural antistress hormones and actually help to slow the degenerative process. It is for this reason that it is a good idea to begin a regular regimen of herbal tonics sometime after the age of 40. Many tonics classified in one category have properties of all other tonic categories as well. For example, while ginseng is classified as a *qi* tonic, it has demulcent nutritive properties; as the king of tonics, it is said to supplement all deficiencies. The same is true of other *qi* tonics, such as dioscorea (*shan yao*) and astragalus. The daily ingestion of astragalus and lycii berries, a combination that mildly nourishes *qi*, blood, yin, and yang, is of great benefit. This can be taken as a tea or cooked with rice or soup.

It is important to realize, however, that yin and yang do not exist independently of each other. In fact, without any yang *qi*, it is impossible to absorb and use yin energy, just as without yin energy, it is impossible to absorb and use yang. A similar relationship exists between blood and *qi*. For this reason, it is often an important strategy to include just enough yin or yang herbs in a formula so that we are able to take in and use that which we truly need. A small amount of yin will attract yang, and vice versa. Each organ has both a yin and a yang aspect. Generally, dryness of the lungs represents lung yin deficiency; inflammation of the mouth and gums is stomach yin deficiency; liver yin deficiency may result in blurred vision, dry eyes, vertigo, or dizziness; and heart yin deficiency produces insomnia, dream-disturbed sleep, mania, and hallucinations. The kidneys, being the root of yin and yang for the body, can exhibit yin deficiency symptoms also, including weakness and soreness of the lower back, knees, and joints; a sensation of heat on any or all of the so-called Five Burning Spaces (the palms, feet, and chest); insomnia; seminal emissions; and afternoon fever.

Treating these conditions requires that appropriate yin tonic herbs be prescribed along with heat-clearing herbs if there are deficient or yin heat signs. Yin heat is an autoinflammatory condition that occurs as a result of an overworked, exhausted body. Special herbs such as Phellodendron, anemarrhena, and moutan peony are used to clear this type of yin heat. Liver yin deficiency can result in hyperactive liver yang with symptoms of hypertension. For this, one might want to add herbs that clear internal liver wind or that calm spirit, such as abalone shell, gastrodia, or uncaria. Each individual has his or her own unique imbalance of yin, yang, *qi,* or blood, so formulas are created that reflect this.

American ginseng (*XI YANG SHEN*)
Radix panacis quinquefolii
COMMON NAME: American ginseng
FAMILY: Araliaceae
PART USED: Root
ENERGY AND FLAVORS: Cool; sweet, slightly bitter
ORGAN MERIDIANS AFFECTED: Lung, heart, kidney, stomach
PROPERTIES: Yin tonic, calmative
EFFECTS AND INDICATIONS: American Ginseng is a yin tonic that benefits the *qi.* It is used for yin deficiency with heat signs and weakness following febrile diseases when the yin has been injured. It is specific for lung yin deficiency with blazing fire when there is blood-streaked sputum, chronic cough, and loss of voice. It is good for counteracting the effects of stress and increasing endurance.
CONTRAINDICATIONS: American ginseng should not be used by those with a cold damp stomach.
DOSE: 3–9 grams
NOTES: American ginseng is the most well known of all North American tonics. It has been imported by the Chinese from North America since the 1700s. It is an important cash crop where it is grown, mostly in the state of Wisconsin.

Asparagus root (*TIAN MEN DONG*)
Tuber asparagi cochinchinensis
COMMON NAME: Asparagus fern tuber
FAMILY: Liliaceae

PART USED: Tuber

ENERGY AND FLAVORS: Very cold; sweet, bitter

ORGAN MERIDIANS AFFECTED: Lung, kidney

PROPERTIES: Yin tonic, nutritive, demulcent, expectorant

EFFECTS AND INDICATIONS: This herb is indicated for yin deficiency of the lung and kidneys when there are signs of false heat because of the yin deficiency. It is used for lung abscesses and hot sputum that may contain blood and is difficult to expectorate. It moistens the dryness of yin deficiency and lubricates the intestines when there is constipation due to dry intestines.

CONTRAINDICATIONS: Asparagus root should not be used by those with deficiency of the spleen and stomach when there is cold accompanied by diarrhea. It should not be used for wind-cold cough.

DOSE: 6–18 grams

NOTE: The asparagus fern grown throughout Western countries as an ornamental is a different species than the asparagus used in TCM. The Chinese often use many species for the same herb and *Asparagus springerii,* the most commonly available Western species, has sweet-flavored gelatinous tubers that I have eaten and found to be effective.

Ophiopogon (*MAI MEN DONG*)

Tuber ophiopogonis japonici

COMMON NAMES: Ophiopogon, Japanese mondo grass, Japanese turf lily

FAMILY: Liliaceae

PART USED: Tuber

ENERGY AND FLAVORS: Cold; sweet, slightly bitter

ORGAN MERIDIANS AFFECTED: Heart, lung, stomach

PROPERTIES: Yin tonic, demulcent, nutritive, expectorant, lowers blood sugar

INDICATIONS: This herb is indicated for lung yin deficiency when there is dry cough or scanty, blood-streaked sputum. It is also used for stomach yin deficiency with dryness of the mouth and lips, possible mouth sores, and inflammation of the gums. It can be used for febrile diseases when the heat is burning up the fluids of the body. It is also good when there is constipation due to fever that has dried the intestines.

CONTRAINDICATIONS: Ophiopogon should not be used by those with weak spleen and stomach with coldness and diarrhea.

DOSE: 6–12 grams

NOTES: Ophiopogon is commonly grown throughout North America as an ornamental. There are several varieties, and so far, every one that I have tried has been pleasant tasting and certainly an effective yin tonic.

Glehnia root (BEI SHA SHEN)
Radix glehniae
COMMON NAME: Glehnia
FAMILY: Umbelliferae
PART USED: Root
ENERGY AND FLAVORS: Cool; sweet, bland
ORGAN MERIDIANS AFFECTED: Lung, stomach
PROPERTIES: Yin tonic, analgesic, regulates body temperature
EFFECTS AND INDICATIONS: Glehnia is a yin tonic that moistens the lungs, making it useful for treating chronic dry cough with difficult-to-expectorate blood-streaked sputum. It helps to generate fluids and benefits the stomach, especially in the aftermath of a febrile disease. It is also useful for treating dry, itchy skin.
CONTRAINDICATIONS: Glehnia should not be used by those with conditions of wind cold or by those with a weak cold spleen.
DOSE: 6–12 grams
NOTE: Glehnia is considered to have properties almost identical to those of American ginseng and can be used as a substitute for it, especially in the treatment of lung yin deficiency.

Dendrobium orchid (SHI HU)
Herba dendrobii
COMMON NAME: Dendrobium orchid
FAMILY: Orchidaceae
PART USED: Leaf
ENERGY AND FLAVORS: Cold; sweet, slightly salty, bland
ORGAN MERIDIANS AFFECTED: Lung, kidney, stomach
PROPERTIES: Yin tonic, anti-inflammatory, digestive
EFFECTS AND INDICATIONS: This herb is used to replenish fluids, especially in the aftermath of febrile diseases, which often leave one feeling weak and dried up. Similarly, it is used to counteract any excess exertion that tends to consume vital body fluids, such as excessive sex and overwork, leaving one feeling exhausted. It is useful when

there is dry mouth, thirst, dry heaves, or a tongue with a shiny or thin coat. It is also effective for aching soreness of the lower back.

CONTRAINDICATIONS: Dendrobium orchid should not be used by those without signs of heat and dryness. Also, it should not be used in the beginning of febrile diseases.

DOSE: 6–18 grams

Solomon's seal rhizome (YU ZHU)

Rhizoma polygonati odorati

COMMON NAME: Solomon's seal

FAMILY: Liliaceae

PART USED: Rhizome

ENERGY AND FLAVOR: Slightly cold; sweet

ORGAN MERIDIANS AFFECTED: Lung, heart, stomach

PROPERTIES: Yin tonic, demulcent, lowers blood pressure

EFFECTS AND INDICATIONS: This herb is used for dryness of the lung and stomach with such symptoms as dry throat, chronic dry cough, thirst, hunger that cannot be satisfied, and irritability. It is used during febrile diseases to nourish the yin while cooling the body. It generates body fluids, extinguishes wind, and can be used during externally contracted febrile diseases associated with wind.

CONTRAINDICATIONS: Solomon's seal rhizome should not be used by those with cold damp phlegm in the stomach.

DOSE: 6–18 grams

Lily bulb (BAI HE)

Bulbus lilii brownii, Lilii pumilum, L. lancifolium

COMMON NAME: Lily bulb

FAMILY: Liliaceae

PART USED: Bulb

ENERGY AND FLAVORS: Slightly cold; sweet, bland

ORGAN MERIDIANS AFFECTED: Heart, lung

PROPERTIES: Yin tonic, demulcent, sedative, expectorant, antitussive

EFFECTS AND INDICATIONS: Lily bulb is used for dry cough and heat in the lung due to yin deficiency. It nourishes the heart and calms the spirit for heart yin and *qi* deficiency, with such symptoms as restlessness, insomnia, and chronic low-grade fever.

CONTRAINDICATIONS: Lily bulb should not be used by those with such wind-cold conditions as the common cold when there is phlegm or by those with spleen deficiency with diarrhea.

DOSE: 9–30 grams

CAUTION: While these lilies are cultivated as ornamentals, they should not be confused with day lilies, of which only the flowers are used in cooking, or calla lilies, which are poisonous.

Black sesame seed (HEI ZHI MA)

Semen sesami indici

COMMON NAME: Black sesame seed

FAMILY: Pedaliaceae

ENERGY AND FLAVOR: Neutral; sweet

ORGAN MERIDIANS AFFECTED: Kidney, liver

PROPERTIES: Tonic, nutritive, demulcent, laxative

EFFECTS AND INDICATIONS: Black sesame seeds nourish the kidney yin, the liver yin, and blood. They are good for such symptoms as dizziness, premature gray hair, tinnitus, blurred vision, and weakness after severe illness. They are also used to moisten the intestines for constipation due to dryness or blood deficiency.

CONTRAINDICATIONS: Black sesame seed should not be used by those with diarrhea.

DOSE: 9–30 grams

Eclipta (HAN LIAN CAO)

Herba ecliptae prostratae

COMMON NAME: Eclipta

FAMILY: Compositae

PART USED: Leaf

ENERGY AND FLAVORS: Cold; sweet, sour

ORGAN MERIDIANS AFFECTED: Liver, kidney

PROPERTIES: Tonic, hemostatic, antibacterial

EFFECTS AND INDICATIONS: Eclipta is used to nourish the yin of the liver and kidney for such symptoms as premature graying of the hair, tooth loss, blurred vision, and dizziness. It also cools the blood and is used for any kind of bleeding that is associated with reckless movement of blood caused by heat.

CONTRAINDICATIONS: Eclipta should not be used by those with cold deficiency symptoms associated with the spleen or kidney.

DOSE: 6–18 grams

Ligustrum berries (NU ZHEN ZI)

Fructus ligustri lucidi

COMMON NAMES: Ligustrum berries, Japanese privet berries, grossy privet fruit

FAMILY: Oleaceae

ENERGY AND FLAVORS: Neutral; sweet, bitter

ORGAN MERIDIANS AFFECTED: Liver, kidney

PROPERTIES: Yin tonic, immune tonic, anti-inflammatory, diuretic, increase the white blood cell count

EFFECTS AND INDICATIONS: This herb is used to nourish the yin of the liver and kidney and is appropriate for such symptoms as premature graying of the hair, weak back and knees, and eye problems, such as blurred vision and spots in the field of vision. It is also used for yin deficiency with internal heat, as it tonifies yin while it cools heat.

CONTRAINDICATIONS: Ligustrum berries should not be used by those with yang deficiency of the spleen with coldness and diarrhea.

DOSE: 6–12 grams

NOTE: It is important to use the indicated species of privet. **Caution:** Some other privet species may be toxic.

Wood ear (BAI MU ER)

Fructificatio tremellae fuciformis

COMMON NAMES: Wood ear, tremella

FAMILY: Tremellaceae

PART USED: The tree mushroom

ENERGY AND FLAVORS: Neutral; sweet, bland

ORGAN MERIDIANS AFFECTED: Lung, kidney, stomach

PROPERTIES: Tonic, demulcent

EFFECTS AND INDICATIONS: Wood ear is a mushroom that can be used as a food as well as a medicine. It nourishes the yin and moistens the lung for cases of chronic dry cough and cough associated with consumptive diseases when there is blood in the sputum. It nourishes the yin of the stomach for conditions of dry mouth and a thin coat—or no coat—on the tongue.

CONTRAINDICATIONS: Wood ear is a very safe herb and can be eaten freely as food.

DOSE: 3–9 grams

Fresh-water turtle shell (GUI BAN)

Plastrum testudinis
COMMON NAME: Fresh-water turtle shell
FAMILY: Testudinidae
PART USED: Primarily the ventral portion
ENERGY AND FLAVORS: Cold; salty, sweet
ORGAN MERIDIANS AFFECTED: Heart, kidney, liver
PROPERTIES: Hemostatic
EFFECTS AND INDICATIONS: Nourishes the yin and holds down the yang, strengthens the kidneys and the bones, cools the blood, stops uterine bleeding, nourishes the heart, and promotes healing. This herb is used to treat hypertension and other symptoms caused by yin deficiency, such as night sweats, dizziness, tinnitus, and steaming bone fever. It is also used to treat facial spasms and tremors of the hands and feet caused by internal wind from liver yin deficiency. It is given to treat aching soreness of the lower back and legs, retarded bone growth in small children, and failure of the fontanel to close. Because it cools the blood, it inhibits excessive menstrual or uterine bleeding. Finally, it is used to treat anxiety, insomnia, and forgetfulness in addition to nonhealing sores and ulcers.
CONTRAINDICATIONS: Fresh-water turtle shell is contraindicated during pregnancy and for individuals with cold and dampness of the spleen.
DOSE: 9–30 grams

Tortoise shell (BIE JIA)

Amydae sinensis
COMMON NAME: Tortoise shell
FAMILY: Trionychidae
PART USED: Carapax (dorsal aspect)
ENERGY AND FLAVOR: Neutral; salty
ORGAN MERIDIANS AFFECTED: Liver, spleen, kidneys
PROPERTIES: Nourishes yin and subdues exuberant yang, resolves hardness
INDICATIONS: This substance is used to treat yin-deficiency patterns, including night sweats and chronic tidal fevers, to reduce abdominal masses, and to treat an enlarged liver and spleen.
CONTRAINDICATIONS: Tortoise shell should not be used during pregnancy or diarrhea.
DOSE: 9–30 grams

Herbs That Stabilize and Bind: Astringents

There is hardly a more common botanical property than that of astringency. The Chinese concept of herbs that stabilize and bind, however, calls for a much deeper understanding. The most common uses for astringents include the following: inhibiting sweating, checking diarrhea, stopping leukorrhea, controlling bleeding, restraining frequent urination, and stopping any leaking or involuntary discharges, such as seminal leakage or premature ejaculation. Some Chinese astringent herbs are also used for nocturnal emissions (wet dreams), involuntary perspiration, night sweats, and chronic cough and asthma. For all of these conditions, one uses astringents to assist the primary therapeutic aim rather than as an aim itself. Some astringents, such as cornus berries and schisandra berries, however, possess tonic properties that support the effect of tonics and assist the body to retain its vital energy. These are generally used along with other tonics to enhance their effects. As a rule, astringents are not indicated so long as there is any sign of an exterior pathogenic influence. For instance, one should not use astringents for acute colds, influenza, or upper-respiratory phlegm and mucus that should be discharged.

Dogwood berries (SHAN ZHU YU)

Fructus corni officinalis
COMMON NAMES: Cornus, dogwood berries
FAMILY: Cornaceae
ENERGY AND FLAVOR: Warm; sour
ORGAN MERIDIANS AFFECTED: Liver, kidney
PROPERTIES: Astringent, diuretic, tonic
EFFECTS AND INDICATIONS: This herb nourishes the liver and kidney and
    astringes essence. It is used for nocturnal emissions, spontaneous
    sweating, sore back and knees, and dizziness. It tonifies essence and
    assists the yang for cases of shock when there has been a collapse of
    both yang and *qi*. It regulates the menses for cases of uterine bleeding
    and excessive menstruation.
CONTRAINDICATIONS: Dogwood berries should not be used by those with
    fire symptoms or those with damp heat and difficult or painful urina-
    tion.
DOSE: 3–12 grams

Schisandra berries (WU WEI ZI)

Fructus schisandrae chinensis

COMMON NAME: Schisandra berries, five-flavored fruit

FAMILY: Magnoliaceae

ENERGY AND FLAVOR: Warm; sour

ORGAN MERIDIANS AFFECTED: Lung, heart, kidney

PROPERTIES: Astringent, adaptogen (immune potentiating), tonic, antitussive, expectorant

EFFECTS AND INDICATIONS: Tonifies heart, lung, and kidney and astringes the essence. This herb is considered useful for chronic cough with deficiency of the lung and kidney. It is used for kidney deficiency and essence leakeage with such symptoms as nocturnal emissions, night sweats, chronic diarrhea, and urinary incontinence. It also calms the spirit when there is deficiency of the heart and kidney with such symptoms as palpitations, insomina, forgetfulness, and dream-disturbed sleep. This herb is said to have the power to help keep one from losing physical, mental, and spiritual energy.

CONTRAINDICATIONS: Schisandra berries should not be used by those with internal heat or by those with an externally contracted disease.

DOSE: 2–9 grams

Mume plum (WU MEI)

Fructus prunus mume

COMMON NAME: Mume plum, black plum

FAMILY: Rosaceae

PART USED: Fruit

ENERGY AND FLAVOR: Warm; sour

ORGAN MERIDIANS AFFECTED: Liver, lung, spleen, large intestine

PROPERTIES: Astringent, anthelmintic

INDICATIONS: This herb is used for chronic cough caused by lung deficiency. It is also commonly used in cases of chronic diarrhea and dysentery, possibly with symptoms of blood in the stool. It can be used when there are diminished fluids due to internal heat and diabetes. It is one of the most important herbs for worms and other intestinal parasites. Finally, it can be applied externally to remove warts and corns.

CONTRAINDICATIONS: Mume plum should not be used by those with excess and stagnation with internal heat or when there is an external pathogenic influence present.

Dose: 3–9 grams

Notes: There is a Greek tradition of eating a few green plums each spring to aid digestion. Similarly, the Chinese gather the unripe fruits in July, baking them—with the stones still inside—at a low temperature until they become black. The stone is then removed.

Lotus seeds (LIAN ZI)

Semen nelumbinis nuciferae

Common Name: Lotus seeds

Family: Nymphaeceae

Energies and Flavor: Astringent, neutral; sweet

Organ Meridians Affected: Heart, spleen, kidney

Properties: Astringent, tonic, sedative

Effects and Indications: This herb is both astringent and tonic and therefore is very useful for chronic diarrhea due to spleen deficiency. It is also useful for kidney deficiency with such symptoms as premature ejaculation and vaginal discharge. It can be used as a tonic for the heart and to calm the spirit in such conditions as insomnia, palpitations, and anxiety.

Contraindications: Lotus seeds should not be used by those with constipation or abdominal distension.

Dose: 6–18 grams

Euryale seeds (QIAN SHI)

Euryales ferocis

Common Name: Foxnuts, euryale seeds

Family: Nymphaeceae

Energies and Flavor: Astringent, neutral; sweet

Organ Meridians Affected: Kidney, spleen

Properties: Antidiarrheal

Effects and Indications: Tonifies the spleen, strengthens the kidneys and restrains essence, dispels dampness and relieves leukorrhea. This herb is especially good for diarrhea in children. It is also used for nocturnal emission, premature ejaculation, spermatorrhea, urinary incontinence, and clear or whitish vaginal discharge.

Contraindications: No contraindications are noted for euryale seeds.

Dose: 9–15 grams.

Notes: This herb is very similar to lotus seeds; the two herbs are frequently used together. Both lotus and euryale seeds are commonly cooked in soups and added to food for their high nutritive tonic properties.

Rose hips (JIN YING ZI)
Rosae laevigatae
COMMON NAME: Rose hips
FAMILY: Rosaceae
ENERGIES AND FLAVOR: Astringent, neutral; sour
ORGAN MERIDIANS AFFECTED: Bladder, kidneys, large intestine
PROPERTIES: Intestinal astringent, antidiuretic
EFFECTS AND INDICATIONS: Controls essence. This herb is combined with euryale seeds and dodder seeds to treat seminal emissions and clear leukorrhea. For the treatment of chronic diarrhea caused by deficient spleen, it is combined with codonopsis, atractylodes, and dioscorea.
CONTRAINDICATIONS: Rose hips should not be used for acute conditions caused by excess heat.
DOSE: 6–9 grams

Chinese raspberries (FU PEN ZI)
Rubi chingii
COMMON NAME: Chinese raspberries
FAMILY: Rosaceae
ENERGIES AND FLAVOR: Astringent, slightly warm; sweet
ORGAN MERIDIANS AFFECTED: Kidney, liver
EFFECTS AND INDICATIONS: Augments the kidneys, restrains essence, supports yang. This herb is used for seminal emissions, premature ejaculation, spermatorrhea, enuresis, and urinary frequency caused by deficient kidneys. It is used to improve eyesight and treats aching lower back and impotence caused by kidney and liver deficiency.
CONTRAINDICATIONS: Use Chinese raspberries with caution for yin deficiency patterns.
DOSE: 6–9 grams

Ephedra root (MA HUANG GEN)
Ephedra sinensis
COMMON NAME: Ephedra root
FAMILY: Ephedraceae
PART USED: Root
ENERGY AND FLAVOR: Neutral; sweet

ORGAN MERIDIAN AFFECTED: Lungs

PROPERTY: Antisudorific

EFFECTS AND INDICATIONS: Stops sweating caused by yin deficiency. This herb is useful for spontaneous sweating, night sweats, and postpartum sweating caused by yin deficiency.

CONTRAINDICATIONS: Ephedra root should not be used for exterior conditions.

DOSE: 3–9 grams

Glutinous rice root (NUO DAO GEN XU)

Radix et rhizoma oryzae glutinosae

COMMON NAME: Glutinous rice root

FAMILY: Gramineae

PARTS USED: Root and rhizome

ENERGY AND FLAVOR: Neutral; sweet

ORGAN MERIDIANS AFFECTED: Kidneys, liver, lungs

PROPERTY: Antisudorific

EFFECTS AND INDICATIONS: Stops sweating caused by yin deficiency. It is used to treat yin deficiency fevers.

CONTRAINDICATIONS: No contraindications for glutinous rice root are noted.

DOSE: 15–60 grams

Cuttlefish bone (HAI PIAO XIAO)

Os sepiae seu sepiellae

COMMON NAME: Cuttlefish bone

FAMILY: Sepiidae

ENERGIES AND FLAVORS: Astringent, slightly warm; salty

ORGAN MERIDIANS AFFECTED: Kidney, liver, stomach

PROPERTIES: Hemostatic, antacid, analgesic

EFFECTS AND INDICATIONS: Astringes and stops bleeding, controls essence and relieves leukorrhea, counteracts stomach acidity and stops pain, and heals ulcers. It is used to stop uterine bleeding and vaginal discharge; the powder can also be applied topically to stop bleeding from wounds and injuries. It controls gastrointestinal acidity and relieves abdominal pains. Cuttlefish bone resolves dampness; its powder can be topically applied to promote the healing of wounds, sores, and weeping eczema. It is also effective for the treatment of diarrhea and dysentery caused by deficiency with pressure sensitivity around the navel.

CONTRAINDICATIONS: Cuttlefish bone should not be used for conditions of deficient yin and excessive heat.

DOSE: 6–12 grams

Light wheat (FU XIAO MAI)
Triticum aestivum
COMMON NAME: Light wheat
FAMILY: Gramineae
PART USED: Sprouted grain
ENERGY AND FLAVOR: Cool; sweet
ORGAN MERIDIANS AFFECTED: Heart
PROPERTY: Antisudorific
EFFECTS AND INDICATIONS: This herb tonifies qi, clears heat and stops sweating.
DOSE: 15–30 grams

Mantis egg case (SANG PIAO XIAO)
Ootheca mantidis
COMMON NAME: Mantis egg case, mantis
FAMILY: Mantidae
ENERGY AND FLAVORS: Neutral; sweet, salty
ORGAN MERIDIANS AFFECTED: Kidney, liver
PROPERTY: Antidiuretic
EFFECTS AND INDICATIONS: Tonifies kidneys and strengthens yang; restrains essence and decreases urination. For seminal emission, nocturnal enuresis, urinary incontinence, premature ejaculation, or clear or whitish leukorrhea, this herb is combined with dragon bone, oyster shell, dodder seeds, and psoralea fruit.
CONTRAINDICATIONS: Mantis egg case should not be used for excessive fire or deficient yin patterns or cystitis.
DOSE: 3–9 grams
RECIPE: For the above conditions, combine 9 grams each of mantis egg case, dragon bone, oyster shell, dodder seeds, and psoralea fruit.

Ginkgo nut (BAI GUO)
Semen ginkgo biloba
COMMON NAME: Ginkgo nut

FAMILY: Ginkgoaceae

ENERGIES AND FLAVORS: Astringent, neutral, slightly toxic; sweet, bitter

ORGAN MERIDIANS AFFECTED: Lung, kidney

PROPERTIES: Antibacterial, astringent, antifungal

EFFECTS AND INDICATIONS: Ginkgo nuts assist the lung *qi* and help with phlegm expectoration, and stop chronic cough and wheezing. They are also used for vaginal discharge and frequent urination, in cases of both deficiency and damp heat.

CONTRAINDICATIONS: Ginkgo nuts should not be used when there is excess or cold and dampness and should be used with caution when there is slimy, difficult-to-expectorate sputum. It should not be used in large doses or for long periods of time.

DOSE: 6–9 grams

NOTE: *Ginkgo biloba* is known as the oldest tree species on the earth today. Its hardiness is exemplified in its ability to survive the exhaust-filled streets of New York City and in the fact that a ginkgo tree was the only tree to survive the Hiroshima atomic blast. (That tree is still living today.) Ginkgo trees have been known to live well over an average of 1,000 years, as long as there has been written history in China. Ginkgo has become one of the most popular herbs in the West because of the unique ability of the concentrated extract of the leaves (24:1) to improve cerebral blood circulation and blood circulation generally. Because of this ability, it has become widely accepted as a treatment to prevent or lessen the effects of senile dementia and Alzheimer's disease. Its circulatory properties have many other practical uses, ranging from strengthening the vascular system and reducing clots to improving hearing and treating tinnitus (ringing in the ears), improving blood circulation in the eye (which helps prevent macular degeneration), reducing the incidence and severity of asthma attacks, and helping to prevent organ transplant rejection. Much of its circulatory powers exist because of its high flavonoid content. Ginkgo is also able to increase acetylcholine levels, which improves the body's ability to transmit electrical impulses. The ancient doctrine of signatures taught that what a thing resembles may be an indication of its use. We have scientifically corroborated the value of the ginkgo tree—as one of the oldest surviving species on the earth—in the treatment of conditions associated with aging and the promotion of human longevity.

Substances That Calm the Spirit

SUBSTANCES THAT ANCHOR, SETTLE, AND CALM THE SPIRIT

Because the spirit represents the mind, herbs that are said to anchor, settle, and calm the spirit are commonly used for heart qi and blood deficiency. In general, symptoms calling for the use of these herbs include restless anxiety, insomnia, irritability, hysteria, dream-disturbed sleep, mania, and psychotic disorders. As with all Chinese herbal treatments, the herbs are generally combined with herbs that treat deficient yin, yang, blood, or qi as indicated. For instance, if there are complications of flaring of heart fire with severe emotional disturbance, herbs such as coptis and cinnabar are combined to relieve this condition. For epilepsy and convulsions, herbs that dissolve phlegm, such as bamboo shavings, are used along with antispasmodic herbs that calm internal wind, such as uncaria stem or gastrodia. Many of the herbs in this category are heavy minerals and are described as weighting the qi to subdue restless energy. This is not unlike the use of lithium in Western medicine, which is used to treat manic depression. Finally, milder tranquilizing herbs in the second part of this category can be used much as valerian, chamomile, hops, and other mild nervines are used in Western herbalism. Some of these, however, such as zizyphus seeds, have special potency that truly feeds the nervous system.

Dragon bone (LONG GU)
Os draconis
COMMON NAME: Dragon bone
ENERGIES AND FLAVOR: Astringent, neutral; sweet
ORGAN MERIDIANS AFFECTED: Liver, heart, kidney
PROPERTIES: Sedative, astringent
EFFECTS AND INDICATIONS: This substance is used to calm the spirit for such symptoms as insomnia, anxiety, restlessness, and fright. It anchors liver yang for such symptoms as irritability, excessive anger, emotional mood swings, and blurred vision. It restrains the leakage of fluids that occur as a result of deficiency, including night sweats, vaginal discharge, nocturnal emissions, and spontaneous sweating.
CONTRAINDICATIONS: Dragon bone should not be used by those with symptoms of damp heat.
DOSE: 15–30 grams

NOTE: Dragon bone originates from the ossified bones of domestic and possibly prehistoric mammals. It should be cooked for 30–45 minutes before any herbs or other substances are added.

Oyster shell (MU LI)

Concha ostrea gigas
COMMON NAME: Oyster shell
FAMILY: Ostreidae
ENERGIES AND FLAVORS: Astringent, slightly cold; salty
ORGAN MERIDIANS AFFECTED: Liver, kidney
PROPERTIES: Sedative, demulcent, antacid, astringent
INDICATIONS: Oyster shell is used to calm the spirit and assist the yin. It is good for such symptoms as anxiety, palpitations, insomnia, irritability, and excessive anger. It is also used as an astringent for spontaneous sweating, night sweats, vaginal discharge, and nocturnal emissions. Finally, it is used to soften hard lumps of all kinds, especially hardening of the lymph nodes.
CONTRAINDICATIONS: Oyster shell should not be used by those who are cold and weak nor by those with high fever without sweating.
DOSE: 15–30 grams; it should be cooked for 30–45 minutes before any herbs or other substances are added.

Cinnabar (ZHU SHA)

Cinnabaris
COMMON NAME: Cinnabar
ENERGIES AND FLAVOR: Cool, toxic; sweet
ORGAN MERIDIAN AFFECTED: Heart
PROPERTIES: Antispasmodic, sedative, antitoxin
INDICATIONS: Depending on the herbs that it is combined with, cinnabar can be used for any pattern associated with disturbance of the spirit. It clears heat, is antispasmodic, and can be used for convulsions caused by epilepsy or very high fever in children. It also relieves toxicity topically, as in from bodily sores, carbuncles, mouth sores, and snakebite.
CONTRAINDICATIONS: Cinnabar should not be used by those without heat signs. It should not be used in large doses or for extended periods of time. **Caution:** Cinnabar is considered toxic and should be taken in powdered form only. *Do not cook.*
DOSE: 0.3–2 grams

NOTE: This substance is included here only for informational purposes. Cinnabar should be used only when dispensed by qualified Chinese herbalists.

Magnetitum (CI SHI)

COMMON NAME: Magnetitum
ENERGY AND FLAVORS: Cold; spicy, salty
ORGAN MERIDIANS AFFECTED: Kidneys, liver, lung, heart
EFFECTS AND INDICATIONS: Calms and sedates the spirit, calms the liver and lowers rising liver yang, helps the kidneys grasp lung qi. It is used for insomnia, restlessness, tremors, convulsions, irritability, dizziness, vertigo, tinnitus, and blurred eyesight. It is also used to treat asthma caused by kidney deficiency.
CONTRAINDICATIONS: Magnetitum should be used for only short periods because of the possible associated presence of heavy metals.
DOSE: 9–30 grams
NOTE: Crush magnetitum into a fine powder and simmer it several hours before adding any herbs to the formula.

Hematitum (DAI ZHE SHI)

COMMON NAMES: Hematite, red ochre
ENERGY AND FLAVOR: Cold; bitter
ORGAN MERIDIANS AFFECTED: Liver, stomach, pericardium, heart
PROPERTY: Hemostatic
EFFECTS AND INDICATIONS: Calms the liver, anchors uprising yang, clears liver fire, moves qi downward, cools the blood. Hematitum is used to treat hyperactive liver yang caused by yin deficiency with symptoms of irritability, dizziness, vertigo, tinnitus, and blurred vision. It is also used to treat acute asthma, vomiting, nausea, and hiccups by causing rebellious qi to descend. In addition hematitum is used to treat nosebleeds, coughing up of blood, and uterine bleeding.
CONTRAINDICATIONS: Use hematitum cautiously during pregnancy. Because it most likely contains traces of arsenic, it should be used for only short periods.
DOSE: 9–30 grams
NOTE: Crush hematite to a fine powder and cook for 2 hours before adding any herbs or other substances to a formula. This substance is included here only for informational purposes. Hematitum should be used only when dispensed by qualified Chinese herbalists.

HERBS THAT TRANQUILIZE AND NOURISH THE HEART AND CALM THE SPIRIT

Zizyphus seeds (SUAN ZAO REN)

Semen zizyphi spinosae

COMMON NAMES: Zizyphus seeds, wild jujube seeds

FAMILY: Rhamnaceae

ENERGY AND FLAVORS: Neutral; sweet, sour

ORGAN MERIDIANS AFFECTED: Liver, heart, spleen, gallbladder

PROPERTIES: Sedative, nutritive, tonic, analgesic, lower body temperature

EFFECTS AND INDICATIONS: This herb is a tonic to the heart and blood and can be used for deficiency patterns with such symptoms as insomnia, irritability, restlessness, and palpitations. It is also used for spontaneous sweating and night sweats. This herb is very tasty and can be used with food. Try it raw in a trail mix with other herbs, such as lycii berries *(Fructus lycii [gou qi zi]),* as a tonic snack.

CONTRAINDICATIONS: Zizyphus seeds should not be used when there is extreme fire in the body or in cases of severe diarrhea.

DOSE: 6–18 grams

Polygala (YUAN ZHI)

Radix polygalae tenuifoliae

COMMON NAMES: Polygala, Chinese senega

FAMILY: Polygalaceae

PART USED: Root

ENERGY AND FLAVORS: Warm; bitter, acrid

ORGAN MERIDIANS AFFECTED: Heart, lung, kidney

PROPERTIES: Expectorant, sedative, antibacterial, lowers blood pressure

EFFECTS AND INDICATIONS: This herb is very effective for disturbance of the spirit when there is phlegm confusing the heart, with such symptoms as insomnia, palpitations, anxiety, mental disturbances, and instances when the emotions have been held in without healthy expression. It is an expectorant and can be used for coughs with sputum that is difficult to expectorate. It also can be used externally or internally for sores and abscesses.

CONTRAINDICATIONS: Polygala should not be used by those with false heat signs in yin deficiency.

DOSE: 3–9 grams

Biota seeds (BAI ZI REN)

Semen biotae orientalis

COMMON NAME: Biota seeds

FAMILY: Cupressaceae

ENERGY AND FLAVOR: Neutral; sweet

ORGAN MERIDIANS AFFECTED: Heart, liver, kidney, large intestine

PROPERTIES: Sedative, mild laxative, emollient, tonic

EFFECTS AND INDICATIONS: This herb is used as a tonic for the heart blood and calms the spirit for symptoms such as insomnia, palpitations, and forgetfulness. It is used as a mild laxative for cases of constipation due to deficiency of either yin or blood, especially for the elderly.

CONTRAINDICATIONS: Biota seeds should not be used by those with diarrhea or for conditions of phlegm.

DOSE: 3–15 grams

NOTES: The fruits are gathered in the autumn. These are then shelled and dried in the shade. The seeds are further crushed and broken for use.

Fleeceflower stem (YE JIAO TENG)

Caulis polygoni multiflori

COMMON NAMES: Fleeceflower stem, *he shou wu* stem

FAMILY: Polygonaceae

ENERGY AND FLAVORS: Neutral; sweet, slightly bitter

ORGAN MERIDIANS AFFECTED: Heart, liver

PROPERTIES: Sedative, tonic

EFFECTS AND INDICATIONS: This herb is used as a tonic to the heart and the blood and to calm the spirit for such symptoms as irritability, insomnia, and dream-disturbed sleep. It can be used externally for itching and rashes.

CONTRAINDICATIONS: Fleeceflower stem should not be used by those with diarrhea.

DOSE: 9–30 grams

Albizzia bark (HE HUAN PI)

Albizzia julibrissin

COMMON NAMES: Albizzia bark, mimosa tree bark

FAMILY: Leguminosae

ENERGY AND FLAVOR: Neutral; sweet

ORGAN MERIDIANS AFFECTED: Heart, liver

PROPERTIES: Sedative, analgesic

EFFECTS AND INDICATIONS: This herb is used to tranquilize the mind and relieve depression, invigorate blood, relieve pain, and reduce swelling.

DOSE: 10–15 grams

NOTE: The flowers have similar properties to those of the bark. The translation of the Chinese name is "happiness bark," perhaps referring to both the tree's beauty when it is in flower and its ability to help counteract feelings of anger and depression.

Aromatic Substances That Revive from Unconsciousness

Chinese reviving herbs are used similarly to Western smelling salts. They can be used for a wide variety of conditions, from simple fainting, called syncope, to delirium, convulsions, coma, and epilepsy. Herbs in this category are strongly stimulating to circulation and are strictly used for first-aid treatment for a short period of time. Because of their strongly aromatic potency, some, such as musk and borneol, can be used in small amounts as carriers to intensify the properties of other herbs that are used topically.

Musk (SHE XIANG)

Secretio moschus

COMMON NAME: Musk

FAMILY: Cervidae

ENERGY AND FLAVOR: Warm; acrid

ORGAN MERIDIANS AFFECTED: Heart, spleen, liver

PROPERTIES: Stimulant (small doses), emmenagogue, carminative, antibacterial, anti-inflammatory

EFFECTS AND INDICATIONS: This is a very powerful substance used for reviving people from loss of consciousness. It can relieve seizures, convulsions, and delirium due to fire entering the pericardium. It moves blood and can be used for pain and swelling from traumatic injuries, obstruction, and tumors. It is also used for assisting delivery of stillborns and placenta that does not descend on its own.

CONTRAINDICATIONS: Musk should not be used by pregnant women or in cases of yin deficiency with heat signs. It should be used with caution by those with high blood pressure.

DOSE: 0.075–0.15 grams

Benzoin (AN XI XIANG)

Benzoinum

COMMON NAME: Benzoin

FAMILY: Styracaceae

ENERGY AND FLAVORS: Neutral; acrid, bitter

ORGAN MERIDIANS AFFECTED: Heart, liver, spleen

PROPERTIES: Stimulant, expectorant, antibacterial, preservative

INDICATIONS: Benzoin is used for loss of consciousness with distension of the chest by moving *qi* and blood. It can be used as an expectorant for sputum that is difficult to expectorate. It is also used for painful obstruction of *qi* or blood in the chest or abdomen.

CONTRAINDICATIONS: Benzoin should not be used by those with yin deficiency with signs of fire.

DOSE: 0.3–1.5 grams

Borneol (BING PIAN)

COMMON NAME: Borneol

FAMILY: Dyptercarpaceae or Compositae

ENERGY AND FLAVORS: Slightly cold; acrid, bitter

ORGAN MERIDIANS AFFECTED: Heart, lung, spleen

PROPERTIES: Antibacterial, analgesic, anti-inflammatory, stimulant

INDICATIONS: This substance is used for reviving people from fainting and convulsions. It is also used externally for inflammation and pain as well as internally for pain and inflammation of the throat and stomach.

CONTRAINDICATIONS: Borneol should not be used by those who are weak or anemic due to *qi* or blood deficiency; it should not be used during pregnancy.

DOSE: 0.03–0.1 grams

NOTE: Do not expose borneol to extreme heat or flame.

Sweetflag (SHI CHANG PU)

Rhizoma acori graminei

COMMON NAMES: Sweetflag, calamus

FAMILY: Araceae

PART USED: Rhizome

ENERGY AND FLAVOR: Warm; acrid

ORGAN MERIDIANS AFFECTED: Heart, liver, stomach

PROPERTIES: Stimulant, carminative, expectorant, lowers body temperature, antispasmodic, antifungal

INDICATIONS: This herb is used for expelling phlegm when it is causing symptoms such as deafness, forgetfulness, or other such obstructions of the senses. It is used when there are disturbances of digestion caused by dampness that interferes with the spleen's function, causing symptoms of pain and abdominal distension. It is also used externally for *bi* (blockage) pain caused by wind-cold damp conditions of obstruction and for trauma.

CONTRAINDICATIONS: Sweetflag should not be used by those with yin deficiency with heat signs and should be used with caution by those with excessive sweating or spermatorrhea.

DOSE: 3–9 grams

Substances That Extinguish Internal Wind and Stop Tremors

Substances that extinguish internal wind and stop tremors comprise one of the most wonderful and powerful categories of TCM. The alternative pharmaceutical drugs, such as dopamine, are often accumulatively toxic. The main use for these herbs is to treat tremors, convulsions, and spasms, which are described as the stirring of liver wind caused by the hyperactivity of liver yang. What does this mean in Western parlance? Envision the neurological system's becoming chronically shorted out, as happens in machinery when bare electric wires are touched together. The result is that certain neurons unintentionally continue to fire, causing a fixed spastic reaction or fixed movement. From the TCM perspective, this is caused by a weakness of both yin substance and blood. The meaning here includes not only neurons but quite possibly also various neurotransmitter hormones whose importance is now being more profoundly understood and appreciated in Western medicine.

The cause of internal liver wind can be biochemical, as a result of inherited factors, prolonged stress, or an accident. A continued spasmodic state can often result in an inflammatory state that ultimately further injures the yin or substance of the body. Antelope horn, a representative substance in the category, is thought to possess a special form of bioavailable calcium and other biochemical constituents that nourish the nerves, counteract inflammation, and quite possibly provide important nutritional precursors for neurotransmitter hormones. Other herbs in this category, such as uncaria stem and gastrodia, are among the most wonderful antispasmodics known. Uncaria is actually related to South American uncaria or South American cat's-claw vine, and they both possess powerful anti-inflammatory properties. In most cases of internal liver wind, it is important to add heat-clearing herbs to the formula to further relieve the cause of the condition. One common internal liver wind disease that displays a prominent inflammatory characteristic is lockjaw as a result of rabies.

Uncaria stem (GOU TENG)
Ramulus cum uncis uncariae
COMMON NAMES: Uncaria stem, gambir, hook vine
FAMILY: Rubiaceae
ENERGY AND FLAVOR: Slightly cold; sweet
ORGAN MERIDIANS AFFECTED: Heart, liver, pericardium
PROPERTIES: Antispasmodic, sedative, anticonvulsant, antipyretic, lowers blood pressure
EFFECTS AND INDICATIONS: This herb is used for convulsions and spasms caused by internally generated wind. It also cools the liver for liver yang rising with such symptoms as irritability, vertigo, headache, and red eyes.
CONTRAINDICATIONS: Uncaria stem should be used with caution by those with heat from excess.
DOSE: 3–15 grams

Gastrodia (TIAN MA)
Rhizoma gastrodiae elatae
COMMON NAME: Gastrodia
FAMILY: Orchidaceae
PART USED: Rhizome
ENERGY AND FLAVOR: Neutral; sweet
ORGAN MERIDIAN AFFECTED: Liver
PROPERTIES: Sedative, analgesic, anticonvulsant, cholagogue
INDICATIONS: This herb is used for liver wind that is generated by either heat or cold and is causing such symptoms as convulsions, dizziness, epilepsy, or intestinal spasms. It is also used for rising liver yang with such symptoms as headache and dizziness. It can also be used for patterns of wind damp painful obstruction with such symptoms as pain in the joints and numbness of the limbs and lower back. This

herb can be used for heat, cold, or deficiency of yin or blood, depending on the other herbs in the formula.

CONTRAINDICATIONS: Gastrodia should not be taken in large doses or for extended periods of time.

DOSE: 3–9 grams

Puncture vine fruit (BAI JI LI)
Fructus tribuli terrestris

COMMON NAMES: Puncture vine fruit, tribulus

FAMILY: Zygophyllaceae

ENERGY AND FLAVORS: Warm; acrid, bitter

ORGAN MERIDIANS AFFECTED: Liver, lung

PROPERTIES: Antispasmodic, calmative, lowers blood pressure, galactagogue

INDICATIONS: This herb is used to soothe the liver and calm rising liver yang with such symptoms as headache and dizziness. It is also used for other stagnant liver *qi* causing lack of mother's milk, pain and distension in the epigastric region, red and painful eyes, dizziness and itching.

CONTRAINDICATIONS: Puncture vine fruit should not be used by women during pregnancy or by those with either yin deficiency or blood deficiency.

DOSE: 3–9 grams

Abalone shell (SHI JUE MING)
Concha haliotidis

COMMON NAME: Abalone shell

FAMILY: Haliotidae

ENERGY AND FLAVOR: Cold; salty

ORGAN MERIDIANS AFFECTED: Liver, kidney

PROPERTIES: Antispasmodic, antipyretic

INDICATIONS: Abalone shell is used for patterns of liver heat with rising yang causing such symptoms as headache, dizziness, spasms of the limbs, and various conditions of the eyes.

CONTRAINDICATIONS: Abalone shell should not be used by those without true heat signs.

DOSE: 9–30 grams.

NOTE: Abalone shell should always be crushed and precooked at least 30 minutes before other ingredients are added.

Antelope horn (LING YANG JIAO)

Cornus saigae tataricae

COMMON NAME: Antelope horn

FAMILY: Bovidae

PART USED: Horn

ENERGY AND FLAVOR: Cold; salty

ORGAN MERIDIANS AFFECTED: Heart, liver

PROPERTIES: Antipyretic, antitoxin

EFFECTS AND INDICATIONS: Clears internal liver wind, subdues yang, clears liver fire, brightens the eyes, eliminates toxins, reduces fever. Antelope horn is used for high fever with spasms, convulsions, delirium, mania, and loss of consciousness. It is also used to treat high blood pressure with dizziness and blurred vision, headache, and eye inflammation and pains.

DOSE: 0.9–3 grams when taken in powders or pills; 1.5–3 grams when taken in decoctions.

NOTES: Antelope horn should be cooked for 1 hour before other ingredients are added. Antelope is perhaps the most representative substance in this important category; however, because of ecological considerations, goat horn (*Cornus naemorhedis [shan yang jiao]*) is commonly being used as a substitute. While having properties similar to those of antelope horn, goat horn is weaker, necessitating the use of a significantly higher dosage of 9–15 grams.

Earthworm (DI LONG)

COMMON NAMES: Earthworm, lumbricus

FAMILY: Megascolecidae

ENERGY AND FLAVOR: Cold; salty

ORGAN MERIDIANS AFFECTED: Liver, spleen, bladder

PROPERTY: Antiasthmatic

EFFECTS AND INDICATIONS: Clears heat and calms internal liver wind, soothes asthma; opens the channels. This substance is used to treat convulsions and spasms caused by high fever. It is also used for asthma, cystitis, and urinary stones.

DOSE: 6–15 grams

RECIPES: For convulsions and spasms, use with 6 grams each of uncaria, silkworm, and scorpion. For asthma, use earthworm with ephedra and apricot seed. For cystitis and urinary stones, combine earthworm with plantain seed, achyranthes, lysimachia, and abutilon seeds.

NOTES: Earthworms have been used as an inexpensive protein food source in many cultures. The use of worms and insects in Traditional Chinese Medicine (TCM) has its counterpart in the traditional medicine of Western Europe as recent as 500 years ago. Insects represent the essence of pure neurological instinct, which mirrors certain aspects of internal wind patterns that have to do with involuntary reflexes, such as spasms, seizures, shaking, toxins, strokes, and so forth. Insects are described as possessing "strange proteins" that seem to have a corrective effect on the nervous system. Today, it is customary to render these into a powder and take them in capsules alone or with an appropriate herbal decoction.

Scorpion (QUAN XIE)

Buthus martensi

COMMON NAMES: Scorpion, buthus

FAMILY: Buthidae

ENERGY AND FLAVORS: Toxic; pungent, neutral

ORGAN MERIDIAN AFFECTED: Liver

PROPERTIES: Antispasmodic, antitoxin, analgesic

EFFECTS AND INDICATIONS: Subdues internal wind; clears toxins; stops pain. Scorpion is used to stop tremors and convulsions in such conditions as opisthotonos, tics, and epilepsy. It detoxifies sores, swellings, and swollen glands. It opens the channels (acupuncture meridians) and is used to treat stubborn headaches, such as migraines and other wind damp pains.

CONTRAINDICATIONS: Scorpion is toxic and overdose should be avoided. It should not be used in those with blood deficiency or during pregnancy.

DOSE: 2–5 grams; 0.6–1 gram of the powder

NOTES: Just as some cultures consume roasted grasshoppers as a food, the Chinese roast scorpions and eat them as a health food. One source informed me that in certain areas of China, people believe that consuming 10 scorpions a month will protect one from all diseases.

Centipede (WU GONG)

Scolopendra subspinipes

COMMON NAME: Centipede, scolopendra

FAMILY: Scolopendridae

ENERGIES AND FLAVOR: Warm, toxic; pungent

ORGAN MERIDIAN AFFECTED: Liver

PROPERTIES: Antispasmodic, antitoxin

EFFECTS AND INDICATIONS: Subdues internal wind, clears toxins, opens the channels, and stops pain. Centipede is used for spasms, tetany, convulsions, and epilepsy. It treats venomous bites and stings, clears toxins, and reduces swollen glands. It also treats stubborn migraine headaches and rheumatic pains.

CONTRAINDICATIONS: Centipede is a toxic substance and the dosage should be conservative. It should not be used during pregnancy. It is taken with the legs removed.

DOSE: 1–3 grams; 0.6–0.9 grams as a powder

Silkworm (JIANG CAN)

Bombyx batryticatus

COMMON NAME: Silkworm, stiff silkworm

FAMILY: Bombycidae

ENERGY AND FLAVORS: Neutral; acrid, salty

ORGAN MERIDIANS AFFECTED: Liver, lung

PROPERTIES: Antispasmodic, antitoxin

EFFECTS AND INDICATIONS: Subdues internal wind, expels wind, stops pain, clears toxins, dissipates nodules. Silkworm is used to treat childhood convulsions, Bell's palsy, epilepsy, and tetanus. It is effective for migraine headaches, sore throat, conjunctivitis, eye pains, and rheumatic pains. It can also be used for toxic swellings and swollen glands.

CONTRAINDICATIONS: Silkworm is traditionally contraindicated with platycodon, poria, dioscorea, hypoglauca, and mantis egg case.

DOSE: 3–10 grams; 0.9–1.5 grams of the powder

Herbs That Expel Parasites

One of the most traditional uses of herbs is for parasites. Today, it may be more convenient to use Western pharmaceuticals prescribed by a medical doctor; however, there are frequent occasions when these may not work and the more traditional methods may work better. Besides, many feel that the side effects of some Western pharmaceuticals are so devastating to the intestinal flora that they severely compromise the body's ability to prevent reinfestation.

Intestinal and other parasites are a common problem in tropical, humid climates. In these areas, it is a good idea to begin each morning with 1 or 2 tablespoons of concentrated bitter syrup or tea of such an herb as mugwort (*Artemisia vulgaris*) and 1 teaspoon of turmeric powder, which can be put into capsules if desired. In addition, the regular ingestion each morning of triphala will be of assistance both in the prevention of and during treatment for parasites. To prepare and administer an herbal compound for intestinal parasites, prepare the mixture by grinding the herbs to a fine powder. This is then mixed with honey to make a pill that contains about 6 to 9 grams of the ingredients. The honey or something sweet taken with the herbal compound is important because it serves as an attractive bait for the parasites to ingest the material. Otherwise, sweets and flour products in all forms should be strictly eliminated from the diet for at least a few days before taking the mixture and 2 weeks afterward. Take the mixture on an empty stomach first thing in the morning. To furnish roughage to aid elimination, chew and eat 2 to 4 tablespoons of uncooked brown rice. Eat only pan-toasted brown rice throughout the course of treatment. Repeat the dose of the herbs twice midday and early evening. In the evening, take an herbal laxative, such as 9 grams rhubarb root, 9 grams mirabilitum, 6 grams citrus peel, and 3 grams of licorice root. Repeat as needed for up to 3 days. Repeat again every 2 weeks for 2 more times (in case the eggs of the worms hatch out to begin infestation again).

Quisqualis (SHI JUN ZI)

Fructus quisqualis indicae

COMMON NAMES: Quisqualis, rangoon creeper

FAMILY: Combretaceae

PART USED: Fruit

ENERGY AND FLAVOR: Warm; sweet

ORGAN MERIDIANS AFFECTED: Spleen, stomach

PROPERTIES: Anthelmintic, antifungal

INDICATIONS: This herb is used to expel parasites and is particularly good for roundworms. It is also used to strengthen the spleen, thus improving digestion, and can be used for malnutrition and other digestive problems in children.

CONTRAINDICATIONS: Quisqualis should not be used by those with weak spleen from cold or by those with diarrhea.

DOSE: 6–12 grams

Chinaberry bark (KU LIAN GEN PI)

Cortex meliae azedarach radicis, Melia toosendan
COMMON NAMES: Chinaberry bark, melia, chinatree
FAMILY: Meliaceae
ENERGIES AND FLAVOR: Cold, toxic; bitter
ORGAN MERIDIANS AFFECTED: Liver, spleen, stomach
PROPERTIES: Anthelmintic, antifungal
INDICATIONS: This herb is used for all kinds of parasites of the intestines, vagina, and skin. It can be taken internally or used topically.
CONTRAINDICATIONS: Chinaberry bark should not be taken for long periods of time and should be used with extreme caution by those with weak constitutions or those with liver problems.
DOSE: 6–12 grams

Torreya (FEI ZI)

Semen torreyae grandis
COMMON NAME: Torreya
FAMILY: Taxaceae
PART USED: Seed
ENERGIES AND FLAVOR: Astringent, neutral; sweet
ORGAN MERIDIANS AFFECTED: Lung, large intestine, stomach
PROPERTIES: Anthelmintic, mild laxative
EFFECTS AND INDICATIONS: This is an important anthelmintic herb because it is not toxic and has a laxative effect. It can be used for most kinds of intestinal parasites, such as tapeworms, hookworms, and roundworms. It can be used for mild constipation and abdominal pain caused by intestinal parasites. It can also be used for mild coughs due to dryness in the lungs.
CONTRAINDICATIONS: No contraindications for torreya have been noted.
DOSE: 6–12 grams

Pumpkin seeds (NAN GUA ZI)

Semen cucurbitae moschatae
COMMON NAME: Pumpkin seeds
FAMILY: Cucurbitaceae
ENERGY AND FLAVOR: Neutral; sweet
ORGAN MERIDIANS AFFECTED: Large intestine, stomach
PROPERTIES: Anthelmintic, nutrient
INDICATIONS: This herb is used for many kinds of intestinal parasites and

has a nutritious value, so it is an important herb to keep in mind when there is deficiency from the parasites. It is also used for post-partum swellings and for lack of mother's milk.

CONTRAINDICATIONS: No contraindications for pumpkin seeds have been noted.

DOSE: 30–60 grams

Garlic (DA SUAN)

Bulbus alli sativi

COMMON NAME: Garlic

FAMILY: Liliaceae

ENERGY AND FLAVOR: Warm; acrid

ORGAN MERIDIANS AFFECTED: Lung, spleen, large intestine, stomach

PROPERTIES: Anthelmintic, nutrient, antibacterial, antifungal, tonic

INDICATIONS: This herb is used for all kinds of intestinal parasites and to fight off colds and influenza in the early stages of these infections. It is also used for issues of the digestive tract such as diarrhea and dysentery.

CONTRAINDICATIONS: Garlic should not be used by those with yin deficiency and heat signs. It should not be applied topically for long periods of time, as it irritates tissue.

DOSE: 6–15 grams

Substances for External Application

The following section includes only a few of the many herbs and substances that are primarily intended for topical application. Some of the most toxic substances have been left out, since it is best that these be administered with the guidance of an experienced Chinese herbalist. Many of these substances, however, such as alumen and calomelas, are well-established in Western herbalism and are even available in over-the-counter medications from Western pharmacies.

Alumen (MING FAN)

COMMON NAME: Alum

ENERGIES AND FLAVOR: Astringent, cold; sour

ORGAN MERIDIANS AFFECTED: Lung, liver, spleen, large intestine

PROPERTIES: Antipruritic, hemostatic

EFFECTS AND INDICATIONS: Stops itching, relieves damp-heat inflammation, kills parasites, stops bleeding, relieves diarrhea, clears heat, and relieves wind-phlegm. It is applied topically for damp-heat itching, rashes, and infestation of parasites. It is also used for blood in the stool, uterine bleeding, and chronic diarrhea and is applied topically for all kinds of bleeding. Finally, it is used for wind-phlegm conditions with such symptoms as convulsions, irritability, and difficult-to-expectorate sputum.

CONTRAINDICATIONS: Alumen should not be used when there is no dampness or heat. This herb should be used with caution when taken internally.

DOSE: 1–3 grams internally

Borax (PENG SHA)

COMMON NAME: Borax
ENERGY AND FLAVORS: Cool; sweet, salty
ORGAN MERIDIANS AFFECTED: Lung, stomach
PROPERTY: Antitoxin
EFFECTS AND INDICATIONS: This substance is applied externally for heat and toxins. It clears hot phlegm in the lungs. It is used for pain and swelling with symptoms of open sores, athlete's foot with associated sores, white draining vaginal lesions, and sores in the mouth and throat. It is also used for hot phlegm in the lungs that is difficult to expectorate.

CONTRAINDICATIONS: Borax should not be used by pregnant women. It should be used with caution internally and should not be used internally for more than 5 days—preferably only 3. Long-term use of more than 1 week or so at a time can cause damage to the kidneys.

DOSE: 2–5 grams internally

Cnidium seeds (SHE CHUANG ZI)

Fructus cnidii monnieri
COMMON NAME: Cnidium seeds
FAMILY: Umbelliferae
ENERGY AND FLAVORS: Warm; acrid, bitter
ORGAN MERIDIANS AFFECTED: Kidney, spleen
PROPERTIES: Antiparasitic, tonic
EFFECTS AND INDICATIONS: Applied topically, the herb clears damp heat on the skin and kills parasites. It tonifies kidney yang and warms and dries wind-damp cold. It is used for external application as a powder,

wash, or ointment for any kind of damp-heat skin affliction, especially in the genital area; for impotence and infertility due to cold in
the kidney or womb; and for damp cold or wind-damp cold with
symptoms of vaginal discharge or sore lower back.

CONTRAINDICATIONS: Cnidium seeds should not be used by those with
conditions of damp heat or by those with yin deficiency with heat
signs.

DOSE: 6–12 grams

Camphor (ZHANG NAO)

COMMON NAMES: Camphor, camphora

FAMILY: Lauraceae

ENERGIES AND FLAVOR: Hot, toxic; acrid

ORGAN MERIDIAN AFFECTED: Heart

PROPERTIES: Anti-inflammatory, antiparasitic

EFFECTS AND INDICATIONS: Moves the blood and reduces inflammation,
opens the orifices and awakens the spirit, and dispels wind damp
and kills parasites. It is applied externally for stagnation of blood of
all kinds, including traumatic injury, and is used for heat-induced
loss of consciousness and coma. Applied topically, it treats itching
associated with sores or parasites.

CONTRAINDICATIONS: Camphor should not be used by pregnant women,
by those who are weak because of qi deficiency, or those with insomnia. This herb should be used with caution when taken internally.

DOSE: .05–.15 grams internally

Tulip bulbs (SHAN CI GU)

Pseudobulbus shancigu Cremastra variabilis, Tulipa edulis

COMMON NAME: Chinese tulip bulbs

FAMILY: Orchidaceae

ENERGIES AND FLAVOR: Cold, slightly toxic; sweet

ORGAN MERIDIANS AFFECTED: Liver, stomach

PROPERTY: Antitoxin

EFFECTS AND INDICATIONS: This herb clears heat and toxicity and dissipates nodules. It is used for swollen glands, nodules, tumors, sores,
ulcers, swellings, and carbuncles.

DOSE: 3–9 grams in decoctions; apply topically as a paste

NOTES: This herb has an antineoplastic effect probably because it contains colchicine. For nodules and tumors, the best application is as a

paste made from the powders of hornet nest, mantis egg case, scorpion, and phytolacca root. The powders are mixed with enough hot water to form a thick paste. It is most likely to be effective for tumors located close to the surface, such as breast tumors. This treatment appears to be similar to approaches in other cultures that employ the topical application of herbal poultices and ointments to draw out moles, nodules and tumors through the skin. **Caution:** Do not use this herb internally without the guidance of an experienced practitioner.

Hornet nest (LU FENG FANG)

Nidus vespae
COMMON NAME: Hornet nest
FAMILY: Vespidae
ENERGIES AND FLAVOR: Neutral, toxic; sweet
ORGAN MERIDIANS AFFECTED: Lung, stomach
PROPERTY: Analgesic
EFFECTS AND INDICATIONS: Clears heat, expels wind, dries damp, and relieves pain. This substance is applied topically as an ointment or a wash for a variety of skin ailments, including rashes with itch, sores, scabies, carbuncles, and wind-damp painful obstruction.
CONTRAINDICATIONS: Hornet nest should not be used by those with *qi* or blood deficiency or when there are open sores.
DOSE: 6–12 grams as a decoction applied externally; 1–3 grams as a powder taken internally.

Calomelas (QING FEN)

COMMON NAME: Calomelas
ENERGIES AND FLAVOR: Cold, toxic; acrid
ORGAN MERIDIANS AFFECTED: Bladder, kidney, liver
PROPERTIES: Antitoxin, antiparasitic
EFFECTS AND INDICATIONS: This substance relieves toxicity, kills parasites, and is used as an external wash for scabies and syphilitic sores. Internally, it is used to expel water, purge the intestines, and reduce edema.
NOTE: Calamine lotion is sold in pharmacies throughout the world to soothe and relieve all kinds of itching.

Sulfur (LIU HUANG)

COMMON NAMES: Sulfur, flower of sulfur
ENERGIES AND FLAVOR: Warm, mildly toxic; pungent

ORGAN MERIDIANS AFFECTED: Spleen, kidneys

PROPERTIES: Antidiuretic, antidiarrheal

EFFECTS AND INDICATIONS: Sulfur is externally applied for the treatment of scabies and tinea infections (fungus infections). It warms kidney and spleen yang, and treats impotence, frequent urination, chronic diarrhea, and constipation caused by coldness.

CONTRAINDICATIONS: Sulfur should not be used for symptoms of yin deficiency or excess yang.

DOSE: 1–3 grams when taken internally.

· NINE ·

CHINESE AND NON-CHINESE HERBS AVAILABLE IN THE WEST

A Chinese herb is a Chinese herb is a Chinese herb is a Chinese herb. . . . Many people express reluctance to use Chinese herbs because they are not Western or local herbs. While basing our diet primarily on locally grown food is beneficial both economically and physiologically (this kind of diet acclimatizes our blood to our particular geographical area's seasonal changes), disease is often an expression of complex emotional and physical stresses as well as exposure to exotic pathogens that go beyond seasonal environment.

Today, not many of the plants that the majority of us see around us are of purely local derivation. Western herbalists commonly use such herbs as the popular African bird, cayenne pepper (as a circulatory stimulant), pau d'arco from South America, buchu leaf from Africa, and kava kava from the South Seas islands that are all used by Western herbalists.

Indeed, there is a veritable pharmacopoeia growing in our immediate natural vicinity, often as common weeds. Many of these may not be the most effective to treat some of the conditions and diseases that arise in our lives, however. It is certainly appropriate that when we are in a state of disease, we select an herb not by where it comes from but whether it can relieve our suffering. Whether an herb or any other substance we use is effective depends more on our diagnosis and subsequent under-standing of what is needed than precisely what that herb or substance may be.

While herbalists prefer to first use foods and then herbs for medicine, practitioners of all traditions have historically felt compelled to reach beyond their countries' boundaries to employ a variety of herbs and treatments that may even extend beyond the realm of the vegetable kingdom to include substances from the animal and mineral kingdoms as well. It is not surprising, then, that the materia medica of our Euro-pean ancestors resembled that of the Chinese materia medica, using a variety of strange animal parts, insects, and minerals, as well as herbs. The *Handbook of Traditional Drugs,* published after the liberation of China in 1949, listed 517 traditional drugs, over 400 of them of plant origin, while 45 are derived from animal sources and 30 are minerals. I'm sure people tried plants first to relieve certain fevers, for instance, before they decided, probably in desperation, to boil into a tea 30 grams of crushed calcium sulfate (gypsum), as is commonly done by Chinese herbalists to lower a high fever. An herb from Africa or from Timbuktu to treat meningitis?—let's have it! The Chinese might use gypsum or an animal-derived substance called *niu huang,* which is the gallstone of a cow.

Officially, there are a minimum of some 250 or so herbs that are commonly used in the official traditional Chinese medicine (TCM) ma-teria medica. Many of these herbs are commonly used in Western herb-alism and include burdock, honeysuckle, teasel, walnut, angelica, lovage, hawthorn berries, horsetail, ginger, garlic, loquat, coltsfoot, kelp, self heal, mugwort, barberry, purslane, malva, plantain, cyperus, and citrus peel. I agree with Yue Chongxi, who said that what is impor-tant is not so much the herb that is used, but that it is used according to the principles of TCM.*

In the introduction to *Herbal Emissaries,* Steven Foster writes of the famous plant hunter, Ernest "Chinese" Wilson (1876–1930), introduc-ing over 1,500 Asian plant species to Western horticulture and men-tions that one of his many books is entitled *China: The Mother of Plants.* He describes the title as fitting because "with an estimated 30,000 flowering plant species, China possesses the most diversified and rich flora in the temperate zones."

---

*Foster, Steven, and Chongxi, Yue. *Herbal Emissaries: Bringing Chinese Herbs to the West* (Healing Arts Press, Rochester, VT, 1992)

Chinese herbs are more available in the United States than is at first obvious. Many Chinese herbs not currently used by Western herbalists are found in nurseries as ornamental garden perennials. These include chrysanthemum (ju hua), daylily (bai he), peony (bai shao), rehmannia (di huang), gardenia (zhi zi), and dianthus (qu mai). Others, such as privet (Ligustrum japonica), forsythia (lian qiao), and hawthorn (shan zha) are used as hedge plants. Various shade and fruit-bearing trees, such as the mulberry (sang shen), mimosa (he huan pi), dogwood (shan zu yu), jujube date (da zao), and ginkgo (bai guo), are also found outside the Orient. Rock-garden enthusiasts commonly use herbs such as ophiopogon (mai men dong), fritillary (chuan bei mu), pinellia (ban xia), and bai-kal skullcap (Scutellaria baicalensis, or huang qin). Indoor ornamentals, such as asparagus fern (tian men dong), have been identified, as have been a wide variety of naturalized and related indigenous species, such as Solomon's seal (Polygonatum species), cuscuta (tu si zi), water plantain (Alisma species), jack-in-the-pulpit (Arisaema species), American ginseng (Panax quinquefolium), and reishi mushrooms (Ganoderma lucidum), that have been found on both sides of the North American continents as well as in the Peruvian Amazon. Finally, there is a wide variety of common spices, such as ginger, cardamom, cinnamon, pepper, and nutmeg, that are an important part of the TCM materia medica.

At present, there are serious efforts to begin cultivation of at least the most popular and important Chinese herbs, such as Schisandra chinensis, Astragalus membranaceus, Chinese scutellaria, Bupleurum falcatum, Dioscorea batatas, and Angelica sinensis. This will necessitate an understanding of how these herbs have been grown and used by the Chinese for thousands of years. Such an understanding will undoubtedly affect the practice of Western herbalism—for the better, one hopes. Western herbalism tends to be too strongly influenced by the dominant Western medical model, which is based on the principle of finding a treatment for a named disease. We see this in the sale of popular Western herbs, such as feverfew (Chrysanthemum parthenium), a diaphoretic with broad application for fevers that is unfortunately being recommended and prescribed solely for migraine headaches; and St.-John's-wort (Hypericum perfoliatum), a specific anti-inflammatory for the healing of nerve pains that is unfortunately being popularly sold only as a mild antidepressant.

The fact remains that the broad classification according to therapeutic properties, such as diuretics, diaphoretics, laxatives, and Western herbalism's alteratives category, remains a far more therapeutically flexible and accurate way to describe how plants work in the body than merely relegating them to the treatment of a specific disease. This also applies to the energetic classifications of TCM, describing the relative heating or cooling nature of medicinal plants, the Five Flavors, and the organ meridians affected.

While certain plants appear to have some specific beneficial effects, we should not limit ourselves to the naive assumption that that is all they do. TCM at least teaches us that all substances have, to varying degrees, variations of two basic energetic effects encompassed by the yin–yang paradigm. This implies that all the complex physiological, neurological, and hormonal responses one would associate with the parasympathetic nervous system are yin cooling, while all the complex physiological, neurological, and hormonal effects associated with the sympathetic nervous system are yang heating. Within this paradigm, TCM classifies the effects of the five flavors as implying more specific biochemical processes and the actual physiological result in terms of what a plant most obviously does—whether it is a laxative, diuretic, diaphoretic, or something else—to specifically effect an organ system, such as the urinary organs, the intestines, or the skin.

For practical purposes, it may be of value to examine the common Western botanicals in terms of their classification and use in TCM.

Common Western Botanicals Used in Chinese Herbalism

Barberry (SHI DA GONG LAO YE)
Mahonia japonica et species
COMMON NAME: Barberry
FAMILY: Berberidacea
PART USED: Rhizome
ENERGY AND FLAVOR: Cold; bitter
PROPERTIES: Anti-inflammatory, antipyretic
EFFECTS AND INDICATIONS: This herb removes fevers, especially those caused by deficiency and weakness. It is used to treat colds, bronchitis, sore throats, toothaches, acute gastroenteritis, dysentery, tuberculosis, pneumonia, infectious hepatitis, rheumatic arthralgia, and cancer of the lungs and liver.
CONTRAINDICATIONS: None
DOSE: 15–30 grams in decoction

Red clover (HONG CHE ZHOU CAO)

Trifolium pratense

COMMON NAME: Red clover
FAMILY: Leguminosae
PART USED: Aerial portion, including flowers
ENERGY AND FLAVOR: Cold; bitter
PROPERTIES: Anti-inflammatory, alterative, blood purifier, diuretic, antipyretic, improves vision
INDICATIONS: This herb is used to treat infections, fevers and influenza, and cancer (especially of the breast).
CONTRAINDICATIONS: Red clover should not be used by someone on blood thinning drugs such as coumarin.
DOSE: 30 grams

Mulberry (SANG BAI PI, SANG YE, SANG SHEN, SANG ZHI)

Morus alba

COMMON NAME: Mulberry
FAMILY: Moraceae
PARTS USED: Roots, branches, leaves, fruits, bark
ENERGIES AND FLAVORS: **Roots**—cool; sweet. **Branches**—cool; bitter. **Leaves**—cool; bitter, sweet. **Fruits**—cool; sweet, sour.
ORGAN MERIDIANS AFFECTED: **Bark:** lungs, spleen. **Fruit:** heart, liver, kidneys. **Leaves:** lungs, liver. **Branch:** liver.
PROPERTIES: **Roots**—antiasthmatic, diuretic, antiswelling. **Branches**—antipyretic, analgesic, antirheumatic. **Leaves**—antipyretic. **Fruit:** yin and blood tonic.
INDICATIONS: The roots are used to treat cough and edema. The branches are used for rheumatic conditions and lumbago. The leaves are used to treat influenza, cough, and conjunctivitis. The fruits are a blood and yin tonic and are used to treat chronic hepatitis, anemia, and nervous collapse.
CONTRAINDICATIONS: None
DOSE: Of roots, 10–15 grams; of branches, 15–30 grams; of leaves, 6–12 grams; of fruit, 10–15 grams

Dandelion (PU GONG YING)

Taraxacum officinale

COMMON NAME: Dandelion
FAMILY: Compositae

PART USED: The whole aerial portion and root

ENERGY AND FLAVORS: Cold; bitter, sweet

ORGAN MERIDIANS AFFECTED: Liver, stomach

PROPERTIES: Anti-inflammatory, cholagogue, diuretic, mild laxative, galactagogue, antimicrobial

EFFECTS AND INDICATIONS: This herb increases the production of mother's milk. It is used to treat jaundice; hepatitis; red, swollen eyes; urinary tract infections; abscesses or firm, hard sores in the breasts; and breast and liver cancer.

CONTRAINDICATIONS: None

DOSE: 10–30 grams

Nettles

Urtica urens

COMMON NAME: Nettles

FAMILY: Urticaceae

PART USED: Aerial portion

ENERGY AND FLAVORS: Cool; bland, slightly bitter

ORGAN MERIDIANS AFFECTED: Small intestines, urinary bladder, lungs

PROPERTIES: Astringent, hemostatic, diuretic, galactagogue, expectorant, tonic, nutritive

INDICATIONS: This herb is used to treat urinary problems, stopped urination, gravel, and inflammatory conditions, such as cystitis and nephritis; asthma and mucous conditions of the lungs, including pleurisy; diarrhea and dysentery; hemorrhoids; bleeding; and edema.

DOSE: 9–30 grams; can be steamed as a pot herb

Yellow dock (*NIU ER DA HUANG*)

Rumex crispus

COMMON NAMES: Yellow dock, broad-leaved dock, curly dock

FAMILY: Polygonaceae

PART USED: Root

ENERGY AND FLAVOR: Cool; bitter

PROPERTIES: Circulatory stimulant, antitoxin, tonic

EFFECTS AND INDICATIONS: Counteracts anemia, tonifies *qi* and blood. It is used to treat skin diseases, such as psoriasis, eczema, herpes, and rashes, and to treat leukemia.

DOSE: 3–9 grams

Horsetail (MU ZEI)
Equisetum hiemalis
COMMON NAME: Horsetail
FAMILY: Equisetaceae
PART USED: Aerial portion
ENERGY AND FLAVORS: Neutral; sweet, bitter
ORGAN MERIDIANS AFFECTED: Lungs, liver
PROPERTIES: Diaphoretic, diuretic, astringent
INDICATIONS: This herb is used to treat conjunctivitis and urinary tract
   infections.
CONTRAINDICATIONS: Horsetail should not be used by pregnant women
   or individuals with frequent urination.
DOSE: 3–9 grams

Garlic (DA SUAN)
Bulbus alli sativi
COMMON NAME: Garlic
FAMILY: Liliaceae
PART USED: Bulbs
ENERGY AND FLAVORS: Warm; spicy, bitter
ORGAN MERIDIANS AFFECTED: Spleen, lungs
PROPERTIES: Detoxifying, reduces swelling, carminative, diaphoretic, di-
   uretic, circulatory stimulant, analgesic, expectorant
EFFECTS AND INDICATIONS: Detoxifies the blood and lymphatic systems;
   treats upper-respiratory tract infections, such as bronchitis, pneumo-
   nia, colds, and influenza; promotes digestion; relieves pain; promotes
   blood circulation; lowers serum cholesterol. It is used to treat heart
   conditions, reduce lumps, and treat cancer.
CONTRAINDICATIONS: None
DOSE: 15–30 grams

Goldenrod (YI ZHI HUANG HUA)
Solidago species
COMMON NAME: Goldenrod
FAMILY: Compositae
PART USED: Aerial portion
ENERGY AND FLAVORS: Neutral; bitter, sweet
PROPERTIES: Alterative, anti-inflammatory, diuretic, circulatory stimu-
   lant, analgesic

EFFECTS AND INDICATIONS: Relieves infections and sore throat. It is used to treat upper-respiratory tract infections, tonsillitis, bronchitis, pneumonia, tuberculosis with hemoptysis, acute and chronic nephritis and cystitis, and cancer.

CONTRAINDICATIONS: Goldenrod should not be taken during pregnancy.

DOSE: 10–30 grams

Hawthorn berries (SHAN ZHA)

Fructus crataegus oxycanthus

COMMON NAMES: Hawthorn, crataegus

FAMILY: Rosaceae

PART USED: Berries

ENERGY AND FLAVORS: Slightly warm; sour, sweet

ORGAN MERIDIANS AFFECTED: Liver, spleen, stomach

PROPERTIES: Digestive, appetite stimulant, circulatory stimulant, regulates blood pressure, lowers cholesterol

EFFECTS AND INDICATIONS: Relieves food stagnation and counteracts fatty foods. It is used to treat low appetite, heart problems, high cholesterol levels, and hypertension. Charred, it is effective for diarrhea and dysentery. It is also used to relieve hernial pain.

CONTRAINDICATIONS: Hawthorn berries should be avoided by those with spleen and stomach deficiency or acid stomach.

DOSE: 9–15 grams

Calamus (SHI CHANG PU)

Rhizoma acorus calamus

COMMON NAMES: Calamus, sweetflag

FAMILY: Araceae

PART USED: Root

ENERGY AND FLAVOR: Neutral to warm; acrid*

ORGAN MERIDIANS AFFECTED: Heart, liver, stomach

PROPERTIES: Stimulant, sharpens mental focus, carminative, expectorant, lowers body temperature, antispasmodic, antifungal

EFFECTS AND INDICATIONS: Aids digestion and relieves dampness, relieves abdominal pain and distension, relieves arthritic and rheumatic conditions and injuries due to trauma. This herb is used to expel phlegm when it is causing such symptoms as deafness, forgetfulness, or other signs of the senses being obstructed by phlegm.

---

*Acrid includes spicy and pungent flavors.

CONTRAINDICATIONS: Calamus should not be used by those with yin deficiency with heat signs and should be used with caution by those with excessive sweating or spermatorrhea.

DOSE: 3–9 grams

Black nightshade (LONG KUI)

Solanum nigri

COMMON NAME: Black nightshade

PART USED: Aerial portion

ENERGIES AND FLAVOR: Cold, slightly toxic; bitter

ORGAN MERIDIANS AFFECTED: Liver, lungs

PROPERTIES: Antipyretic, detoxifying, antifungal, anticancer

INDICATIONS: This herb is used to treat acute hepatitis, acute conjunctivitis, and tonsillitis; high fever, possibly with convulsions; abscesses, boils, and vaginal and scrotal itching; fungal infections; and cancer.

CONTRAINDICATIONS: Should not be used for cold conditions

DOSE: 3–9 grams in decoction

Chenopodium (LI)

Chenopodium ambrosiodes

COMMON NAME: Chenopodium

FAMILY: Chenopodiaceae

PART USED: Leaves

ENERGIES AND FLAVORS: Slightly warm, slightly toxic; acrid, bitter

ORGAN MERIDIANS AFFECTED: Lungs, large intestine

PROPERTIES: Insecticidal, vermifuge, digestive, antipruritic

EFFECTS AND INDICATIONS: This herb is used to treat hookworm, roundworm, and threadworm infestations. When it is cooked with beans, it promotes digestion and prevents gas. It is used externally as a wash or poultice for eczema, pruritus, tineas, head lice, and ringworm of the feet and is a maggoticide.

DOSE: 3–6 grams taken internally for parasites; externally, make into a wash and apply

Thistles (DA JI)

Cirsium japonicum

COMMON NAME: Thistles

PART USED: Aerial portion.

ENERGY AND FLAVOR: Cool; bitter

ORGAN MERIDIAN AFFECTED: Liver

PROPERTIES: Hemostatic, counteracts swelling, antitoxin

EFFECTS AND INDICATIONS: Thistles resolve blood clots. They are used to treat functional uterine bleeding and all other types of bleeding, hepatitis, jaundice, nephritis, hypertension, contusions, and boils.

DOSE: 15–30 grams in decoction

NOTES: Other thistle species can be used, such as the Western blessed thistle (*Cnicus benedicta*) or milk thistle (*Sylamarin*). For best results in treating bleeding, use the ashes of the calcined herb, 1–2 teaspoons in 1 cup of water, repeated as needed.

Shepherd's purse (*JI CAI*)

Capsella bursa-pastoris

COMMON NAME: Shepherd's purse

FAMILY: Cruciferae

PART USED: Aerial portion

ENERGY AND FLAVORS: Cold; bitter, sour

PROPERTIES: Hemostatic, astringent, alterative

EFFECTS AND INDICATIONS: Stops bleeding. This herb is used to treat bacillary dysentery.

CONTRAINDICATIONS: None found

DOSE: 3–15 grams

Chelidonium (*BAI GU CAI*)

Chelidonium majus

COMMON NAME: Chelidonium, Greater Celandine

FAMILY: Papaveraceae

PART USED: Whole herb

ENERGY AND FLAVORS: Cool; bitter, acrid

ORGAN MERIDIANS AFFECTED: Liver, large intestines

PROPERTIES: Alterative, diuretic, purgative, antispasmodic, diaphoretic, anodyne, narcotic

INDICATIONS: This herb is used for acute hepatitis, jaundice, and cirrhosis.

CONTRAINDICATIONS: Not for prolonged usage alone

DOSE: 3–9 grams

Fennel (*XIAO HUI XIANG*)

Fructus foeniculum vulgares

COMMON NAME: Fennel seed

FAMILY: Umbelliferae
PART USED: Seeds
ENERGY AND FLAVOR: Warm; acrid
ORGAN MERIDIANS AFFECTED: Liver, kidney, spleen, stomach
PROPERTIES: Carminative, stomachic, analgesic
EFFECTS AND INDICATIONS: Aids digestion, alleviates hernia and testicle
   pains caused by coldness. This herb is used to relieve vomiting, nau-
   sea, cramping, or abdominal pains caused by coldness.
CONTRAINDICATIONS: Fennel should not be used by those with yin defi-
   ciency with heat signs or by those with excess heat.
DOSE: 3–9 grams

Wild carrot (HE SHI FENG)
Daucus carota
COMMON NAME: Wild carrot
FAMILY: Umbelliferae
PART USED: Root
ENERGY AND FLAVOR: Hot; sweet
PROPERTIES: Digestive, diuretic.
EFFECTS AND INDICATIONS: Promotes the circulation of *qi*. This herb is
   used to treat gastrointestinal congestion, fluid retention, vitamin A
   deficiency, and cancer, including leukemia.
DOSE: 9–15 grams
NOTE: For leukemia and liver cancer, drink fresh carrot juice (it can be
   the yellow domestic carrot). **Caution:** Be aware that poison hemlock
   often grows in the same areas as wild carrot and can be fatally mis-
   taken for it.

Walnuts (HU TAO REN)
Juglandis regiae
COMMON NAME: Walnut
FAMILY: Juglandaceae
PART USED: Nut meats
ENERGY AND FLAVOR: Warm; sweet
ORGAN MERIDIANS AFFECTED: Lung, kidney, large intestine
PROPERTIES: Yang tonic, nutrient, dissolves stones, mild laxative, emol-
   lient
EFFECTS AND INDICATIONS: This herb is used to treat kidney-yang defi-
   ciency signs, such as lower back pain and urinary incontinence. It

astringes essence and therefore can be used when there is premature ejaculation or other similar reproductive issues. It is also used for chronic coughing caused by lung and kidney deficiency and constipation caused by kidney-yang deficiency and dryness and for constipation in the elderly.

CONTRAINDICATIONS: Walnuts should not be used by those with yin deficiency when there are heat signs present or by those with heated phlegm and a hot cough.

DOSE: 9–30 grams

Impatiens

Impatiens chinensis

COMMON NAMES: Impatiens, jewel weed

FAMILY: Balsaminaceae

PART USED: Whole herb

ENERGY AND FLAVORS: Neutral; bitter, acrid

PROPERTIES: Anti-inflammatory, circulatory stimulant

ORGAN MERIDIAN AFFECTED: Liver

EFFECTS AND INDICATIONS: Reduces swelling, ripens abscesses and boils. This herb is used to treat pulmonary tuberculosis, sore throats, dysentery, and cancer, especially Hodgkin's disease and leukemia

CONTRAINDICATIONS: Impatiens should not be taken during pregnancy.

DOSE: 30–60 grams in decoction

Rue (CHOU CAO)

Ruta graveolens

COMMON NAMES: Rue, garden rue

FAMILY: Rutaceae

PART USED: Aerial portion

ENERGY AND FLAVORS: Cool; acrid, slightly bitter

PROPERTIES: Antipyretic, anti-inflammatory, circulatory stimulant, analgesic

INDICATIONS: This herb is used to treat colds, fever, infantile convulsions, epigastric pains, hernia, toothache, irregular menses, amenorrhea, infantile eczema, furunculosis, traumatic injuries, pyodermas, and snake and insect bites.

CONTRAINDICATIONS: Rue should not be used during pregnancy.

DOSE: 10–15 grams

Knotweed (BIAN XU)

Polygonum aviculare
COMMON NAME: Knotweed
FAMILY: Polygonaceae
PART USED: Whole herb
ENERGY AND FLAVOR: Neutral; bitter
PROPERTIES: Antipyretic, diuretic, vermifuge, insecticide
INDICATIONS: This herb is used for urinary stones, jaundice, weeping eczema and mucous and blood-tinged vaginal discharge
DOSE: 9–15 grams

Malva (DONG KUI ZI)

Malva verticillata
COMMON NAME: Malva
FAMILY: Malvaceae
PART USED: Aerial portion
ENERGY AND FLAVORS: Slightly cold; pleasant, bland
ORGAN MERIDIANS AFFECTED: Lungs
PROPERTIES: Diuretic, mild laxative, galactagogue
INDICATIONS: This herb is used to treat edema and difficult urination, constipation, and low supply of mother's milk.
CONTRAINDICATIONS: None noted
DOSE: 9–15 grams in decoction.
NOTE: The seeds can also be used.

Purslane (MA CHI XIAN)

Herba portulacae oleraceae
COMMON NAMES: Purslane, portulaca
FAMILY: Portulacaceae
PART USED: Whole herb
ENERGY AND FLAVORS: Cold energy; sour, bitter
ORGAN MERIDIANS AFFECTED: Bladder, liver
PROPERTIES: Antipyretic, antitoxin, diuretic, quenches thirst
INDICATIONS: This herb is used to treat dysentery and enteritis, urinary tract infections, cystitis, and leukorrhea; hemorrhoids, erysipelas, boils, and ulcers (taken internally or applied externally as a poultice); and snake and insect bites.
CONTRAINDICATIONS: Purslane should not be used for cold conditions or by someone with weak digestion.
DOSE: 9–15 grams

Motherwort (YI MU CAO)

Leonurus cardiaca

COMMON NAMES: Motherwort, lion's-tail

FAMILY: Labiatae

PART USED: Leaves

ENERGY AND FLAVORS: Slightly cold; acrid, bitter

ORGAN MERIDIANS AFFECTED: Heart, liver, urinary bladder

PROPERTIES: Emmenagogue, antihypertensive, antispasmodic, diuretic, antibacterial, antifungal

EFFECTS AND INDICATIONS: Regulates menses, relieves hypertension. Motherwort is used to treat nephritis, edema, oliguria, hematuria, and uterine and breast cancers.

CONTRAINDICATIONS: Motherwort should not be used during pregnancy.

DOSE: 10–30 grams

Prunella (XIA KU CAO)

Spica prunella vulgaris

COMMON NAMES: Prunella, self heal, all heal

FAMILY: Labiatae

PART USED: The spike

ENERGY AND FLAVOR: Cool; bitter

ORGAN MERIDIANS AFFECTED: Liver, gallbladder

PROPERTIES: Detoxifies the liver, relieves congestion, diuretic

INDICATIONS: This herb is used to treat swollen lymph glands, goiter, hypertension, conjunctivitis, edema, difficult urination, abscesses, and swellings.

DOSE: 6–15 grams

Sarsaparilla (TU FU LING)

Smilax chinensis

COMMON NAME: Sarsaparilla

FAMILY: Liliaceae

PART USED: Rhizome

ENERGY AND FLAVORS: Cool; mildly acrid, pleasant

ORGAN MERIDIANS AFFECTED: Spleen, stomach, liver

PROPERTIES: Carminative, antitoxin, diuretic

EFFECTS AND INDICATIONS: Strengthens the bones and muscles, removes dampness. This herb is used to treat boils and abscesses, rheumatoid arthritis, urinary tract infections, enteritis, and diarrhea. It also neutralizes mercury toxicity.

CONTRAINDICATIONS: Not for someone with yin deficiency

DOSE: 30–60 grams in decoction

Aralia (SONG MU BAI PI)

Aralia chinensis

COMMON NAME: Aralia

FAMILY: Aralaciae

PART USED: Root

ENERGY AND FLAVOR: Warm; acrid

ORGAN MERIDIANS AFFECTED: Liver, spleen

PROPERTIES: Analgesic, antirheumatic, carminative, diuretic

EFFECTS AND INDICATIONS: Mild Qi Tonic. This herb is used to treat arthritis, rheumatoid arthritis, headaches, edema, gas, and fatigue.

CONTRAINDICATIONS: Not for inflammatory conditions or Yin deficiency

DOSE: 15–30 grams in decoction

Castor-oil plant (BI MA ZI)

Ricinus communis

COMMON NAMES: Castor-oil plant, castor bean, Palma Christi

FAMILY: Euphorbiaceae

PART USED: Oil from the seeds

ENERGY AND FLAVOR: Neutral; sweet

ORGAN MERIDIAN AFFECTED: Liver

PROPERTIES: Laxative, antirheumatic, analgesic

EFFECTS AND INDICATIONS: Loosens and draws out toxins, relieves pain. This herb is also used for constipation. Externally, it is used to heal gunshot wounds, boils, abscesses, and enlarged lymph nodes. The leaves can be applied externally for swollen, painful joints.

CONTRAINDICATIONS: Castor-oil plant should not be used during pregnancy.

DOSE: 1–2 tablespoons of the oil at a time

Burdock (NIU BANG ZI)

Arctium lappa

COMMON NAMES: Burdock, lappa, beggar's buttons

FAMILY: Compositae

PARTS USED: Seeds and root

ENERGY AND FLAVORS: Cold; bitter, acrid

ORGAN MERIDIANS AFFECTED: Lung, stomach

PROPERTIES: Antibiotic, antifungal, diaphoretic, diuretic, mild laxative, antipyretic

EFFECTS AND INDICATIONS: **Seeds**—These are used to treat wind-heat fevers and sore throat. They help erupt rashes and other eruptive skin diseases, such as measles, in the early stage; they are also effective for hives, mumps, boils, carbuncles, and furuncles. **Root**—This is used as a food and a general detoxifier of the blood and lymphatic system. It is effective for the treatment of cancer, especially lymphoma.

CONTRAINDICATIONS: Burdock should not be used by those with diarrhea.

DOSE: 3–9 grams

Black cohosh (SHENG MA)

Cimicifuga foetidae et species

COMMON NAMES: Black cohosh, cimicifuga, Chinese cohosh

FAMILY: Ranunculaceae

PART USED: Root

ENERGY AND FLAVORS: Cool; spicy, sweet, acrid, slightly bitter

ORGAN MERIDIANS AFFECTED: Lung, spleen, stomach, large intestine

PROPERTIES: Diaphoretic, antipyretic, antifungal, antibacterial

EFFECTS AND INDICATIONS: Clears wind heat and fever, regulates the circulation of *qi,* relieves pain and headaches, and hastens the completion of eruptive skin diseases, such as measles, in the early stages. It is used to treat gingivitis and hives caused by wind heat, diarrhea, and prolapsed internal organs, such as the anus and the uterus.

CONTRAINDICATIONS: Black cohosh should not be used during pregnancy or when measles are fully developed.

DOSE: 3–9 grams

Scrophularia (XUAN SHEN)

Radix Scrophulariae ningpoensis

COMMON NAME: Scrophularia, Chinese figwort

FAMILY: Scrophulariaceae

PART USED: Root

ENERGY AND FLAVORS: Cold; bitter, sweet, salty

ORGAN MERIDIANS AFFECTED: Lung, stomach, kidney

PROPERTIES: Anti-inflammatory, antihypertensive, antibacterial, antifungal, vasodilator

EFFECTS AND INDICATIONS: Nourishes the yin and relieves irritability and constipation. This herb is used to treat warm febrile diseases possibly associated with bleeding; sore throats; swollen, inflamed lymph glands; burning urination; and tumors.

CONTRAINDICATIONS: Should not be used by someone with diarrhea

DOSE: 9–30 grams

Solomon's seal (YU ZHU)

Rhizoma polygoni odorati

COMMON NAME: Solomon's seal

FAMILY: Liliaceae

PART USED: Root

ENERGY AND FLAVOR: Slightly cold; sweet

ORGAN MERIDIANS AFFECTED: Lungs, heart, stomach

PROPERTIES: Qi and yin tonic, antitussive, demulcent

INDICATIONS: This herb is used for debilitating chronic cough, body weakness and dryness, and thirst with heat intolerance.

CONTRAINDICATIONS: Not for qi stagnation, dampness in the stomach

DOSE: 15–30 grams

Agrimony (XIAN HE CAO)

Herba agrimoniae pilosulae

COMMON NAME: Rosaceae

FAMILY: Rosaceae

PART USED: Aerial portion

ENERGIES AND FLAVOR: Neutral, astringent; bitter

ORGAN MERIDIANS AFFECTED: Lung, liver, spleen

PROPERTIES: Hemostatic, astringent, antiparasitic, anti-inflammatory, anthelmintic, antibacterial, increases blood pressure, tonic, analgesic

INDICATIONS: This herb is used for all types of bleeding anywhere in the body to treat diarrhea, and to kill parasites.

CONTRAINDICATIONS: Not for cold damp stagnation

DOSE: 6–15 grams

NOTE: This herb can be used externally as a wash.

Aloe (LU HUI)

Aloe vera

COMMON NAMES: Aloe, aloe vera

FAMILY: Liliaceae

PARTS USED: Leaves and flowers

ENERGY AND FLAVOR: Cold; bitter

ORGAN MERIDIANS AFFECTED: Liver, lung

PROPERTIES: Anti-inflammatory, laxative, vulnerary, parasiticide

INDICATIONS: Internally, this herb is used for headaches, dizziness, constipation, infantile convulsions, malnutrition, and pertussis and as a women's tonic. Externally, the juice of the leaves is used for burns and scalds.

CONTRAINDICATIONS: Aloe should not be used during pregnancy.

DOSE: 10–15 grams of the leaf; 1.5–3 grams of the concentrated powder (which is a laxative), taken in pill form

Mugwort (AI YE)

Artemisia vulgaris

COMMON NAMES: Mugwort, moxa

FAMILY: Compositae

PART USED: Aerial portion

ENERGY AND FLAVORS: Warm; bitter, fragrant

ORGAN MERIDIANS AFFECTED: Lung, liver, spleen, kidney

PROPERTIES: Hemostatic, antitoxin, carminative, cholagogue, vermifuge

EFFECTS AND INDICATIONS: 1. Irregular menstruation, vomiting blood; 2. Abdominal pains caused by Coldness; 3. Quiets a restless fetus; 4. Skin conditions.

CONTRAINDICATIONS: Mugwort should not be taken internally during pregnancy.

DOSE: 9–15 grams

Plantain (CHE QIAN ZI)

Plantago major

COMMON NAMES: Plantain, Englishman's foot, ribwort, greater plantain

FAMILY: Plantaginaceae

PARTS USED: Whole herb, seeds

ENERGY AND FLAVOR: Cold; sweet

ORGAN MERIDIANS AFFECTED: Bladder, small intestine, gallbladder

PROPERTIES: Anti-inflammatory, diuretic, expectorant, antitussive

INDICATIONS: This herb is used to treat urinary tract infections, stones, edema, colds, cough, bronchitis, enteritis, dysentery, hepatitis, and conjunctivitis.

CONTRAINDICATIONS: Not for cold deficient conditions
DOSE: 15–30 grams of herb; 3–10 grams of seeds

Passionflower
Passiflora edulis
COMMON NAME: Passionflower
FAMILY: Passifloraceae
PART USED: Fruits
ENERGY AND FLAVORS: Neutral; sweet, sour
PROPERTIES: Anti-inflammatory, sedative
EFFECTS AND INDICATIONS: Relieves dryness. Passionflower is used to treat cough, dry throat, hoarseness, dysentery, constipation, insomnia, and dysmenorrhea.
CONTRAINDICATIONS: None noted
DOSE: 9–15 grams

Poke *(SHANG LU)*
Phytolacca acinosa et species
COMMON NAMES: Poke, poke root, phytolacca
FAMILY: Phytolaccaceae
PART USED: Roots
ENERGIES AND FLAVOR: Cold, toxic; bitter
ORGAN MERIDIANS AFFECTED: Spleen, kidney
PROPERTIES: Alterative, detoxifier, diuretic
INDICATIONS: This herb is used to treat edema, ascites, abdominal distension, cervical dysplasia, cancer, leukorrhea, boils, furuncles, and pyodermas.
CONTRAINDICATIONS: Poke should not be used during pregnancy.
DOSE: 3–10 grams in decoction
NOTE: Cook the herb at least 1 hour when making a decoction.

Ground ivy *(DI CHIEN TSAO)*
Glechoma hederacea
COMMON NAMES: Ground ivy, ivy
FAMILY: Labiatae
PART USED: Whole herb
ENERGY AND FLAVORS: Cool; acrid, slightly bitter
PROPERTIES: Antibiotic, anti-inflammatory, diuretic
EFFECTS AND INDICATIONS: Dispels stones, dispels blood stagnation, re-

duces swelling. This herb is used to treat urinary tract infections, hepatitis, gallstones, influenza, cough, rheumatic conditions, and irregular menstruation

CONTRAINDICATIONS: Not for cold conditions

DOSE: 60 grams

Morning glory (QIAN NIU ZI)

Semen pharbitidis nil

COMMON NAMES: Morning glory, pharbitidis

FAMILY: Convolvulaceae

PART USED: Seeds

ENERGIES AND FLAVOR: Cold, slightly toxic; bitter

ORGAN MERIDIANS AFFECTED: Lung, kidney, large intestine

PROPERTIES: Laxative, diuretic, vermifuge

EFFECTS AND INDICATIONS: Reduces swelling. This herb is used to treat nephritic edema, cirrhosis, ascites, constipation, ascariasis, taeniasis.

CONTRAINDICATIONS: Morning glory seeds should not be taken during pregnancy.

DOSE: 3–5 grams crushed in decoction

Jasmine

Jasmine lanceolarium

COMMON NAME: Jasmine

FAMILY: Oleaceae

PART USED: Stem

ENERGY AND FLAVOR: Warm; bitter

ORGAN MERIDIANS AFFECTED: Liver

PROPERTIES: Antirheumatic, circulatory stimulant

EFFECTS AND INDICATIONS: Moves stagnant blood. This herb is used to treat rheumatic arthralgia.

DOSE: 30–60 grams in decoction or soaked in wine

Coriander (HU SUI)

Coriandrum sativum

COMMON NAMES: Coriander, cilantro

FAMILY: Umbelliferae

PARTS USED: Whole herb or the fruits

ENERGY AND FLAVOR: Warm; acrid

ORGAN MERIDIANS AFFECTED: Stomach

PROPERTIES: Diaphoretic, stomachic

EFFECTS AND INDICATIONS: **Herb**—promote the eruption of measles. It is used to treat influenza in which there is no sweating. **Fruits**—used to treat indigestion, anorexia, and stomachache.

CONTRAINDICATIONS: None noted

DOSE: 10–15 grams

Gota kola

Hydrocotyle species

COMMON NAME: Gota kola

FAMILY: Umbelliferae

PART USED: Whole herb

ENERGY AND FLAVORS: Cool; sweet, bland, slightly acrid

ORGAN MERIDIANS AFFECTED: Liver, bladder

PROPERTIES: Anti-inflammatory, antibiotic, diuretic

EFFECTS AND INDICATIONS: 1. Reduces swelling and is used to treat infectious hepatitis; 2. Liver cirrhosis, ascites, gallstones; 3. Urinary tract infections, stones; 4. Influenza, cough, pertussis; 5. Stomatitis, pharyngitis, tonsillitis; 6. Leprosy and skin conditions caused by heat.

DOSE: 15–30 grams in decoction

Camellia (SHAN CHA HUA)

Camellia japonica

COMMON NAME: Camellia

FAMILY: Theacea

PART USED: Flowers

ENERGY AND FLAVORS: Cold; acrid, bitter

PROPERTIES: Astringent, blood purificant, hemostatic

EFFECTS AND INDICATIONS: Controls all types of bleeding. This herb can be used externally for bleeding, scalds, burns, cracked nipples, and boils.

CONTRAINDICATIONS: Not for cold conditions

DOSE: 6–9 grams

Hibiscus (FU SANG HUA)

Hibiscus rosa-sinensis

COMMON NAME: Hibiscus

FAMILY: Malraceae

PARTS USED: Roots, leaves, flowers

ENERGY AND FLAVORS: Neutral; sweet
ORGAN MERIDIANS AFFECTED: Bladder, liver
PROPERTIES: Anti-inflammatory, diuretic, emmenagogue
INDICATIONS: **Root**—used to treat swollen glands, conjunctivitis, bronchitis, urinary tract infections, leukorrhea, irregular menses, and amenorrhea. **Flowers**—used as a blood purifier and to treat irregular menses.
DOSE: 15–30 grams of root or leaves; 30 grams of flowers
NOTE: Leaves can be crushed and applied topically.

Rose (MEI GUI HUA)
Rosa chinensis
COMMON NAME: Rose
FAMILY: Rosaceae
PART USED: Flowers
ENERGY AND FLAVORS: Warm; sweet
ORGAN MERIDIAN AFFECTED: Liver
PROPERTIES: Circulatory stimulant, emmenagogue, anti-inflammatory
EFFECTS AND INDICATIONS: Counteracts swelling. This herb is used to treat irregular menses, boils and pyodermas, and depression.
CONTRAINDICATIONS: Not during pregnancy or with weak digestion
DOSE: 3–10 grams in decoction

Loquat (PI PA YE)
Folium eriobotryae japonica
COMMON NAME: Loquat tree
FAMILY: Rosaceae
PART USED: Leaves (rub the hair from the leaves and then dry them)
ENERGY AND FLAVOR: Neutral; bitter
ORGAN MERIDIANS AFFECTED: Lungs, stomach
PROPERTIES: Antitussive, expectorant, stomachic, antiemetic
INDICATIONS: This herb is used to treat bronchitis, cough, gastritis, and vomiting.
DOSE: 10–15 grams

Valerian (XIE CAO)
Valeriana officinalis
COMMON NAME: Valerian
FAMILY: Valerianaceae

PART USED: Roots
ENERGY AND FLAVORS: Warm; bitter, acrid
ORGAN MERIDIANS AFFECTED: Liver
PROPERTIES: Carminative, antispasmodic, antipyretic, sedative
INDICATIONS: This herb is used to treat influenza, rheumatism, neuras-
thenia, insomnia, and traumatic injuries.
CONTRAINDICATIONS: None noted
DOSE: 9–15 grams

St.-John's-wort (DI ER CAO)

Hypericum perfoliatum, H. japonicum
COMMON NAME: St.-John's-wort
FAMILY: Guttiferae
PART USED: Whole herb
ENERGY AND FLAVOR: Slightly cold; bitter
ORGAN MERIDIANS AFFECTED: Liver
PROPERTIES: Antipyretic, antitoxin
EFFECTS AND INDICATIONS: Promotes resolution of pus and tissue healing.
This herb is used to treat boils, abscesses, stomachache, vomiting,
and headaches.
CONTRAINDICATIONS: Not for individuals with sun sensitivity
DOSE: 9–15 grams

Sedum

Sedum spectabile
COMMON NAME: Sedum
FAMILY: Crassulaceae
PART USED: Whole herb
ENERGY AND FLAVORS: Neutral; bitter
ORGAN MERIDIANS AFFECTED: Liver, lung
PROPERTIES: Anti-inflammatory, antitoxin, sialagogue
EFFECTS AND INDICATIONS: Quenches thirst. This herb is used to treat sore
throat, abscesses, erysipelas, and redness and swelling from injuries.
CONTRAINDICATIONS: Not for cold conditions or with digestive weakness
DOSE: 30–60 grams

Prickly Ivy (GOU GU YE)

Ilex cornuta
COMMON NAME: Prickly ivy

FAMILY: Aquifoliacea
PART USED: Roots, leaves, fruits
ENERGY AND FLAVOR: Cool; bitter
ORGAN MERIDIANS AFFECTED: Liver
PROPERTIES: **Roots**—anti-rheumatic, analgesic, anti-inflammatory; **leaves**—anti-inflammatory; **fruits**—anti-inflammatory, astringent.
INDICATIONS: **Roots**—used to treat rheumatic and arthritic pains, lumbago, headaches, toothaches, and hepatitis. **Leaves**—used to treat pulmonary tuberculosis. **Fruit**—used to treat leukorrhea, chronic diarrhea, and dysentery.
DOSE: 6–15 grams of roots and fruits; 30 grams of leaves
NOTE: Use the young leaves to make an anti-inflammatory tea.

Violet (ZI HUA DI DING)

Viola japonica et species
COMMON NAME: Violet
FAMILY: Violaceae
PART USED: Leaves
ENERGY AND FLAVOR: Cold; slightly bitter
ORGAN MERIDIANS AFFECTED: Liver, Lung
PROPERTIES: Anti-inflammatory, antitoxin, demulcent, analgesic
EFFECTS AND INDICATIONS: Relieves pain. This herb is used to treat boils, ulcers, abscesses, conjunctivitis, laryngitis, acute jaundice, and hepatitis. It is also used to soften and dissolve cancers and tumors.
CONTRAINDICATIONS: Not for cold conditions, weak digestion
DOSE: 30 grams

Japanese elderberry

Sambucus japanica
COMMON NAME: Javanese elderberry
FAMILY: Caprifoliaceae
PART USED: Leaves, stems, roots; **not** the berries
ENERGY AND FLAVOR: Neutral; bitter
ORGAN MERIDIANS AFFECTED: Lungs, bladder
PROPERTIES: Analgesic, Carminative, diuretic
EFFECTS AND INDICATIONS: This herb is used to treat traumatic injuries, broken bones, rheumatoid arthritis, and acute and chronic nephritis.
CONTRAINDICATIONS: Only use the ripe Blueberried Elder, the red berries are poisonous.

DOSE: 30–60 grams in decoction (boil 1 hour)
NOTE: Use as an external wash for contusions, pruritis, and eczema.

Corn silk (YU MI XU)
Zea mays
COMMON NAME: Corn silk, stigmata maydis
FAMILY: Gramineae
PART USED: Silk tassels
ENERGY AND FLAVOR: Neutral to cool; mildly sweet
ORGAN MERIDIANS AFFECTED: Bladder, small intestine, liver
PROPERTIES: Diuretic
EFFECTS AND INDICATIONS: Dissolves urinary stones. This herb is used to treat urinary tract infections, edema, hepatitis, gallstones, gallbladder pains, diabetes, and hypertension.
DOSE: 90–150 grams
NOTE: The corncob can also be used; the dose is 25–30 grams.

Elecampane (XUAN FU HUA)
Flos inula japonica et species
COMMON NAMES: Elecampane, inula
FAMILY: Compositae
PART USED: Flowers
ENERGY AND FLAVORS: Warm; salty, acrid
ORGAN MERIDIANS AFFECTED: Lung, spleen, stomach, liver, large intestine
PROPERTIES: Expectorant, antiemetic
INDICATIONS: This herb is used to treat bronchitis, coughing, shortness of breath, chest congestion, pleurisy, and ascites.
CONTRAINDICATIONS: Not for persons with TB, or wind heat (inflammation) type cough
DOSE: 3–9 grams

Forsythia (LIAN QIAO)
Forsythiae suspensae
COMMON NAME: Forsythia
FAMILY: Oleaceae
PART USED: Fruits
ENERGY AND FLAVORS: Cool; bitter
ORGAN MERIDIANS AFFECTED: Heart, liver, lung, gallbladder

PROPERTIES: Antibacterial, antiemetic, parasiticide, antipyretic, anti-inflammatory

INDICATIONS: This herb is used to treat wind-heat fevers, sore throats, common colds, influenza, and for toxic sores, carbuncles, and swollen lymph nodes.

CONTRAINDICATIONS: Forsythia should not be used by those with weak and cold spleen/stomach conditions. It should not be used for sores that are already open or are caused by yin deficiency.

DOSE: 3–12 grams

Some Chinese Herbs That Commonly Grow in the West

Asparagus fern root (TIAN MEN DONG)
Asparagus conchinsinensis

COMMON NAMES: Asparagus fern root, asparagus fern tuber, asparagus root

FAMILY: Liliaceae

PART USED: Tubers

ENERGY AND FLAVORS: Cool; sweet, bitter

ORGAN MERIDIANS AFFECTED: Lung, kidney

PROPERTIES: Demulcent, anti-inflammatory, sialagogue

EFFECTS AND INDICATIONS: Acts as a lung yin tonic. This herb is used to treat pulmonary tuberculosis, dry cough, chronic bronchitis, dry throat, thirst, diphtheria, pertussis, rhinitis, diabetes mellitus, and breast cancer

CONTRAINDICATIONS: Not for diarrhea, or coughs caused by the common cold

DOSE: 15 grams

NOTES: This herb is highly respected in both Chinese and Ayurvedic herbalism, the latter of which calls it *shatavari*. It is used as a female hormone tonic in much the same way as angelica *dang gui* is by the Chinese. There are many species; In the West, a species called *Asparagus sprengeri* seems to have the same characteristic demulcent tubers on the roots as the Asian species. I have eaten *A. sprengeri* and find it to be quite satisfactory.

Epimedium (YIN YANG HUO)
Epimedium grandiflorum, Herba epimedii

COMMON NAMES: Epimedium, epimedium leaf, horny goat herb

FAMILY: Berberidaceae
PART USED: Aerial portion
ENERGY AND FLAVOR: Warm; pleasant
ORGAN MERIDIANS AFFECTED: Kidneys, liver
PROPERTIES: Yang tonic
EFFECTS AND INDICATIONS: Removes dampness, relieves flatulence. This herb is used to treat impotence, weakness of the lower back and knees, rheumatic and arthritic conditions, and numbness.
DOSE: 15 grams
NOTES: There are a few species of this herb and they all seem to have similar properties. It is commonly available from nurseries. It should be grown in a shaded, moist environment.

Astragalus (HUANG QI)

Membranaceus Astragalus
COMMON NAME: Astragalus
FAMILY: Leguminosae
PART USED: Root
ENERGY AND FLAVOR: Slightly warm; sweet
ORGAN MERIDIANS AFFECTED: Lung, spleen
PROPERTIES: Diuretic, lowers blood pressure
EFFECTS AND INDICATIONS: Qi tonic, immune tonic. Astragalus is the primary herb used in Chinese medicine to tonify the immune system, or *wei qi*, of the lungs. It is useful for conditions of immunodeficiency that causes spontaneous sweating. It is also used for spleen *qi* deficiency with symptoms of weak and low metabolism, edema, and prolapse of internal organs, as it raises the spleen yang and *qi*. It can be used for *qi* and blood deficiency caused by loss of blood or childbirth.
CONTRAINDICATIONS: Astragalus should not be used with excess heat or yin deficiency with heat signs. It should not be used when there is stagnation of *qi* or dampness, especially when there is painful obstruction.
DOSE: 9–30 grams; much more can be used when indicated
NOTE: This herb is being cultivated in many areas of the West. Seeds are commercially available.

Codonopsis (DANG SHEN)

Codonopsis pilosulae
COMMON NAME: Codonopsis

FAMILY: Campanulaceae

PART USED: Roots

ENERGY AND FLAVOR: Neutral; sweet

ORGAN MERIDIANS AFFECTED: Spleen, lungs

PROPERTIES: Tonic, growth stimulant for white and red blood cells.

EFFECTS AND INDICATIONS: Acts as a *qi* tonic, lowers blood pressure, regulates blood sugar. It is used to treat low energy, fatigue and weakness of the limbs, lung *qi* deficiency causing shortness of breath or chronic cough, lack of appetite, and organ prolapse.

CONTRAINDICATIONS: Codonopsis should be used with caution when there is acute illness.

DOSE: 9–30 grams

NOTE: This herb is being cultivated with good success in this country. It is a delicate vinelike plant that prefers protection from direct sunlight.

American ginseng (XI YANG SHEN)

Panacis quinquefolii

COMMON NAME: American ginseng

FAMILY: Araliaceae

PART USED: Root

ENERGY AND FLAVORS: Cool; sweet, slightly bitter

ORGAN MERIDIANS AFFECTED: Lung, heart, kidney, stomach

PROPERTIES: Tonic, sedative

EFFECTS AND INDICATIONS: Yin tonic, counteracts the effects of stress and nervous exhaustion. This herb is used to treat lung yin deficiency, pulmonary tuberculosis, and febrile disease with chronic cough, blood-streaked sputum, and loss of voice.

CONTRAINDICATIONS: American ginseng should not be used by those with a cold damp stomach.

DOSE: 3–9 grams

Ginkgo biloba (BAI GUO)

Ginko biloba

COMMON NAMES: Ginkgo biloba, ginkgo nut

FAMILY: Ginkgoaceae

PARTS USED: Nuts, leaves

ENERGIES AND FLAVORS: **Nut**—neutral slightly toxic, astringent; sweet, bitter. **Leaf**—warm; bitter (most of the studies have been done on a 24% extract)

ORGAN MERIDIANS AFFECTED: Lung, kidney

PROPERTIES: **Nut**—antibacterial, astringent, antifungal. **Leaves**—circulatory stimulant, antirheumatic

EFFECTS AND INDICATIONS: **Nut**—aids expectoration of phlegm, assists lung qi, stops chronic cough, stops wheezing. The nut is used for vaginal discharge and frequent urination, and can be used for cases of both deficiency and damp heat. **Leaves**—improve cerebral blood circulation and blood circulation generally, lessen and help to prevent the effects of senile dementia and Alzheimer's disease, strengthen the vascular system and reduce clots, improve hearing and treat tinnitus, improve blood circulation to the eye and help prevent macular degeneration, reduce asthma attacks, and help to prevent organ transplant rejection.

CONTRAINDICATIONS: Ginkgo biloba should not be used when there is excess or cold and dampness and should be used with caution when there is slimy, difficult-to-expectorate sputum. This herb should not be used in large doses or for long periods of time.

DOSE: 6–9 grams

NOTE: This is a beautiful but slow-growing tree and the only living member of the oldest living tree species on the earth. It is easily grown in most areas and seems to have an extraordinary ability to withstand climatic and environmental stress.

Japanese knotweed

Polygonum cuspidatum

COMMON NAME: Japanese knotwood, "Kiss me over the fence"

FAMILY: Polygonaceae

PART USED: Roots, leaves

ENERGIES AND FLAVORS: Cool, slightly toxic; bitter, sour

ORGAN MERIDIANS AFFECTED: Bladder, liver

PROPERTIES: Antipyretic, antitoxin, vulnerary

EFFECTS AND INDICATIONS: Moves blood. This herb is used to treat burn injuries, boils, abscesses, venomous bites and stings, acute hepatitis, appendicitis, traumatic injuries, and menstrual irregularities.

DOSE: 9–15 grams

NOTE: The leaves can be crushed and powdered for external application.

Lily bulb (BAI HE)
Bulbus lilii brownii
COMMON NAMES: Lily bulb, Easter lily bulb
FAMILY: Liliaceae
PART USED: Bulb (not of the calla lily, however)
ENERGY AND FLAVORS: Cool; sweet, slightly bitter
ORGAN MERIDIANS AFFECTED: Lungs, heart
PROPERTIES: Tonic, demulcent, antitussive, sedative
EFFECTS AND INDICATIONS: Acts as a yin tonic. This herb is used to treat
  lung yin deficiency with dryness and chronic cough, chronic bron-
  chitis, hemoptysis, hematemesis, restlessness, nervousness, and in-
  somnia.
CONTRAINDICATIONS: Not for diarrhea, or coughs caused by wind-cold
  conditions with chills
DOSE: 10–30 grams in decoction
NOTE: Calla Lily Bulbs are poisonous.

Imperata (BAI MAO GEN)
Imperata cylindrica
COMMON NAMES: Imperata, woolly grass, white grass
FAMILY: Gramineae
PART USED: Aerial portion
ENERGY AND FLAVOR: Cool; sweet
PROPERTIES: Antipyretic, diuretic, hemostatic
INDICATIONS: This herb is used to treat urinary tract infections, all types
  of bleeding, fever, cough, and hypertension.
CONTRAINDICATIONS: Not for cold conditions
DOSE: 15–30 grams
NOTE: This is sold as an ornamental grass.

Fleeceflower (HE SHOU WU, YI JIAO TENG)
Polygonum multiflorum
COMMON NAME: Fleeceflower
FAMILY: Polygonaceae
PARTS USED: Roots, stems
ENERGIES AND FLAVORS: **Root**—Slightly warm, astringent; sweet, bitter.
  Stem—sweet, slightly bitter; neutral energy.
ORGAN MERIDIANS AFFECTED: Liver, kidney

PROPERTIES: Tonic, lowers cholesterol, laxative, antibacterial. **Stems and Leaves**—sedative

EFFECTS AND INDICATIONS: This herb is used to treat liver and kidney blood and yin deficiency. It helps to retain essence and so is used for such symptoms as premature graying of the hair, anemia, dizziness, weak lower back and knees, nocturnal emissions, and vaginal discharge. It is also used as a tonic because it has no tendency to stagnate, and it is especially good for treating constipation in the elderly.

CONTRAINDICATIONS: Fleeceflower should not be used by those with diarrhea or when there are phlegm conditions associated with spleen deficiency.

DOSE: 9–30 grams

NOTE: Fleeceflower is widely cultivated and available in some garden catalogs. It is easily grown from cuttings. Being a vine, it grows very fast and should be given plenty of room in which to spread. Normally, this herb is preprocessed by cooking with black soybeans.

Houttuynia (YU XING CAO)

Houttuynia cordata

COMMON NAME: Houttuynia

FAMILY: Sauruaceae

PART USED: Aerial portion

ENERGY AND FLAVORS: Cool; sour, acrid

ORGAN MERIDIANS AFFECTED: Lungs, liver

PROPERTIES: Antipyretic, antitoxin, diuretic

INDICATIONS: This herb is used to treat lung inflammation, mastitis, cellulitis, middle-ear infections, urinary tract infections, edema, enteritis, and dysentery.

DOSE: 15–30 grams

Begonia

Begonia laciniata et species

COMMON NAME: Begonia

FAMILY: Begoniaceae

PART USED: Whole herb

ENERGY AND FLAVOR: Cool; sour

ORGAN MERIDIANS AFFECTED: Lungs, liver

PROPERTIES: Antipyretic, antitoxin, antiedema

INDICATIONS: This herb is used to treat influenza, acute bronchitis, rheumatic arthritis, hematoma, amenorrhea, enlarged liver, snakebites, and cancer

CONTRAINDICATIONS: Not for cold conditions or weak digestion

DOSE: 10–15 grams in decoction

NOTE: This herb is commonly available as an ornamental in most nurseries. It prefers to be in semishade and near water.

Lantana

Lantana camara

COMMON NAME: Lantana

FAMILY: Verbenaceae

PARTS USED: Roots, flowers, leaves

ENERGIES AND FLAVORS: **Roots**—cool; bland. **Flowers**—cool; sweet. **Leaves**—Cool, mildly toxic; bitter (have foul odor)

ORGAN MERIDIANS AFFECTED: Lungs, liver

PROPERTIES: **Roots**—antipyretic, antitoxin, analgesic. **Flowers**—hemostatic, anti-inflammatory. **Leaves**—antipruritic, antitoxin, antiedema

INDICATIONS: **Roots**—used to treat influenza, high fever, swollen glands, rheumatism, and traumatic injury. **Flowers**—used to treat bleeding from the lungs. **Leaves**—used to treat dermatitis, eczema, tinea (skin fungus and athlete's foot), boils, and furuncles.

CONTRAINDICATIONS: Not for cold conditions or those with weak digestion

DOSE: 30–60 grams of roots; 6–10 grams of flowers; leaves are mostly used externally for traumatic injury and wound bleeding.

NOTE: This common ornamental comes in many colors and is used as a hedge. **Caution:** Overdose can cause vomiting and dizziness.

Cocklebur fruit (CANG ER ZI)

Xanthium sibiricum

COMMON NAMES: Cocklebur fruit, xanthium

FAMILY: Compositae

PART USED: Fruits.

ENERGIES AND FLAVORS: Warm, slightly toxic; sweet, bitter, pungent

ORGAN MERIDIAN AFFECTED: Lungs

PROPERTIES: Decongestant, antirheumatic, analgesic, antifungal

INDICATIONS: This herb is used to treat upper-respiratory allergies, sinus congestion, chronic nasal discharge, respiratory allergies, loss of smell, and arthritic and rheumatic pains aggravated by cold, wind, and damp.

CONTRAINDICATIONS: Cocklebur fruit should not be used by those with blood deficiency (anemia).

DOSE: 3–9 grams

NOTE: This is a common and somewhat noxious wayside weed found in many parts of the country. **Caution:** Overdose can result in vomiting, abdominal pain, and diarrhea.

Rehmannia (SHU DI HUANG)

Rehmanniae glutinosae

COMMON NAMES: Rehmannia, prepared rehmannia

FAMILY: Scrophulariaceae

PART USED: Processed root

ENERGY AND FLAVOR: Slightly warm; sweet

ORGAN MERIDIANS AFFECTED: Heart, liver, kidney

PROPERTIES: Blood tonic, yin nutritive tonic, cardiotonic, antihypertensive, diuretic, nutritive, demulcent

EFFECTS AND INDICATIONS: Lowers blood sugar, lowers blood pressure, nourishes essence. This herb is used to treat blood and yin deficiency and deficiency of the liver and kidney with such symptoms as night sweats, nocturnal emissions, and wasting disorders. It is a blood tonic for such conditions as irregular menses, pale complexion, and dizziness. It is also used to treat lower back pain, weakness in the lower extremities, premature graying of the hair, and general exhaustion.

CONTRAINDICATIONS: Rehmannia should be used with caution by those with weak digestion and spleen *qi*; it should be avoided by those with stagnation of *qi* or phlegm.

DOSE: 9–30 grams

Scutellaria (HUANG QIN)

Scutellaria baicalensis

COMMON NAMES: Scutellaria, scute, Chinese skullcap, baikal scull cap

FAMILY: Labiatae

PART USED: Root

ENERGY AND FLAVOR: Cold; bitter

ORGAN MERIDIANS AFFECTED: Liver, lung, heart, gallbladder, large intestine

PROPERTIES: Anti-inflammatory, antibiotic, cholagogue, antihypertensive, calmative

EFFECTS AND INDICATIONS: This herb is an anti-inflammatory, especially for damp heat of the upper body. It is used for symptoms of yellow phlegm, including phlegm with blood; diarrhea, dysentery, and jaundice; urinary tract infections; skin diseases; to calm fetal restlessness; and for hypertension with symptoms of irritability, red eyes, and flushed face.

CONTRAINDICATIONS: Scutellaria should not be used by those with deficiency heat in the lungs, with coldness in the Middle Warmer, such as diarrhea, or by those mothers with restless fetus due to cold conditions.

DOSE: 3–9 grams

NOTE: This herb is often grown as an ornamental in rock gardens.

Platycodon (JIE GENG)

Platycodon grandiflorum

COMMON NAMES: Platycodon, balloon flower, balloon flower root

FAMILY: Campanulaceae

PART USED: Root

ENERGY AND FLAVORS: Neutral; acrid, bitter

ORGAN MERIDIAN AFFECTED: Lungs

PROPERTIES: Expectorant, demulcent, anti-inflammatory

EFFECTS AND INDICATIONS: Aids expectoration of phlegm and stops cough, eliminates pus, reduces inflammation, and promotes healing. This herb is used to treat both hot and cold phlegm symptoms, especially when there is dryness, and to treat pulmonary abscesses, throat inflammations, and loss of voice.

CONTRAINDICATIONS: Because of its ascending energy, platycodon is generally contraindicated for hemoptysis (blood in the sputum).

DOSE: 3–9 grams

NOTE: This herb is a common ornamental, easily grown, coming in either blue or white flowers. Both can be used.

Pinellia (BAN XIA)

Pinellia ternata

COMMON NAME: Pinellia

FAMILY: Araceae

PART USED: Processed root

ENERGIES AND FLAVOR: Warm, toxic; acrid

PROPERTIES: Antitussive, expectorant, antiemetic, antitoxin, anodyne

INDICATIONS: This herb is used to treat cough with cold phlegm, damp spleen, nausea and vomiting, swollen glands, and goiter.

CONTRAINDICATIONS: Pinellia should not be taken during pregnancy or with any symptoms associated with bleeding. **Caution:** Do not take this herb with aconite. Pinellia must be used only in its prepared form, as the raw, unprepared roots are poisonous.

DOSE: 3–12 grams

Ophiopogon (MAI MEN DONG)

Ophiopogon japonicum et species

COMMON NAMES: Ophiopogon, Japanese mondograss, Japanese turf lily.

FAMILY: Liliaceae

PART USED: Root

ENERGY AND FLAVORS: Cold; sweet, slightly bitter

ORGAN MERIDIANS AFFECTED: Heart, lung, stomach

PROPERTIES: Yin tonic, demulcent, nutritive, expectorant, lowers blood sugar

INDICATIONS: This herb is used to treat dry cough with or without blood-streaked sputum, dryness of the mouth and lips, mouth sores, inflammation of the gums, febrile diseases where heat is burning up the fluids of the body, and constipation due to fever that has dried the intestines.

CONTRAINDICATIONS: Ophiopogon should not be used by those with weak spleen and stomach with coldness and diarrhea.

DOSE: 6–12 grams

NOTE: Ophiopogon, most commonly known as Japanese mondo grass, is often used in landscape gardening and is readily available.

Rhubarb root (DA HUANG)

Rheum palmatum

COMMON NAME: Rhubarb root

FAMILY: Polygonacea

PART USED: Root

ENERGY AND FLAVOR: Cold; bitter

ORGAN MERIDIANS AFFECTED: Liver, spleen, large intestine, stomach, and pericardium

PROPERTIES: Purgative, antibacterial, antitumor, antifungal, diuretic, hemostatic, cholagogue, antihypertensive, lowers serum cholesterol, anti-inflammatory

EFFECTS AND INDICATIONS: This herb is an anti-inflammatory that can be used both internally and topically on infections. It also kills blood flukes. It is used to treat constipation; blood stagnation with symptoms of acute, stabbing pain and bruises, for which it can be taken both internally and externally (for the latter, in a liniment); and dysentery with symptoms of bleeding in the stool.

CONTRAINDICATIONS: Rhubarb root should be used only when there is excess heat and dampness. Nursing mothers should use it with extreme caution.

DOSE: 3–12 grams

NOTE: The common Western cultivated species is not the variety used in traditional Chinese medicine (TCM); however, the TCM variety is becoming increasingly available. This herb, also known as "turkey rhubarb," is used in Western herbalism for the same purposes.

Perilla (SEEDS: *ZI SU ZI*; LEAVES: *ZI SU YE*)

Perillae frutescentis

COMMON NAME: Perilla

FAMILY: Labiatae

PARTS USED: Leaves, seeds

ENERGY AND FLAVOR: Warm; acrid

ORGAN MERIDIANS AFFECTED: **Leaf**—lung, spleen. **Seeds**—Lung, large intestine

PROPERTIES: **Leaves**—diaphoretic, carminative, antiemetic. **Seeds**—antitussive, expectorant, emollient, antiasthmatic, mild laxative

INDICATIONS: **Leaves**—used to treat the common cold, cough, chest congestion, bloated stomach and abdomen, nausea and vomiting, and seafood poisoning. **Seeds**—used to treat cold and copious phlegm with wheezing, chest constriction with labored breathing, and constipation due to dryness in the intestines.

CONTRAINDICATIONS: Perilla leaves should not be used by those who have external diseases when there is already sweating or by those who have a damp-heat condition. Perilla leaves should not be used when there is diarrhea or cough due to weakness.

DOSE: 3–9 grams of either the leaf or seeds

NOTE: This is a commonly grown condiment similar to sweet basil. It is used in Japanese cooking, in which it is called *shiso*.

Peony (BAI SHAO)

Paeonia alba or *P. lactiflora*
COMMON NAME: Peony
FAMILY: Ranunculaceae
PART USED: Root
ENERGY AND FLAVORS: Slightly cold; bitter, sour
ORGAN MERIDIANS AFFECTED: Liver, spleen
PROPERTIES: Blood tonic, antispasmodic, analgesic, sedative, anti-inflammatory, diuretic, antibacterial
INDICATIONS: This herb is used to treat anemia and blood deficiency, irregular menstruation, uterine bleeding, and abdominal spasms and pain.
CONTRAINDICATIONS: White peony should not be used by those with diarrhea and spleen and stomach deficiency or those with an exterior condition. **Caution:** Avoid using white peony rhubarb.
DOSE: 3–12 grams
NOTE: Peony is commonly grown in many Western gardens. It is hard to conceive of destroying the plant—along with its beautiful flowers—by digging up the root. Another species, called tree peony, is also grown and commonly used in TCM. White peony is the cultivated variety and is used as a tonic, while red peony is uncultivated and is more blood-moving.

Pueraria (GE GEN)

Puerariae lobata
COMMON NAMES: Pueraria, kudzu, kuzu
FAMILY: Leguminosae
PART USED: Root
ENERGY AND FLAVORS: Cool; acrid, sweet
ORGAN MERIDIANS AFFECTED: Spleen, stomach, urinary bladder
PROPERTIES: Diaphoretic, antispasmodic, muscle relaxant, antipyretic
EFFECTS AND INDICATIONS: This herb is used to treat wind-heat colds, influenza, and fevers; hypertension; dysentery and colitis; and sudden nerve deafness. Relieves muscular tension and spasms, especially of the neck and shoulders; vents eruptive skin diseases, such as measles.
CONTRAINDICATIONS: Pueraria should not be used by those with cold in the stomach and excessive sweating.
DOSE: 9–15 grams
NOTE: Kudzu is considered the scourge of the South because of its fast-

growing invasiveness. It is not one to plant in a home garden, as it is very difficult to control. The flowers are used in the treatment of alcoholism effectively to lessen the desire for alcohol.

Artemisia annua (QING HAO)

Artemesiae annuae

COMMON NAMES: Artemisia annua, sweet Annie

FAMILY: Compositae

PART USED: Leaves

ENERGY AND FLAVORS: Cold; acrid, bitter

ORGAN MERIDIANS AFFECTED: Liver, kidney, gallbladder

PROPERTIES: Antipyretic, antibacterial, antifungal, antimalarial

INDICATIONS: Specific anti-inflammatory for symptoms associated with wasting and yin deficiency. This herb is used to treat heatstroke and other inflammatory conditions, including all kinds of fevers; malaria; and bacterial and fungal infections (herb is applied topically).

CONTRAINDICATIONS: Artemisia annua should be avoided by those with diarrhea due to weak, cold spleen and stomach and by those without heat signs due to yin deficiency.

DOSE: 3–9 grams

NOTE: This is the only artemisia species that is an annual. It is easily grown from seed, which is available from many suppliers in the West.

Day lily (XUAN CAO)

Hemerocallis fulva

COMMON NAME: Daylily

FAMILY: Liliaceae

PART USED: Flower buds

ENERGY AND FLAVORS: Cool; mildly sweet, mucilaginous

PROPERTIES: Diuretic, alterative, anti-inflammatory

INDICATIONS: Daylily is used to treat the pain of childbirth and tumors.

CONTRAINDICATIONS: None noted

DOSE: Only a few of the unopened flower buds are used in stir-fried preparations.

NOTES: Daylilies are commonly grown throughout American gardens. The flower buds are considered edible, while the roots are considered toxic. **Caution:** Overdose can cause urinary incontinence, respiratory arrest, dilated pupils, and even blindness. Traditionally, coptis and phellodendron have been used to counteract toxicity of the root. Generally, the root is not used; however, the unopened flower buds are commonly dried and used in Chinese cooking. They are believed to lighten the mind and clear heat.

Blackberry lily (SHE GAN)

Belamcanda chinensis

COMMON NAME: Blackberry lily

FAMILY: Iridaceae

ENERGY AND FLAVOR: Cold; bitter

PROPERTIES: Anti-inflammatory, antitoxin, expectorant, circulatory stimulant

INDICATIONS: 1. Sore throat, swelling, chronic bronchitis, mumps, excessive phlegm; 2. Irregular menstruation, swollen breasts; 3. Boils, contusions, rheumatic complaints.

CONTRAINDICATIONS: Blackberry lily should not be used during pregnancy.

DOSE: 3–9 grams decocted

NOTE: This is a type of iris that is grown as an ornamental in many gardens. It can also be powdered and applied externally as a poultice. **Caution:** Like other members of the iris family, blackberry lily is potentially toxic, so it should be used with care.

Jujube date (DA ZAO)

Zizyphus spinosa

COMMON NAME: Jujube date

FAMILY: Rhamnaceae

PART USED: Fruit

ENERGY AND FLAVOR: Neutral; sweet

ORGAN MERIDIANS AFFECTED: Spleen, stomach

PROPERTIES: Qi tonic, sedative, nutrient, antihepatotoxin

INDICATIONS: This herb is used to treat fatigue, loose stools, and lack of appetite; anemia; and restlessness, insomnia, and emotional instability associated with blood deficiency.

CONTRAINDICATIONS: Jujube date should not be used in the presence of conditions of dampness or food stagnation or in the presence of intestinal parasites or dental diseases.

DOSE: 6–30 dates in decoction

NOTES: There are literally hundreds of cultivated species of jujube in

China. The tree is easily cultivated and is increasingly found in gardens of those interested in the cultivation of Chinese herbs. In China, it is considered both a fruit and a medicine. I have been able to special-order jujube from a local nursery.

From the above partial lists, we learn that, for increasing numbers of Chinese herbs, we need not look very far. First, many of the so-called Western herbs are used both in the TCM materia medica as well as in folk medicine. In fact, many Chinese herbalists seek to use some of these more common herbs that are also used by Western herbalists. Furthermore, with the increasing acceptance of TCM throughout the West, we are finding even more Chinese herbs being grown from both imported seeds and stock as well as becoming some of the most common Western ornamentals.

· T E N ·

SOME USEFUL PATENT HOME REMEDIES*
CHINESE HERBAL PATENT MEDICINES

Chinese patents are herbal formulas made into a more convenient form for usage than teas. They typically come as pills, syrups, powders, and liniments. Patents are effective, convenient, and economical. Furthermore, they may be easily carried and taken throughout the day. They can be stored for long periods of time and the pills have no taste, so they substitute well for bad-tasting teas. Patents have generally been used for hundreds of years (the first known use of patents is over 2,000 years ago) and have proven themselves in clinical application. When taken properly, most patents have significant benefits, without side effects, for a variety of health complaints. Many are quite effective for acute conditions, such as colds, flus, fevers, trauma, and pain. For chronic conditions, their convenience often makes them the best therapy for modern life.

General Information

How Chinese Patents Are Created

Chinese patents are carefully grown, harvested, and processed in China. Often, entire villages work together to cultivate the plants. Many

---

*Modified from *Healing with Chinese Herbs*, by Lesley Tierra, Crossing Press (Freedom, CA), 1997, with permission.

highly respected U.S. practitioners have personally viewed the production process of patents and can attest to the high quality of manufacturing practices employed. Most patents are made from concentrated extracts by boiling the herbs down in a tea and then drying it. The resulting pills may then be sugar-coated to preserve them and prevent them from melting together.

How to Take Patents

Patents are best taken at least 30 minutes before or after meals with room-temperature or warm water or tea. They are best absorbed when chewed, if taste permits. Sometimes certain foods must be avoided; for example, beans and seafood must be avoided if you are taking any patents for arthritis and rheumatism. Chinese patents are generally packaged in glass bottles with corks to seal them, topped by plastic twist caps. A good way to remove the cork is to use a small knife and carefully ease it into the side of its top at an angle to gently pull it out. Corkscrews also work well. Other patents come as large soft balls in wax "eggs." The eggs are pressed so they pop open and the balls are chewed or cut into smaller pieces and swallowed. Patents may be taken alone or in combination, which can enhance their effects. For example, a cold may be treated with *Ganmaoling* along with a syrup, such as *Hsiao Keh Chuan,* for an accompanying cough; a woman with irregular periods, premenstrual syndrome (PMS), poor digestion, phlegm in the lungs, and abdominal fullness may take *Hsiao Yao Wan* along with *Er Chen Wan.*

Length of Time to Take Patents

Most patents are only taken until the symptoms being treated subside. The exceptions are for tonics, such as those to increase energy or build blood, and in chronic conditions, when the patents are taken for extended periods. Their effects should be periodically reevaluated to see if the formula should be discontinued or changed.

Doses

In the sections that follow, the usual dose is given for each formula; however, it is not uncommon for this to be increased by 50% to 100% in acute cases for short periods or for faster effects. When taking the patent as the principle therapy, use up to twice the dosage for a few days to a week, then go back to the indicated dosage. Dosages for children are reduced according to age as follows: 0 to 3 years, less than one third of the adult dose; 3 to 7 years, one third of the adult dose; 7 to 15 years, one half of the adult dose; over 15 years, adult dose.

Cautions

When there is an important contraindication or caution regarding the use of a patent, it is listed here. Pregnancy is the most common reason for caution; however, certain formulas may impair digestion or cause diarrhea with prolonged or improper use. It is extremely important, therefore, to heed the cautions listed.

Obtaining Patents

Patents may be obtained from Chinese pharmacies, generally located in the Chinatowns of major cities, in certain health-food stores, from many acupuncture practitioners, and from Chinese herbal patent distributors. Many suppliers sell by mail order, and some of these are listed in Herbal Resources (pages 453–56).

Animal Products

Several patents contain animal products because of their potent effects. This is because their constituents contain substances quite similar to those found in our own bodies. Some examples are rhinoceros or antelope horn, gecko lizard, deer antler, human placenta, tiger bone, and oyster shell. For ecological reasons, we should all *strictly avoid purchasing any products that contain animal parts of endangered species or are taken from wild animals, such as bears, whose existence would be threatened.* Furthermore, vegetarians may object to products with such ingredients; generally, substitute patents may be found. The use of both rhinoceros horn and tiger bone is restricted in North America, and thus any patents containing either of these items are not included here.

Western Drugs in Chinese Patents

In general, the Chinese do not mix Western drugs into Chinese herbal patents. Occasionally, one hears of an occasional case of certain pharmaceutical drugs being mixed with a specific patent; however, this is comparatively rare, and any patents known to contain Western drugs are noted here. Some remedies, such as *Gan Mao Ling, Bi Yan Pian, Pe Min Kan Wan,* and Margarite Acne Pills, are available both ways. In these cases, Plum Flower brand manufactures the same formulas without food coloring or drugs. It is available from Mayway (see Herbal Resources).

Note

The patents listed here are generally safe and without side effects. They are only a few of the hundreds available—a visit to a Chinese pharmacy can be eye-opening. It is always wise to seek the advice of a professional, however, when seeking the appropriate patents for your condition.

To identify the form of a patent, use the following guidelines: *wan* means "round pill," *san* means "powder," *gao* means "plaster," and *dan* refers to a form of patent medicine containing minerals.

The Chinese herbal patents in this section are divided among the following categories.

Chinese Patent Medicines

- Colds and influenza
- Coughs, phlegm, and labored breathing
- Headaches
- Allergies and sinus infections
- Sore throats, mouth disorders, and ear problems
- Eyes
- Genitourinary conditions
- Hemorrhoids
- Gynecological conditions
- Digestive disorders
- Liver and gallbladder disorders
- Heart disorders
- Skin disorders
- Arthritis and rheumatism
- Restlessness and insomnia
- Hypertension

- Energy tonics
- Infants' and young children's disorders
- Pain
- First aid

This is not a traditional classification, but it is used for easier identification. Again, not all of the most common patents are included here, as those with prohibited substances, such as tiger bone, and most of those with animal parts have not been listed here. For differentiating the many patents in any one category, see Chapter 10, Commonly Used Formulas.

Colds and Influenza

PILLS

Ganmaoling

INDICATIONS: One of the most commonly known and used Chinese herbal patents, this remedy is excellent for colds and influenza with chills, high fever, swollen lymph glands, sore throat, and stiffness of the upper back and neck. It may also be taken for a few days to prevent the onset of a cold or influenza.

DOSAGE: Bottle of 36 tablets. Take 3–6 tablets, 3 times a day. For prevention of colds: 2 tablets, 2–3 times a day, for 3 days.

NOTE: Use Plum Flower brand; the other brand contains food coloring and drugs.

Yin Chiao (Tianjin)

EFFECTS AND INDICATIONS: Like *Ganmaoling*, *Yin Chiao* is one of the most common Chinese herbal patents, useful for the first 1 or 2 days of influenza, colds, measles, tonsillitis, pneumonia, swollen lymph nodes, sore throat, aching body, fever with chills, headache, thirst, sore shoulders, stiff neck, skin itching (when there is aversion to heat), and hives. It promotes sweating.

DOSAGE: Boxes of 12 bottles, 8 pills to the bottle; also bottles of 100 pills. Take 5–6 pills every 2–3 hours for the first 9 hours, then every 4–5 hours as needed. Discontinue by the third day.

NOTE: There are several types of *Yin Chiao* tablets. The brand Superior Quality–Sugar Coated has a sugar coating, contains antelope horn, and includes Western chemicals. This brand should be avoided. The others are fine and differ only in amount of herbs in the formula. The

Tianjin brand has more herbs. Planetary Formulas makes a pure *Yin Chiao* and *Yin Chiao Plus with Echinacea.*

Huo Hsiang Cheng Chi Pien (Lophanthus Antifebrile Pills)

INDICATIONS: This patent is excellent for colds and influenza with diarrhea, vomiting, abdominal pain with gurgling and a lot of gas, nausea, fever, chills, and headache. Often, diarrhea is the predominant symptom.

CONTRAINDICATIONS: Do not use if there is dry mouth, thirst, and fever without chills.

DOSAGE: Bottles of 100 pills or vials of 12 tablets. Take 10 pills or 4–8 tablets, 3 times a day.

Chuan Xiong Chao Tiao Wan

INDICATIONS: For sudden headache due to a cold with chills, nasal congestion, sinusitis, and rhinitis.

DOSAGE: Bottles of 200 pills. Take 8 pills, 3–5 times a day.

OTHER

For stomach flu with sudden and violent abdominal cramping, bloating with pain, vomiting, headache, constipation, or diarrhea, use Pill Curing, under Digestive Disorders.

Coughs, Phlegm, and Labored Breathing

PILLS

Bronchitis Pills (compound)

EFFECTS AND INDICATIONS: These are useful for acute and chronic bronchitis, chronic asthma, and cough and phlegm brought on by colds and influenza. They resolve coughs, phlegm, and labored breathing due to weakness of the lungs and retention of phlegm.

DOSAGE: Bottles of 60 capsules. Take 2–3 capsules, 3 times a day.

Ching Fei Yi Huo Pien

INDICATIONS: For toxic heat with profuse or sticky yellow phlegm, dry or raspy cough, swollen and painful throat, fever, concentrated urine, constipation, mouth or nose sores, bleeding gums, and toothache.

CONTRAINDICATIONS: Prohibited during pregnancy. **Caution:** Discontinue after heat symptoms subside or if diarrhea develops.

DOSAGE: Tubes of 8 tablets, 12 tubes to a box. Take 4 tablets, 2–3 times a day.

Pulmonary Tonic Pills

EFFECTS AND INDICATIONS: Strengthens the lungs for symptoms of chronic lung weakness with heat, dry cough, and sticky yellow phlegm.

DOSAGE: Bottles of 60 pills. Take 5 pills 3 times a day.

Er Chen Wan

EFFECTS AND INDICATIONS: This is the primary formula for dissolving phlegm congestion in the stomach, lungs, or face with symptoms of nausea, abdominal fullness, a sensation of chest fullness, dizziness, vertigo, phlegm in the lungs, some instances of postnasal drip and nasal mucus, phlegm in the throat, excessive salivation, and alcoholic hangover.

DOSAGE: Bottle of 200 pills. Take 8 pills, 3 times a day.

Ping Chuan

INDICATIONS: A very useful remedy for chronic asthma, bronchitis, and emphysema, along with cough and shortness of breath that worsens in the evening or with overexertion, with additional symptoms of low back pain, frequent and/or night time urination, and weakness.

DOSAGE: Bottles of 120 pills. Take 10 pills 3 times a day.

NOTE: Contains gecko lizard.

Hsiao Keh Chuan

INDICATIONS: An excellent remedy for acute and chronic bronchitis and asthma, cough with copious clear to white mucus, coldness, lung congestion, and difficulty in breathing.

DOSAGE: Bottles of 18 capsules. Take 2 capsules, 3 times a day.

Qing Qi Hua Tan Wan (Pinellia Expectorant Pills)

INDICATIONS: For heat and mucus in the lungs, throat, and sinuses; bronchial congestion; sinus congestion; and asthma with excessive yellow, thick, and sticky phlegm or nasal discharge.

CONTRAINDICATIONS: Do not use if there are chills, or a dry cough with no phlegm.

DOSAGE: Bottles of 200 pills. Take 6 pills 3 times a day.

OTHER

For coughs with accompanying nasal congestion, see *Bi Yan Pian,* under Allergies and Sinus Infections.

For coughs with accompanying poor digestion, poor appetite, loose stools, or diarrhea, see *Liu Jun Zi* tablets, under Digestive Disorders.

SYRUPS

Hsiao Keh Chuan (Special Medicine for Bronchitis)

EFFECTS AND INDICATIONS: Very useful for acute and chronic bronchitis, cough, and asthma with clear to white watery phlegm; coldness; weakness of the lungs; and possible low-back pain or frequent clear urination. It also increases the body's resistance to disease.

DOSAGE: Bottles of 100 milliliters of liquid. Take 1–2 tablespoons, 3 times a day with water.

Natural Herb Loquat-Flavored Syrup

INDICATIONS: For acute and chronic cough due to weak lungs, heat, or lung dryness with sticky phlegm. Useful in emphysema, acute bronchitis, and accompanying sinus congestion.

DOSAGE: Bottles of 5 ounces, 10 ounces, and 25 ounces of liquid (10- or 25-ounce size recommended). Adults: 1 tablespoon 3 times a day. Children: 1 teaspoon, 3 times a day.

TEA

Lo Han Kuo

INDICATIONS: Useful for coughs with sticky or bloody phlegm, thirst, itchy throat, and stubborn chronic coughs, such as those associated with whooping cough or tuberculosis. It is pleasant to taste and easy to prepare.

DOSAGE: Boxes of 12 smaller boxes, each with 2 doses. Take 1 cube at a time and dissolve in 1 cup of hot water. Take 3–6 times a day.

Headaches

For headaches with:

- Fever, use *Yin Chiao* tablets, under Colds and Influenza
- Allergies or sinusitis, use *Bi Yan Pian,* under Allergies and Sinus Infections
- Indigestion, use Pill Curing, under Digestive Disorders
- Muscle tension or spasm, use *Hsiao Yao Wan,* under Gynecological Conditions
- Migraine pain, use *Corydalis Yan Hu Suo* Analgesic tablets, under Pain
- Migraine with a cold, use *Tian Ma Wan,* under Arthritis and Rheumatism
- With chills or cold, use *Chuan Xiong Chao Tiao Wan,* under Colds and Influenza

Allergies and Sinus Infections

PILLS

Bi Yan Pian

INDICATIONS: Good for sneezing, itchy eyes, facial congestion, and sinus pain. Useful in acute and chronic rhinitis, sinusitis, hayfever, nasal allergies, stuffy nose with yellowish thick discharge and foul smell, and general facial mucosal congestion.

DOSAGE: Bottle of 100 tablets. Take 4–6 tablets, 3–5 times a day.

NOTE: Use Plum Flower brand; the other brand contains food coloring and drugs.

Pe Min Kan Wan

INDICATIONS: Very useful for hay fever, sinus infections, rhinitis and acute or chronic sinusitis, and facial congestion during colds with sneezing; runny nose; itchy, watery eyes; and postnasal drip, for which it is specific.

DOSAGE: Bottles of 50 pills. Take 3 pills, 3 times a day.

NOTE: Use Plum Flower brand; the other brand contains food coloring and drugs.

OTHER

For sinus congestion with thick, sticky yellow mucus, use *Qing Qi Hua Tan Wan* (Pinellia Expectorant Pills), under Coughs, Phlegm, and Labored Breathing.

For headaches with sinusitis, rhinitis, nasal congestion, and coldness, use *Chuan Xiong Chao Tiao Wan* under Colds and Influenza.

Sore Throats, Mouth Disorders, and Ear Problems

PILLS

Huang Lien Shang Ching Pien

INDICATIONS: Good for conditions of heat, including high fever, headaches, sore throats, ear infections, itching, hives, swollen gums, toothaches, nosebleeds, insomnia, red eyes, constipation, diarrhea, and concentrated, scanty urine.

CONTRAINDICATIONS: Stop taking *Huang Lien Shang Ching Pien* when the heat symptoms listed above subside. Discontinue the pills if frequent loose stools develop. **Caution:** Use of *Huang Lien Shang Ching Pien* is prohibited during pregnancy.

Chuan Xin Lian (Antiphlogistic Pills)

INDICATIONS: Excellent for acute throat inflammations with swollen glands and fever, including strep infections. Also used to treat viral infections causing fever, such as measles, influenza, and hepatitis, and for furuncles, mastitis, and abscesses.

DOSAGE: Bottles of 60 pills. Take 3 pills, 3 times a day, for 1 or 2 days at most.

Laryngitis Pills

INDICATIONS: Used for laryngitis due to heat and for acute tonsillitis, acute mumps, or lingering sore throat with heat.

CONTRAINDICATIONS: Take Laryngitis Pills only for a short time—1 or 2 doses. **Caution:** Use of Laryngitis Pills is prohibited during pregnancy.

DOSAGE: Small boxes of 3 vials, each with 10 pills. Take 3 times a day as follows: infants to 1 year, 1 pill; 1–2 years, 2 pills; 2–3 years, 3–4 pills; 4–8 years, 5–6 pills; 9–15 years, 8–9 pills; adults, 10 pills.

NOTE: If there is a strep infection involved, combine this patent with *Chuan Xin Lian* (Antiphlogistic Pills). This product contains animal parts.

Superior Sore Throat Powder Spray

INDICATIONS: Use for sore throat, mouth ulcers, ulcerative skin lesions, inflamed sinuses, and middle-ear infections when there is heat.

DOSAGE: Bottles of powder (2.2 grams) in spray form. For throat and mouth, spray once, 3 times a day; for sinusitis, spray in nose, 5 times a day; for oozing middle-ear inflammations, wash the ear with hydrogen peroxide and spray, 1 time daily; for ulcerative skin lesions, spray 1 time daily.

NOTE: This formula is effective but tastes bad.

Tso-Tzu Otic Pills

INDICATIONS: These are used for ear ringing, headache, eye pressure, insomnia, thirst, eye irritation and pressure, and high blood pressure.

DOSAGE: Bottles of 200 pills. Take 8 pills, 3 times a day.

POWDER

Xi Gua Shuang

INDICATIONS: This is watermelon "frost." It is excellent for mouth sores and ulcers or toothaches. It also treats burns on the skin.

Caution: Do not eat greasy, oily food when taking this formula.

DOSAGE: Box of 10 vials, each containing 2 grams of powder. Mix 1–2 grams of powder with water and take this amount 2–3 times a day. For the skin, mix 2 vials of powder with some cooking oil and apply topically for a few days until the burn is healed.

OTHER

For painful and swollen sore throat, nose or mouth sores, toothache, nosebleeds, and swollen gums, use *Ching Fei Yi Huo Pien,* under Coughs, Phlegm, and Labored Breathing.

For sore throat, fever blisters on the mouth, red and burning eyes, headache, scanty urine, or constipation, use *Lung Tan Xie Gan* pills, under Genitourinary Conditions.

Eyes

PILLS

Ming Mu Shang Ching Pien

INDICATIONS: For red, itching, and tearing eyes; swelling of the eyes associated with conjunctivitis; vertigo; photophobia; and night blindness.

Symptoms may also include scanty, dark urine; constipation; night sweats; fatigue; dry throat or mouth; and fever.

Caution: Prohibited during pregnancy.

DOSAGE: Boxes of 12 vials, each with 8 tablets—take 4 tablets, 2 times a day, or in bottles of 200 pills—take 10 pills, 3 times a day.

Dendrobium Moniliforme Night Sight Pills

INDICATIONS: This formula is used for improving vision, especially eyesight that is beginning to diminish with blurriness or dizziness; photophobia; the early stages of cataracts; eye tearing; red, itchy, or dry eyes; and hypertensive pressure behind the eyes. Other symptoms of night sweats, fatigue, low-back pain, and insomnia may be present.

DOSAGE: Boxes of 10 pills, each 6 grams—Take one pill, 2 times a day, or boxes of 10 honey pills—take 1 honey pill, 2 times a day.

NOTE: This formula contains some animal parts.

OTHER

For red and burning eyes, sore throat, fever blisters on the mouth, headache, scanty urine, or constipation, use *Lung Tan Xie Gan* pills, under Genitourinary Conditions.

Genitourinary Conditions

PILLS

Chien Chin Chih Tai Wan

INDICATIONS: Extremely useful for leukorrhea with white discharge, trichomonas, and vaginal infections with anemia or weakness, such as low-back pain, fatigue, and abdominal distensions and pain.

DOSAGE: Bottles of 120 pills. Take 10 pills, 1–2 times a day.

Yudai Wan

INDICATIONS: This formula is used for dark and odorous leukorrhea and acute vaginitis with lower-back ache, fatigue, abdominal distension, and pain. It is also good for bladder infections from yeast.

DOSAGE: Bottles of 100 pills. Take 8 pills, 3 times a day.

Lung Tan Xie Gan

INDICATIONS: This formula is excellent for urinary bladder infections, oral and genital herpes, prostatitis, urethritis, red and burning eyes, sore throat, fever blisters on the mouth, scanty urine, constipation, and leukorrhea with yellow discharge.

DOSAGE: Bottles of 100 pills. Take 6 pills, 2 times a day.

Specific Drug *Passwan*

EFFECTS AND INDICATIONS: This formula is used for acute and chronic urinary calculi (stones) in the kidney, bladder, or ureters. It will dissolve the crystalization and stop bleeding and pain.

DOSAGE: Bottles of 120 capsules. Take 6–8 capsules, 3 times a day.

Kai Kit Wan

INDICATIONS: This formula is a specific remedy for enlarged prostate gland with painful or difficult urination, pain in the groin, frequent and nighttime urination, fatigue, and possible weakness. It is especially good for chronic conditions in which swelling is pronounced.

DOSAGE: Bottles of 54 pills. Take 3–6 pills, 2–3 times a day.

TEA

Chih Pai Di Huang Wan (Eight–Flavor Tea)

INDICATIONS: This formula is used for bladder or vaginal infections with dry throat, thirst, hot flashes, night sweating, heat in soles of feet or palms, insomnia, and restless sleep.

DOSAGE: Bottles of 200 pills. Take 8–16 pills, 3 times a day.

Hemorrhoids

PILLS

Fargelin for Piles

INDICATIONS: This formula is used for acute and chronic hemorrhoids with heat signs, such as itching, bleeding, burning, prolapsed anus, and possible constipation.

DOSAGE: Bottles of 36 or 60 tablets. Take 3 tablets, 3 times a day.

NOTE: This formula may contain some animal parts.

OTHER

For hemorrhoids with bleeding, use *Yunnan Paiyao,* under First Aid.

Gynecological Conditions

PILLS

Hsiao Yao Wan (Bupleurum Sedative Pills)

INDICATIONS: This is a specific formula for PMS; menstrual disorders, such as cramps, irregular periods, infertility, breast distension, depression, and irritability; and vertigo, headaches, fatigue, blurred vision, and red, painful eyes. It also aids digestive dysfunction with abdominal bloating and fullness, hiccups, and poor appetite. It may also be used for food allergies, chronic hay fever, and hypoglycemia.

DOSAGE: Bottles of 100 or 200 pills. Take 8 pills, 3 times a day.

NOTE: This product also comes labeled as *Xiao Yao Wan*. It is the same formula.

Butiao

INDICATIONS: This formula is used for irregular periods, menstrual pain and cramps, and excessive uterine bleeding accompanied with fatigue and possible anemia. Not to be used during pregnancy.

DOSAGE: Bottles of 100 tablets. Take 3 pills, 3 times a day.

Wu Chi Pai Feng Wan (White Phoenix Pills)

INDICATIONS: This formula is used for menstrual disorders with possible anemia, cramps, headaches, amenorrhea, pain with ovulation, fatigue, low-back pain, poor appetite, or prolonged or irregular periods. May also be used for postpartum fatigue or bleeding.

DOSAGE: Boxes of 10 large chewable pills or bottles of 120 pills. Take ½–1 chewable pill, 2 times a day. Chew the pills or cut them into smaller pieces and swallow them. The pills may also be dissolved in warm water. Take 5 regular pills, 3 times a day.

NOTE: This formula contains animal parts. A similar formula, called *Pai Feng Wan*, is available that involves a shorter regimen.

An Tai Wan (For Embryo)

INDICATIONS: This formula is used to calm a restless fetus, premature uterine contractions, and threatened miscarriage with lower abdominal pains during pregnancy.

Caution: Use of any Chinese herbal patent medicines during pregnancy should be monitored by a qualified practitioner of traditional Chinese medicine (TCM).

DOSAGE: Bottles of 100 pills. Take 7 pills, 3 times a day.

Shih San Tai Pao Wan

INDICATIONS: This formula is used in the first trimester of pregnancy for threatened miscarriage, fatigue, anemia, and nausea.

Caution: Use of any Chinese herbal patent medicines during pregnancy should be monitored by a qualified practitioner of TCM.

DOSAGE: Boxes of 10 waxed egg pills. Take 1 pill, 2 times a day.

He Che Da Zao Wan (Placenta Compound Restorative Pills)

INDICATIONS: This formula is useful for menopausal night sweats and hot flashes in women and for spermatorrhea in men when the semen is lost at night, during a dream. For both men and women, accompanying symptoms are dizziness, tinnitus, weak and tired legs, aching lower back, low-grade afternoon fever, and fatigue, red cheeks, or hot, flushed face.

DOSAGE: Bottles of 100 pills. Take 8 pills, 3 times a day.

NOTE: This formula contains animal parts.

TONIC

Tang Kwei Gin

INDICATIONS: This is a widely used liquid tonic for improving the quality of the blood, for both men and women, as in possible anemia or fatigue following illness, surgery, or trauma. It is also good for palpitations, dizziness, poor memory, irregular menses with pale blood, amenorrhea, and postpartum weakness due to excess blood loss.

DOSAGE: Bottles of 100 or 200 milliliters. Take 1–2 tablespoons, 2 times a day.

OTHER

Men suffering from impotence, infertility, sexual dysfunction with coldness, such as cold hands and feet, frequent urination, diarrhea, undigested food in the stools, and fatigue, can use Golden Book Tea or Sexoton Pills, under Energy Tonics.

Women have additional choices:

• For uterine bleeding, habitual miscarriage, prolapse of the uterus or bladder, low energy, and digestive weakness, use *Bu Zhong Yi Qi Wan* (Central *Qi* Pills), under Energy Tonics.

- For abnormal uterine bleeding, irregular or heavy menses, palpitations, fatigue, night sweats, insomnia, dizziness, and restless dreaming, see *Gui Pi Wan*, under Restlessness and Insomnia.
- For light or irregular menses with dizziness, poor memory, pale face, and fatigue, use Eight Treasure Tea, under Energy Tonics.
- For acute vaginitis use *Yudai Wan,* under Genitourinary Conditions.
- For severe menstrual cramps and excessive bleeding, use *Yunnan Paiyao,* under First Aid.
- For menstrual pain use Corydalis *Yan hu suo* Analgesic Tablets, under Pain.
- For vaginal or menstrual infections, hot flashes, night sweats, a burning sensation in the palms or soles, or insomnia, use Eight-Flavor Tea, under Genitourinary Conditions.

Digestive Disorders

PILLS

Ren Shen Jian Pi Wan (Ginseng Stomachic Pills)

INDICATIONS: This formula is used for chronically poor digestion with abdominal bloating and pain, diarrhea or loose stools, loss of appetite, low energy, pale face, and inability to gain or maintain weight.

CONTRAINDICATIONS: Avoid eating cold foods when taking *Ren Shen Jian Pi Wan.* **Caution:** Nursing mothers should not use this formula.

DOSAGE: Bottles of 200 pills. Take 6 pills, 3 times a day.

NOTE: This product is most commonly available without the ginseng, in a form called *Jian Pi Wan.*

Liu Jun Zi tablets

INDICATIONS: This formula is used for poor digestion with poor appetite, loose stools or diarrhea, indigestion, acid regurgitation, and nausea.

CONTRAINDICATIONS: Avoid eating cold foods when taking *Liu Jun Zi.*

DOSAGE: Bottles of 96 tablets. Take 8 tablets, 3 times a day, after meals.

Fu Zi Li Zhong Wan (Carmichaeli Tea Pills)

INDICATIONS: This formula is used for watery, pale diarrhea or loose stools; nausea; vomiting; poor digestion; clear urine; abdominal fullness; and cold hands or feet.

DOSAGE: Bottle of 200 pills. Take 8–12, 3 times a day.
NOTE: This patent contains aconite.

Mu Xiang Shun Qi Wan (Aplotaxis Carminative Pills)

INDICATIONS: This formula is used for food congestion with a "stuck" feeling in the abdomen or abdominal distension, poor digestion, erratic stools, constipation, foul belching, and foul breath. It is useful for hypoacidity.
CONTRAINDICATIONS: Avoid eating cold foods when taking this formula.
DOSAGE: Bottles of 200 pills. Take 8 pills, 2 times a day.

Pill Curing (Planetary Formula is *Digestive Comfort*)

INDICATIONS: This formula is useful for food congestion or food poisoning as well as stomach flu with sudden and violent abdominal cramping, bloating with pain, vomiting, headache, constipation, or diarrhea. It is also excellent for general nausea, motion sickness, and morning sickness. It is safe in pregnancy and for children.
DOSAGE: Boxes of 10 bottles or packets. Take 1–2 bottles at a time as needed.

Ping Wei Pian

EFFECTS AND INDICATIONS: This formula soothes gastric disturbance, gas, abdominal cramping or bloating, poor appetite, diarrhea, nausea, and pain. It maintains digestive function.
DOSAGE: Bottles of 48 tablets. Take 4 tablets, 2 times a day.

Shu Kan Wan (condensed)

INDICATIONS: This formula is used for abdominal gas, hiccups, belching, or flatulence with abdominal pain, poor digestion, loose or erratic stools, poor appetite with nausea, vomiting, and regurgitation associated with hyperacidity. It is also used for limb coldness accompanied by facial flush.
Caution: The use of *Shu Kan Wan* is prohibited during pregnancy.
DOSAGE: Bottles of 120 pills. Take 8 pills, 3 times a day.

Fructus persica

INDICATIONS: This formula is used for habitual constipation with dryness or heat.
DOSAGE: Bottles of 200 pills. Take 4–8 pills, 3 times a day.

Sai Mei An (Internal Formula)

EFFECTS AND INDICATIONS: This formula is used for hyperacidity, gastritis with hyperacidity in the stomach, duodenal and gastric stomach ulcers without bleeding, and for irritation and inflammation of the stomach lining with pain following meals. This remedy promotes regeneration of tissue in the stomach.

CONTRAINDICATIONS: Take *Sai Mei An* for only a short time, as prolonged use can damage the stomach and digestion. **Caution:** Discontinue use of the formula 2 weeks after symptoms subside.

DOSAGE: Bottles of 50 pills. Take 3 pills, 3 times a day, before meals on an empty stomach.

NOTE: If there is also bleeding, add *Yunnan Paiyao,* under First Aid.

Wei Te Ling

INDICATIONS: This formula is used to relieve the pain and bleeding of gastric and duodenal ulcers, gastritis with hyperacidity, stomach distension, and gas.

DOSAGE: Bottles of 120 tablets. Take 4–6 tablets, 3 times a day, before meals or when necessary.

JELLY

Rensheng Feng Wang Jiang (Ginseng Royal Jelly)

EFFECTS AND INDICATIONS: This product promotes appetite and stimulates the absorption of foods. It is beneficial following illness or childbirth, in hypoglycemia, and in older people.

CONTRAINDICATIONS: Avoid eating citrus and cold foods or drinking caffeinated drinks.

DOSAGE: Boxes of 10 glass vials, 10 milliliters each. Take 1–2 vials per day, alone or with water.

OTHER

For stomach pain or gastric or duodenal ulcer pain, use Corydalis *Yan Hu Suo* Analgesic Tablets, under Pain.

For poor digestion with:

- Abdominal bloating and fullness, hiccups, poor appetite, and food allergies, use *Hsiao Yao Wan,* under Gynecological Conditions
- Abdominal bloating, pain, gas and erratic stools, chronic diarrhea,

hypoglycemia, and low energy, use *Bu Zhong Yi Qi Wan* (Central *Qi* Pills), under Energy Tonics

- Undigested food in the stools, coldness, low-back pain, and diarrhea, use Golden Book Tea, under Energy Tonics.
- Low appetite, hypoglycemia, pale face, anemia, fatigue, and dizziness, use Eight Treasure Tea, under Energy Tonics
- Nausea, vertigo, headache, pasty loose stools or diarrhea, and flatulence, use *Huo Hsiang Cheng Chi Pien,* under Colds and Influenza. (This remedy can be used without signs of a cold or influenza.)

Liver and Gallbladder Disorders

PILLS

Lidan Tablets

INDICATIONS: This formula is specific for acute and chronic gallstone or bile-duct inflammation. In China, it is used to dissolve and remove gallstones.

DOSAGE: Bottles of 120 tablets. Take 6 tablets, 3 times a day.

Li Gan Pian (Liver Strengthening Tablets)

EFFECTS AND INDICATIONS: This formula decreases pain in the liver area. It can be taken with Lidan Tablets. It is used for acute and chronic jaundice, hepatitis, and gallstones and to regulate bile.

DOSAGE: Bottles of 100 tablets. Take 2–4 tablets, 3 times a day with meals.

Ji Gu Cao

INDICATIONS: This formula is used for acute and chronic hepatitis with jaundice. It is reported to have excellent results without side effects.

DOSAGE: Bottles of 50 pills. Take 4 pills, 3 times a day.

NOTE: In acute hepatitis, combine this formula with *Li Gan Pian.*

OTHER

For hepatitis or gallbladder pain, use Corydalis *Yan Hu Suo* Analgesic Tablets, under Pain.

Heart Disorders

PILLS

Dan Shen *Tablet Co.*

INDICATIONS: This formula reduces blood cholesterol and lipids. It is used for angina pectoris with pain radiating down the left arm, heart palpitations, and chest pains.

Caution: As with any potentially dangerous health condition, it is important to seek the aid of a qualified health practitioner.

DOSAGE: Bottles of 50 pills. Take 3 pills, 3 times a day.

Ren Shen Zai Zao Wan (Ginseng Restorative Pills)

Aids symptoms related to stroke such as hemiplegia, speech disturbances and contractive, spastic or flaccid muscle tone in the extremities. Also useful for facial paralysis (Bell's Palsy). This remedy contains some animal parts.

CONTRAINDICATIONS: Do not use *Ren Shen Zai Zao Wan* if there is bleeding. **Caution:** Use of this formula is prohibited during pregnancy.

DOSAGE: Boxes of 10 pills in wax eggs or bottles of 50 pills. Take 1 wax egg pill 2 times a day or 10 bottle pills 1 time a day.

OTHER

For stroke symptoms of paralysis, Bell's palsy with migraines, or rheumatic pain, use *Tian Ma Wan,* under Arthritis and Rheumatism.

Skin Disorders

PILLS

Margarite Acne Pills

INDICATIONS: This formula is used for acne, furuncles, skin itching, rashes, and hives. It is excellent for adolescent acne.

Caution: Reduce dosage if diarrhea develops.

DOSAGE: Bottles of 30 pills. Take 6 pills, 2 times a day.

NOTE: Use Plum Flower brand; the other brand contains food coloring and drugs.

Lien Chiao Pai Tu Pien

INDICATIONS: This formula is used for acute inflammations and infections, ulcerated abscesses and carbuncles with pus, and skin itching with rash and redness.

Caution: The use of Lien Chiao Pai Tu Pien is prohibited during pregnancy.

DOSAGE: Boxes of 12 vials, 8 tablets to a vial. Take 2–4 tablets, 2 times a day.

OTHER

For furuncles and abscesses, use Chuan Xin Lian, under Sore Throats, Mouth Disorders, and Ear Problems.

For ulcerative skin lesions, spray once daily with Superior Sore Throat Powder Spray, under Sore Throats, Mouth Disorders, and Ear Problems.

For itching and hives, use Huang Lien Shang Ching Pien, under Sore Throats, Mouth Disorders, and Ear Problems.

For boils, nose and mouth sores, toothaches, sore throats, or nosebleeds, use Ching Fei Yi Huo Pian, under Coughs, Phlegm, and Labored Breathing.

Arthritis and Rheumatism

PILLS

Specific Lumbaglin

INDICATIONS: This formula relieves inflammation, pain, and achiness of lower-back pain, muscular strain, and sciatic inflammation. It also strengthens the waist and kidneys.

CONTRAINDICATIONS: Avoid eating beans and seafoods while taking Specific Lumbaglin. **Caution:** Avoid taking this formula during pregnancy.

DOSAGE: Boxes of 24 capsules. Take 1–2 capsules, 3 times a day.

Du Huo Jisheng Wan

EFFECTS AND INDICATIONS: This classic Chinese formula aids lower-back and knee pain accompanied by weakness, stiffness, and numbness due to cold (frequent and/or nighttime urination producing clear urine, feelings of coldness, and aversion to cold). Conditions for which it is used include chronic sciatica, arthritis, and rheumatism.

CONTRAINDICATIONS: Avoid eating beans, seafoods, and cold foods while taking *Du Huo Jisheng Wan*. **Caution:** Avoid using this formula during pregnancy.

DOSAGE: Bottles of 100 pills. Take 9 pills, 2 times a day.

Xiao Huo Luo Dan

INDICATIONS: This formula is used for rheumatic pain, numbness, difficulty in moving joints, stiff joints, limb numbness, sharp joint pain or aching in joints or muscles, and chronic low-back pain from coldness (frequent and/or nighttime urination producing clear color, feelings of coldness, and aversion to cold).

CONTRAINDICATIONS: Do not use *Xiao Huo Luo Dan* if joints are red and swollen and fever is present. Avoid eating beans, seafoods, and cold foods while taking this formula. **Caution:** Use of this formula is prohibited during pregnancy.

DOSAGE: Bottles of 100 pills. Take 6 pills, 2–3 times a day.

Feng Shih Hsiao Tung Wan

INDICATIONS: This formula is used for rheumatism causing lower-back aches, chronic sciatica, or pain in the fingers, shoulder, knees, and hips with a feeling of cold in the limbs. It is especially used with chronic rheumatoid arthritis or osteoarthritis or for older people with debility of the legs and difficulty walking due to pain and stiffness in the joints.

CONTRAINDICATIONS: Avoid eating beans, seafoods, and cold foods while taking *Feng Shih Hsiao Tung Wan*. **Caution:** Avoid taking this formula during pregnancy.

DOSAGE: Bottles of 100 pills. Take 10 pills, 2 times a day.

Tian Ma Wan

CONTRAINDICATIONS: This formula is used for rheumatic or arthritic pain with coldness; migraines; paralysis of the face, arm, or leg; and Bell's palsy. It is well suited for the elderly.

DOSAGE: Bottles of 100 pills. Take 6–8 pills, 3 times a day.

OTHER

For rheumatic pain, use Corydalis *Yan Hu Suo* Analgesic Tablets, under Pain.

For rheumatism with difficulty in movement, painful joints, and numbness and tingling of the limbs, use *Ren Shen Zai Zao Wan,* under Heart Disorders.

Restlessness and Insomnia

PILLS

An Mien Pien

INDICATIONS: This formula is used for insomnia with mental agitation or exhaustion, anxiety, red or irritated eyes, excessive dreaming, too much thinking, poor memory, and difficulty falling asleep.

CONTRAINDICATIONS: Avoid eating hot, greasy foods when taking *An Mien Pien.*

DOSAGE: Bottles of 60 tablets. Take 4 tablets, 3 times a day.

Ding Xin Wan

INDICATIONS: This formula is used for restlessness, anxiety, insomnia, palpitations, poor memory, dizziness, hot flashes, dry mouth, and difficulty falling asleep or staying asleep.

CONTRAINDICATIONS: Avoid eating hot, greasy foods when taking *Ding Xin Wan.*

DOSAGE: Bottles of 100 pills. Take 6 pills, 2–3 times a day.

Shen Ching Shuai Jao Wan

INDICATIONS: This formula is used for insomnia, nightmares, restless sleep, night sweating, vertigo, tinnitus, palpitation, and fatigue.

CONTRAINDICATIONS: Avoid eating cold foods when taking *Shen Ching Shuai Jao Wan.* **Caution:** Excessive or prolonged use of this formula can impair the digestion.

DOSAGE: Bottles of 200 pills. Take 20 pills, 2 times a day. Discontinue after 2 weeks and wait 1–2 weeks before resuming.

NOTE: This formula contains some animal parts.

An Shen Bu Xin Wan

EFFECTS AND INDICATIONS: This formula is calming, soothing, and tranquilizing. It is used for insomnia, palpitations, poor memory, uneasiness, excessive dreaming, restlessness, and dizziness.

Caution: Discontinue use of *An Shen Bu Xin Wan* after 2 weeks and wait 1–2 weeks before resuming.
DOSAGE: Bottles of 300 pills. Take 15 pills, 3 times a day.

Gui Pi Wan (Kwei Be Wan)

INDICATIONS: This formula is used for insomnia, palpitations, dizziness, nightmares or restless dreaming, poor memory, fatigue, and night sweating. It is also used for irregular menstrual cycles and abnormal uterine bleeding.
DOSAGE: Bottles of 200 pills. Take 8 pills, 3 times a day.

TEA

Tian Wang Bu Xin Wan (Emperor's Tea)

INDICATIONS: This formula is used for insomnia, restlessness, anxiety, palpitations, vivid dreaming, and nocturnal emission with possible night sweats. It may also be used in hyperactive thyroid and is excellent for students during prolonged studying.
CONTRAINDICATIONS: Avoid eating hot, greasy foods when taking *Tian Wang Bu Xin Wan*. **Caution:** Do not take this formula for longer than 2 weeks at a time. Discontinue use for 1 week and then resume for 2 weeks.
DOSAGE: Bottles of 200 pills. Take 8 pills, 3 times a day.

OTHER

For insomnia due to pain, use Corydalis *Yan Hu Suo* Analgesic Tablets, under Pain.

Hypertension

PILLS

Fu Fang Du Zhong Pian (Compound Cortex Eucommia Tablets)

INDICATIONS: This formula is used for hypertension in people with a flushed or pale face, who feel cold and have low-back pain, palpitations, headache, dizziness, possible frequent urination, and tiredness.

CONTRAINDICATIONS: Avoid eating cold foods when taking *Fu Fang Du Zhong Pian*.

DOSAGE: Bottles of 100 tablets. Take 5 tablets, 3 times a day.

Jiang Ya Ping Pian (Hypertension Repressing Tablets)

INDICATIONS: This formula is used for hypertension with dizziness, ear ringing, headache, and flushed face with heat signs, such as thirst, yellow phlegm, dark yellow urine, and constipation. It may also be used to lower blood cholesterol and prevent hardening of the arteries. The hypertension should begin to lessen within 2 weeks.

Caution: Avoid eating hot, greasy foods while taking *Jiang Ya Ping Pian*.

DOSAGE: Boxes of 12 bottles, each with 12 tablets. Take 4 tablets, 3 times a day, in 3 courses of 14 days each.

NOTES: This formula can be used for long periods with no side effects. It contains some animal parts.

OTHER

For hypertension with tinnitus, thirst, eye irritation and pressure, insomnia, and headache, use *Tso-Tzu* Otic Pills, under Sore Throats, Mouth Disorders, and Ear Problems.

Energy Tonics

PILLS

Bu Zhong Yi Qi Wan (Central Qi Pills)

INDICATIONS: This formula is used for low energy, poor digestion with abdominal bloating, pain, gas and erratic stools; for prolapse of the rectum, uterus, or colon; and for hemorrhoids, varicose veins, and hernia. It is also useful in treating uterine bleeding, habitual miscarriage, chronic diarrhea, and hypoglycemia.

CONTRAINDICATIONS: *Bu Zhong Yi Qi Wan* is not to be used by those who feel hot or have an aversion to heat, are thirsty, sweat easily, or have strong body odor, dark yellow scanty urine, or discharges that are yellow to red in color. **Caution:** Avoid eating cold foods while taking this formula.

DOSAGE: Bottles of 100 pills. Take 8 pills, 3 times a day.

Yang Rong Wan (Ginseng Tonic Pills)

EFFECTS AND INDICATIONS: This formula is good for promoting longevity. It is used to promote or maintain health and is good for general weakness in chronic illnesses or following childbirth, surgery, or trauma.

Caution: Avoid eating cold foods when taking *Yang Rong Wan.* This formula should not be taken by those with heat, an aversion to heat, thirst, yellow discharges, or phlegm.

DOSAGE: Bottles of 200 pills. Take 8 pills, 3 times a day.

TEAS

Eight Treasure Tea

EFFECTS AND INDICATIONS: This classical formula nourishes the blood and strengthens energy. It is an excellent general tonic, particularly for women with a pale face, fatigue, dizziness, shortness of breath, heart palpitations, anemia, hypoglycemia, low appetite, irregular menstruation, amenorrhea, or general weakness during pregnancy or recovery from childbirth or illness.

DOSAGE: Bottles of 200 pills. Take 8 pills, 3 times a day.

Golden Book Tea or Sexoton Pills

INDICATIONS: This formula is used for lowered energy with coldness, including cold hands or feet, lower-back ache, poor digestion with gas or undigested food in stools, persistent diarrhea, poor circulation, frequent voiding of clear urine, edema, impotence, infertility, and sexual dysfunction.

CONTRAINDICATIONS: Golden Book Tea should not be taken by those with heat, an aversion to heat, thirst, yellow discharges, or phlegm.

Caution: Avoid eating cold foods when taking this formula.

DOSAGE: Bottles of 120 and 200 pills. Take 8–10 pills, 3 times a day.

Liu Wei Di Huang Wan (Six-Flavor Tea)

INDICATIONS: This formula is used for lowered energy with sore throat, thirst, mild night sweats, dizziness, burning on the soles or palms, impotence, tinnitis, restlessness, insomnia, and lower-back pain.

DOSAGE: Bottles of 200 pills. Take 8–12 pills, 3 times a day.

OTHER

For fatigue with dizziness, palpitations, irregular menses, amenorrhea, poor memory, and possible anemia, use *Tang Kwei Gin,* under Gynecological Conditions.

For fatigue with dizziness, palpitations, irregular menses, poor memory, night sweats, insomnia, and abnormal uterine bleeding, use *Gui Pi Wan,* under Restlessness and Insomnia.

Infants' and Young Children's Disorders

PILLS

Bo Ying

INDICATIONS: This formula is used for a wide range of children's diseases, including fever, coarse respiration, productive cough, teething, stomachache, diarrhea, vomiting, restlessness, and night crying.

Caution: Use *Bo Ying* for a short time only, giving 1–2 doses.

DOSAGE: Tins of 6 vials of powder, which may be mixed with a favorite food or placed on the mother's nipple. Infants younger than 1 month old, give ½ bottle, 1–2 times a day; infants over 1 month old to children up to 3 years old, give 1 bottle, 1–2 times a day; children 3–10 years old, give 2–3 bottles, 1–2 times a day. Preventative: 2 times a month of the age-appropriate dosage.

NOTE: This formula contains some animal parts.

Hui Chun Tan

INDICATIONS: This formula is used for fever, cough with phlegm, colds, fitfulness, measles, stomachache, vomiting, diarrhea, and difficult respiration.

Caution: Use *Hui Chun Tan* for a short time only, giving 1–2 doses.

DOSAGE: Boxes of 10 bottles, each containing 3 pills. For children under 1 year old, give 1 pill, 3 times a day; for children between 1 and 5 years old, give 3 pills, 3 times a day; for children between 5 and 9 years old, give 5 pills, 3 times a day.

NOTE: This formula contains some animal parts.

Tao Chih Pien (For Babies)

INDICATIONS: This formula is used for sore throat, mouth sores, swollen gums, fevers, red eyes, constipation, stomachache, and scanty dark urine.

Caution: Use *Tao Chih Pien* for a short time only, giving 1–2 doses. Reduce the dosage or discontinue the formula if diarrhea develops.

DOSAGE: Tubes of 8 tablets, 12 tubes to a box. Infants younger than 1 year, 1–2 tablets, 2 times a day; for children 1–7 years old, give 2–4 tablets, 2 times a day.

NOTE: This formula contains some animal parts.

OTHER

For acute tonsillitis, acute mumps, and strep throat, use Laryngitis Pills, under Sore Throats, Mouth Disorders, and Ear Problems.

Pain

Corydalis *Yan Hu Suo* Analgesic Tablets

INDICATIONS: This formula is used for pain—especially dull pain— including dysmenorrhea, postpartum pain, stomachache, gastric or duodenal ulcer, abdominal pain, liver or gallbladder pain, chest pain, pain due to rheumatism or injury, and insomnia caused by pain. It is also good for treating tremors, spasms, and seizures.

DOSAGE: Bottles of 20 tablets. Take 4–6 tablets, 3 times a day or as needed.

First Aid

PILLS

Yunnan Paiyao

EFFECTS AND INDICATIONS: Based mainly on *tian qi* ginseng root, this formula stops internal and external bleeding and pain, including that from wounds, cuts, hemorrhaging, vomiting of blood, blood in the stools, coughing up of blood, serious nosebleeds, and menstrual flooding. It eases traumatic swelling from injuries, including fractures, sprains, tears of ligaments and muscles, dislocations, bone breaks, and bruising from falls or blows. It is commonly used for excessive menstrual bleeding, severe menstrual cramps, ulcer bleeding, insect bites, and carbuncles. It may be taken internally or applied externally.

Caution: Internal use of *Yunnan Paiyao* is prohibited during pregnancy.

DOSAGE: Boxes of 10 bottles, 4 grams each, or packets of 20 capsules. Internally, take 0.2–0.5 gram or 1–2 capsules, 4 times a day; externally, apply directly to bleeding wound (clean first, bandage after). For deep or wide wounds, squeeze the edges of the cut together, pour the powder on the wound, and keep the wound closed for 1–2 minutes.

LINIMENT

Zheng Gu Shui

EFFECTS AND INDICATIONS: This formula is a liniment for external use only that relieves pain, relaxes tendons and muscles, and promotes healing from traumatic injuries, including fractures, sprains, dislocated joints, tears to ligaments and muscles, and bruising. It is effective for sports and martial arts injuries.

CONTRAINDICATIONS: If there is a serious skin reaction, discontinue use of *Zheng Gu Shui*. **Caution:** Do not get the liniment into the eyes. Wash hands thoroughly after use. Keep the liniment away from flame, as it is volatile. Do not rub into open wounds.

DOSAGE: Bottles of 30 and 100 milliliters. Apply the liniment often with light massage or on gauze and a bandage. It will stain clothes, but it can be removed with rubbing alcohol.

OTHER

For pain due to trauma or injury, use Corydalis *Yan Hu Suo* Analgesic Tablets, under Pain.

· E L E V E N ·

SPECIFIC DISEASES AND TREATMENTS

[Following are a number of diseases and possible herbal treatments. Because of the depth and complexity of Traditional Chinese Herbal medicine, the treatments are only offered as suggestions and not intended to replace the assistance of qualified medical practitioners. Some of the treatments recommend classical Chinese formulas and Planetary herb formulas based on my own experience. These are available either from Chinese pharmacies or Chinese herbalist practitioners and suppliers from throughout the country or from other sources mentioned in the appendix.]

Acquired Immunodeficiency Syndrome (AIDS)

CHINESE FOOD THERAPY: Astragalus congee
Combination (Bu Zhong Yi Qi Tang), Minor Bupleurum Combination, Energetics Yin, and Energetics Yang (equal amounts, 3 times daily)

Allergies (Upper Respiratory)

CHINESE FOOD THERAPY: Avoid allergenic foods such as dairy, wheat, and sugar.
CHINESE PATENTS:

- *Bi Yan Pian:* The most commonly used Chinese patent for chronic rhinitis, sinusitis, hayfever, nasal allergies, stuffy nose with yellowish thick discharge. Use Plum Flower brand to avoid additives.
- *Pe Min Kan Wan:* Used for hay fever, sinus infections, rhinitis, acute or chronic sinusitis, and facial congestion during colds with sneezing, runny nose, itchy and watery eyes, and postnasal drip, for which it is specific. Use Plum Flower brand to avoid additives.

Altitude Sickness

GENERAL HERBAL TREATMENT: For altitude sickness, suck on a few slices of honey-cured ginseng *ren shen*. It works even better than coca leaves, which, in any case, are not available in Western countries.

Asthma

GENERAL HERBAL TREATMENTS:

- For asthma and wheezing caused by kidney–adrenal deficiency, combine 9 grams each of prepared rehmannia, cornus berries, dioscorea, poria, alisma, and moutan peony; 6 grams each of prepared aconite and cinnamon bark; and 3 grams of aquilaria. Make the mixture into a decoction and have 2 cups daily.
- For asthma caused by lung and kidney deficiency, combine 15 grams of hematite with 9 grams each of ginseng and cornus.

CHINESE FOOD THERAPY: Pearl barley congee

CHINESE FORMULAS: *Ma Xing Shi Gan Tang* (Ephedra, Apricot, Gypsum, and Licorice Combination), *Xiao Qing Long Tang* (Minor Blue-Green Dragon Combination), *Ba Wei Di Huang Wan* (Rehmannia Eight)

CHINESE PATENTS: *Ge Jie Jiu (Gecko Wine)*, Bronchitis Pills (Compound), Pulmonary Tonic Pills, Asthmawan

Bleeding and Hemorrhage

GENERAL HERBAL TREATMENTS:

- *Tienchi* ginseng is commonly taken alone for bleeding and hemorrhage. The most famous Chinese trauma medicine is called *Yunnan Baiyao,* and it is commonly available at all Chinese pharmacies.
- For coughing of blood, combine 9 grams each bletilla and loquat leaf tea in which 12 grams of donkey-skin gelatin has been dissolved.
- For hemorrhage caused by external injury, apply powdered eclipta topically.

Blood Deficiency (Anemia)

GENERAL HERBAL TREATMENTS:

- For blood deficiency and anemia, combine 9 grams each of prepared rehmannia, angelica *dang gui,* white peony, and ligusticum. This is called Dang Gui Four *(Si Wu Tang).*

- For soup of chicken or bone marrow, combine 6 grams of angelica *dang gui,* and 15 grams of astragalus.
- For blood deficiency, anemia, dizziness, vertigo, premature graying of hair, or aching soreness of the lower back and knees, combine 9 grams each of fleeceflower root, prepared rehmannia, ligustrum fruit, lycii berries, dodder seed, eclipta root, and loranthes.
- For deficient blood and yin with the yang floating to the surface with symptoms of night sweats and spontaneous sweating, combine 9 grams of white peony root with 15 grams each of crushed oyster shell and dragon bone and 20 grams of light wheat.

CHINESE PATENTS: *Tang Kwei Gin, Butiao* pills, *Wu Chi Pai Feng Wan* (White Phoenix Pills), *Shih San Tai Pao Wan*

Cancer

GENERAL HERBAL TREATMENT: For cancers of all kinds, combine 9 grams of burdock root, 6 grams of phytolacca, 6 grams of yellow dock, 9 grams of scrophularia, and 9 grams of barberry root.
CHINESE FORMULA: *San Huang Xie Xin Tang* (Three Yellows)
PLANETARY FORMULAS: River of Life, The Complete Pau d'Arco

Chapped Hands

GENERAL HERBAL TREATMENT: For chapped hands and feet, apply a mixture of powdered bletilla and sesame oil.

Childhood Convulsions

GENERAL HERBAL TREATMENT: For chronic childhood convulsions with diarrhea caused by spleen deficiency, combine 6 grams of silkworms with 9 grams each of codonopsis and atractylodes *bai zhu* and 6 grams of gastrodia.

Cholesterol (to Lower)

GENERAL HERBAL TREATMENT: To lower cholesterol and other blood lipid levels; take 30 grams of cattail pollen daily.
CHINESE PATENT: *Dan Shen* Tablet Co.

Colds, Influenza, Fevers

GENERAL HERBAL TREATMENTS:

- For the initial stages of the common cold, influenza, and fevers, steep 6 grams each of chrysanthemum flowers, and honeysuckle flowers and 3 grams of licorice in 2 cups of boiling water. Take 1–2 cups before retiring to induce perspiration.
- For external wind-cold syndrome with symptoms of colds, influenza, fever, and chills with no perspiration, combine 10 grams of black soybeans with 9 grams of green onion in decoction.
- For external wind-heat syndrome with symptoms of colds, influenza, fever, sore throat, and perspiration, combine 9 grams each of black soybean, burdock seed (crushed), forsythia fruit, and platycodon.
- For the initial stage of colds and influenza, combine 10 grams of green onion and 4 slices of fresh ginger with brown sugar to make a tea.
- For boils and carbuncles, mash green onions, mix with honey, and apply directly to the affected area.
- For the common cold, influenza, fever, sore throat, boils, carbuncles, and furuncles, combine 9 grams each of isatis leaf, isatis root, scrophularia, honeysuckle flowers, and forsythia with 6 grams of licorice.

CHINESE FOOD THERAPY: Garlic congee, scallions and glutinous sweet rice congee

CHINESE FORMULAS: *Chai Hu Gui Zhi Tang* (Bupleurum and Cinnamon Combination), *Sang Ju Yin* (Mulberry Leaf and Chrysanthemum Flower Tea), *Bai Hu Tang* (White Tiger Decoction), *Yin Qiao San* (Lonicera and Forsythia Powder)

CHINESE PATENTS: *Ganmaoling* tablets (Plum Flower brand), *Yin Chiao* tablets (*Tianjin* brand), *Huo Hsiang Cheng Chi Pien* (Lophanthus Antifebrile Pills)

Constipation

GENERAL HERBAL TREATMENTS:

- For constipation caused by excess heat, combine 6 grams each of rhubarb, mirabilitum, and citrus peel with 3 grams each of ginger and licorice.
- For acute constipation, combine 6 grams of senna leaf with 3 grams each of ginger and licorice.

- Another combination for acute constipation is 3 grams of aloe, 6 grams of rhubarb, 4 grams of ginger, and 3 grams of licorice.
- For constipation caused by dryness, combine 9 grams each of trichosanthes fruit, hemp (Cannabis sativa), or flaxseed, psyllium seed husks, and green citrus peel.
- For dry constipation caused by blood deficiency, combine 9 grams each peach seed, apricot seed, angelica *dang gui,* and hemp seed.
- For constipation caused by dryness and blood deficiency, combine 9 grams each of fleeceflower root and angelica *dang gui* and 15 grams of cannabis seed.
- For dry constipation in the elderly, combine 9 grams of cistanche and 15 grams of cannabis seeds.
- For constipation caused by dryness, combine 9 grams each of asparagus root, angelica *dang gui,* and cistanche.
- For constipation in postpartum women or the elderly, combine 15 grams each of biota seeds, cannabis seeds, and Walnut kernels.
- For constipation and toxicity, use *San Huang Xie Xin Tang* (Coptis, Scutellaria and Rhubarb Combination).

Coughs

GENERAL HERBAL TREATMENTS:

- For cough with yellow mucus caused by damp heat in the lungs, combine 9 grams each of plantain seeds, trichosanthes, bamboo shavings, scutellaria, and fritillary.
- For unproductive cough with yin deficiency, make a powder of equal parts processed fritillary bulb, ophiopogon, and elecampane root. Take 3 grams of the mixture with warm water.
- For phlegm-heat cough with thick yellow mucus and a full feeling in the chest, combine 9 grams each trichosanthes fruit and pinellia and 1 crushed clove of garlic. Make the mixture into a decoction and have 2 cups daily.
- Another combination for phlegm heat is 9 grams each of trichosanthes (fruit or seed), scutellaria, and platycodon and 6 grams each of green citrus and coptis. Make the mixture into a decoction and have 2 cups daily.
- For cough with swollen sore throat, combine 9 grams each of platycodon, and forsythia, lonicera and 6 grams of licorice. Make the mixture into a tea and have 2–3 cups daily.

- For cough and difficult breathing caused by cold-phlegm congestion in the chest, combine 9 grams each of magnolia bark, *ma huang* ephedra and apricot seed and 3 grams of licorice.
- For excessive phlegm with symptoms of cough, bronchitis, asthma, or emphysema, make a powder of 9 grams each of radish seed, perilla seed, and white mustard seed. Take 2–5 grams of the powder twice a day with boiled warm water.
- To stop cough and resolve phlegm, combine 9 grams each of aster root (Aster tataricus), coltsfoot flowers, pinellia, and citrus peel and 6 grams each of licorice and apricot seed.
- For cough and asthma with symptoms of heat in the lungs with yellow phlegm, combine 9 grams each of loquat leaves, mulberry bark, platycodon, and bamboo shavings and 6 grams of licorice.
- For elderly patients with chronic cough caused by weak digestion and deficient spleen and stomach *qi,* use *San Zi Yang Qing Tang* (Decoction of Three Seeds Nursing the Parents).
- For whooping cough, combine 9 grams each of stemona root, glehnia root, fritillary, and aristolochia and 6 grams of Licorice.
- For cough with the common cold, combine 9 grams each of stemona, schizonepeta, platycodon, and aster root and 3 grams of licorice.
- For cough associated with tuberculosis (TB), combine 9 grams each of ophiopogon root, stemona root, American ginseng, and unprepared rehmannia root.
- For chronic cough caused by lung *qi* deficiency, combine 9 grams each of dioscorea, glehnia root, ophiopogon, and schisandra berries.
- For deficient lung yin (dryness) with dry cough and low energy, combine 9 grams each of pseudostellaria root, glehnia, and ophiopogon.
- For cough and asthma caused by lung *qi* and yang deficiency, prepare 9 grams of ginseng *ren shen* with 15 grams of walnuts.
- For yin deficiency of the lungs and kidneys with lung dryness, cough with blood-streaked phlegm, and TB, combine 9 grams each of asparagus root, ophiopogon, glehnia root, unprepared rehmannia, dioscorea, and ginseng *ren shen.*
- For lung yin deficiency with cough and scanty, blood-streaked phlegm that is difficult to expectorate, combine 9 grams each of ophiopogon, glehnia, asparagus root, fritillary, and unprepared rehmannia.
- For dry cough with difficult-to-expectorate blood-streaked phlegm,

combine 9 grams each of Solomon's seal, asparagus root, ophiopogon, glehnia, anemarrhena, and fritillary.

- For yin deficiency of the lungs with dryness, spitting of blood, and inflammation, combine 9 grams each of lily bulb, scrophularia, fritillary, and unprepared rehmannia.
- For chronic cough, asthma, and emphysema caused by deficiency of the lungs and kidneys, combine 6 grams of schisandra berries and 9 grams each of prepared rehmannia, ophiopogon, and dioscorea.
- For cough caused by rebellious *qi*, possibly with vomiting, belching, or hiccuping, combine 15 grams of hematite with 9 grams each of inula flowers, pinellia, and fresh ginger.
- For cough with thick phlegm that is difficult to expectorate, combine 9 grams each of polygala, platycodon, apricot seed, pinellia, citrus, and licorice root.

CHINESE FOOD THERAPY: Garlic congee

CHINESE FORMULAS: *Chai Hu Gui Zhi Tang* (Bupleurum and Cinnamon Combination), *Sang Ju Yin* (Mulberry Leaf and Chrysanthemum Flower Tea)

CHINESE PATENTS: Bronchitis Pills (Compound), *Ching Fei Yi Huo Pien,* Pulmonary Tonic Pills, *Qing Qi Hua Tan Wan* (Pinellia Expectorant Pills), *Bi Yan Pian Hsiao Keh Chuan* (Special Medicine for Bronchitis), *Lo Han Kuo* tea, Natural Herb Loquat-Flavored Syrup

Dentifrice for Gum Disease

GENERAL HERBAL TREATMENT: Brush teeth with a combination of Turmeric and a half part each of cloves and cinnamon.

Diabetes

GENERAL HERBAL TREATMENTS:

- For diabetes with symptoms of extreme thirst, excessive drinking, excessive appetite, profuse urination, and fatigue, combine 9 grams each of dioscorea, astragalus, unprepared rehmannia, pueraria root, and trichosanthes root in the formula *Yu Ye Tang.*
- For diabetes, combine 9 grams each of Solomon's seal, ophiopogon, lycii berries, astragalus, trichosanthes root, and unprepared rehmannia.
- For diabetes with excessive thirst and fluid intake, general weakness, and *qi* deficiency, combine 6 grams of schisandra berries with 9 grams

each of astragalus, unprepared rehmannia, ophiopogon, and trichosanthes root.

- For diabetes, eat dioscorea and lycii berry soup. This is made by cooking a soup with lean meat, 30 grams of dioscorea, and 20 grams of
lycii berries.

CHINESE FOOD THERAPY: Dioscorea (shan yao) congee or soup, water
chestnut congee

CHINESE FORMULA: Liu Wei Di Huang Tang (Rehmannia Six Combination)

Diarrhea and Dysentery

GENERAL HERBAL TREATMENTS:

- For diarrhea and dysentery, combine 9 grams each of philodendron,
pulsatilla, and scutellaria and 6 grams of coptis (or goldenseal).
- For damp-heat dysentery and jaundice with abdominal pain, combine
9 grams each of saussurea, rhubarb root, and areca seed and 3 grams
of licorice. Make a tea and take 2 cups of it daily.
- For dysentery, combine 9 grams each of honeysuckle flowers and pulsatilla root and 6 grams of coptis (or hydrastis).
- For diarrhea caused by deficient yang of the spleen and kidneys, combine 9 grams each of psoralea seeds and evodia, 3 grams of nutmeg,
and 4 grams of schisandra berries.
- For chronic diarrhea caused by spleen and kidney deficiency, combine 6 grams each of schisandra berries and evodia and 4 grams of
nutmeg.
- For chronic diarrhea caused by spleen deficiency, combine 18 grams
of lotus seeds, 10 grams of euryale seeds and 9 grams each of atractylodes bai zhu and poria.
- For diarrhea and dysentery caused by damp heat, combine 9 grams
each of gentian, plantain seeds, poria, alisma, and atractylodes.

CHINESE FOOD THERAPY: Carrot congee, preroasted brown rice
CHINESE FORMULA: Wu Mei San (Mume Plum Combination)
CHINESE PATENT: Curing Pills

Digestive Disorders

GENERAL HERBAL TREATMENTS:

- For stomach heat with symptoms of acid belching, indigestion, nausea, and vomiting, combine 9 grams each of phragmites, fresh ginger juice, bamboo shavings, and loquat leaves.

- For stomach congestion, with distension, acid belching, and possible nausea and vomiting, combine 9 grams each of magnolia bark, atractylodes, and pinellia and 6 grams of citrus peel. Make the mixture into a tea or powder.
- For abdominal congestion, combine 9 grams each of black atractylodes, magnolia bark, pinellia, and citrus peel and 2 or 3 slices of fresh ginger. Make the mixture into a decoction and take 2–3 cups of it daily or sip it throughout the day.
- For abdominal congestion with pain, bloating, and nausea, combine 9 grams each of magnolia bark, pinellia, and citrus peel and 5 grams of ground cardamon seed. Grind this into a fine powder and take 1.5–3 grams as a single dose 2–3 times daily.
- For gastrointestinal discomfort caused by food stagnation, combine 10 grams each of powdered hawthorn berries, barley sprouts, and medicated leaven. Steep 1–2 tablespoons of the powder in 1 cup of boiling water and have 2–3 cups of it daily.
- For food stagnation with lack of appetite and abdominal distension and pain, combine 9 grams each of barley sprouts, hawthorn berries, and chicken gizzards. Make the mixture into a decoction and drink it as needed.
- For food stagnation, weak digestion, and loss of appetite, make a powder of *equal parts* rice sprouts, ginseng, atractylodes, citrus peel, and a quarter part licorice. Take 2–3 grams of the powder in warm water 15 minutes before eating.
- For food stagnation, use hawthorn berries, sprouted barley, and possibly chicken gizzards. Grind this mixture into a powder and take approximately 1.5–3 grams for each dose as needed.
- For food stagnation and retention with abdominal fullness and pain, acid regurgitation, and diarrhea, make a powder of 9 grams each of radish seed, hawthorn berries, medicated leaven, and citrus peel. Take 2–3 grams of the powder with warm water as needed.
- For dampness obstructing the spleen and stomach, combine equal parts of citrus peel, black atractylodes, magnolia bark, and poria and make the mixture into a powder. Take 2–3 grams of the powder twice daily or as needed.
- For excessive dampness, combine pinellia, poria, and licorice with citrus to make *Er Chen Tang* (Pinellia Combination).

- For digestive coldness and weakness, especially from eating too much cold or raw food, combine 4 grams each of dry ginger powder and cinnamon bark with 9 grams each of powdered codonopsis, atractylodes *bai zhu*, poria, and licorice. Take approximately 6–9 grams of the powder mixed with warm honey 2–3 times daily before meals.
- For cold attacking the spleen and stomach with symptoms of stomachache and epigastric pain, combine 6 grams each of evodia, saussurea, dry ginger, and atractylodes *bai zhu*. All the herbs should be simmered only lightly in a covered container for no longer than 20 minutes.
- As a warming condiment, a few slices of dried galangal can be cooked in soups. Used in this way, it is a common spice in Thai cuisine, along with lemongrass.

CHINESE FOOD THERAPY: Ginger tea with meals.

CHINESE FORMULAS: *Chai Hu Gui Zhi Tang* (Bupleurum and Cinnamon Combination); *Si Jun Zi Tang* (Four Gentlemen Combination); *Liu Jun Zi Tang* (Six Gentlemen Combination)

CHINESE PATENTS: *Ren Shen Jian Pi Wan* (Ginseng Stomachic Pills); *Liu Jun Zi* pills, *Mu Xiang Shun Qi Wan* (Aplotaxis Carminative Pills); *Fu Zi Li Zhong Wan* (Carmichaeli Tea Pills); *Rensheng Feng Wang Jiang* (Ginseng Royal Jelly vials); Pill Curing, *Ping Wei Pian*, *Shu Kan Wan* (condensed)

Dizziness and Vertigo

GENERAL HERBAL TREATMENT: For dizziness and vertigo caused by yin deficiency with upflaring yang, combine with dragon bone (*long gu*) and oyster shell (*mu li*).

Edema

GENERAL HERBAL TREATMENTS:

- For edema as well as blood in the urine, diarrhea, or dysentery, combine 20 grams of coix with 9 grams each of alisma, poria, and atractylodes.
- For edema, possibly with ascites and phlegm caused by spleen and stomach deficiency, combine 9 grams each of atractylodes *bai zhu*, areca seed, and poria.

- For phlegm symptoms associated with cough, asthma, a full feeling in the chest, and possibly palpitations, combine 9 grams each of atractylodes *bai zhu,* cinnamon twigs, and poria with 3 grams of licorice.

CHINESE FOOD THERAPY: Coix and brown rice congee with poria

CHINESE FORMULAS: *Wu Ling San* (Poria Five Herb Combination) and *Yi Yi Ren Tang* (Coix Combination) or *Ba Wei Di Huang Wan* (Rehmannia Eight Combination) if the condition is caused by kidney yang deficiency.

CHINESE PATENT: Golden Book Tea or Sexoton Pills if the condition is caused by kidney yang deficiency

Eye Disorders

GENERAL HERBAL TREATMENTS:

- For blurred vision, dry eyes, dizziness, and cataracts, combine 9 grams each of buddleia, lycii berries, and chrysanthemum flower.
- For conjunctivitis, photophobia, excessive tearing, and cataracts, combine 9 grams each of buddleia, chrysanthemum flowers, and tribulus fruit, 15 grams of abalone shell, and 6 grams of cassia seeds.
- For eyesight problems, blurred vision, photophobia, and cataracts, combine 9 grams each of plantain seeds, lycii berries, and chrysanthemum flowers with 12 grams of unprepared rehmannia.
- For cataracts, glaucoma, night blindness, and photophobia, make a powder of 9 grams of black atractylodes and 20 grams each of black sesame seeds and lycii berries. Take 1 tablespoon of the mixture 3 times daily.
- For conjunctivitis and opthalmia, make an eyewash with turmeric root, strain through a fine cloth, and rinse the eyes with the solution using a small eyecup.
- For blurred vision with dryness of the eyes caused by deficiency of liver blood, combine 20 grams of crushed abalone shell with 9 grams each of prepared rehmannia and lycii berries.

CHINESE PATENT: *Ming Mu Di Huang Wan*

Fevers

GENERAL HERBAL TREATMENTS:

- For fevers with thirst, aversion to cold and wind, and sore throat, combine 9 grams each of honeysuckle flowers, forsythia fruit, and burdock seeds (crushed).

- For very high fever with extreme dehydration and thirst, combine 9 grams each of honeysuckle flowers and anemarrhena with 30 grams of gypsum.
- For symptoms of high fever, vomiting of blood, nosebleeds, and blood in the urine with deep red tongue, combine 9 grams each of moutan peony and red peony, 15 grams of unprepared rehmannia, and 40 grams of powdered cow horn in decoction.
- For diseases with fever, irritability, and thirst, combine 9 grams each of bamboo leaves and anemarrhena with 30 grams of gypsum.
- For high fever, combine 9 grams each of isatis leaves and moutan peony.

CHINESE FORMULA: *Bai Hu Tang* (White Tiger Decoction)
CHINESE PATENTS: *Yin Chiao San, Ganmaoling*

Fish Bone Stuck in the Throat

GENERAL HERBAL TREATMENT: To remove fish bones, take a decoction of clematis root with apple cider vinegar.

Flexibility (to Increase)

GENERAL HERBAL TREATMENT: One of the traditional turmeric preparations is golden milk. Boil ¼ cup of turmeric powder in ½ cup of water until a thick paste is formed. This can be refrigerated and stored for use. Then bring to a boil 1 cup of milk to which is added ¼ teaspoon of the turmeric paste, 1 teaspoon of clarified butter (ghee) or sesame oil, and honey to taste. This is used for general health purposes as well as for maximizing flexibility for the practice of yoga.

Frigidity and Infertility

GENERAL HERBAL TREATMENT: For female frigidity and infertility, combine 9 grams each of cistanche root, antler glue, human placenta, angelica *dang gui*, and prepared rehmannia.
CHINESE FORMULA: *Si Wu Tang* (Dang Gui Four Combination)

Gallstones and Cholecystitis

GENERAL HERBAL TREATMENT: For gallstones or gallbladder inflammation, take 1 teaspoon of turmeric root 3 times daily with a glass of warm water.

Gynecological Disorders

GENERAL HERBAL TREATMENTS:

- For amenorrhea (stopped menses), combine 9 grams each of dianthus, peach seed, safflower, and leonurus.
- For leukorrhea, trichomonas, and genital itching, combine 9 grams each of gentian, philodendron, sophora root, and plantain seed. Use the mixture as a tea as well as a douche.
- For painful and irregular menstruation with tender breasts caused by irregular liver Qi, combine 9 grams each of cyperus, angelica *dang gui*, and ligusticum (*chuan xiong*) in a decoction.
- For painful menstruation, combine 9 grams each of angelica *dang gui*, ligusticum (*chuan xiong*), prepared rehmannia, and white peony with 6 grams each of lindera and cyperus.
- For Blood and *qi* stagnation with symptoms of irregular menstruation or blocked or painful menstruation, combine 6 grams each ligusticum, red peony, cyperus, achyranthes, and angelica *dang gui*.
- For stopped menstruation, irregular menstruation, or postpartum pain, combine 9 grams each of red sage root, angelica *dang gui*, motherwort, red peony, and safflower and 6 grams of ligusticum (*chuan xiong*).
- For irregular or stopped menstruation, take 1 teaspoon of equal parts turmeric root and motherwort in a powder 3 times daily.
- For painful and irregular menstruation, combine 9 grams each of motherwort, cyperus, angelica *dang gui*, ligusticum (*chuan xiong*), and red peony root.
- For blood stagnation associated with menstrual irregularities and postpartum pain, combine 9 grams each of bugleweed, angelica *dang gui*, ligusticum (*chuan xiong*), and red peony root.
- For blood stagnation with irregular and painful menstruation, combine 9 grams each of red peony root, angelica *dang gui*, and ligusticum (*chuan xiong*).
- For irregular and painful menstruation, combine 9 grams each of

peach seed, angelica *dang gui*, ligusticum *(chuan xiong)*, and red peony root.
- For painful and/or irregular menstruation, combine 9 grams each of safflowers, peach seed, angelica *dang gui*, ligusticum *(chuan xiong)*, and red peony root. This same combination can also be used externally as a liniment for injuries and traumas.
- For painful and irregular menstruation, combine 9 grams each of achyranthes root, peach seed, safflower, angelica *dang gui*, and corydalis with 6 grams of ligusticum *(chuan xiong)*.
- For uterine bleeding, combine 9 grams each of angelica *dang gui*, unprepared rehmannia, and mugwort leaf. After the tea is prepared, dissolve 15 grams of donkey-skin gelatin into the tea.
- For gynecological conditions, including menstrual irregularities, anemia, infertility, and frequent threatened miscarriage in weaker women, use *Dang Gui Shao Yao San* (Dang Gui and Peony Formula).

CHINESE FOOD THERAPY: Angelica *dang gui* with lamb. Cook 15 grams of angelica *dang gui* with lamb and several slices of ginger to taste.

CHINESE PATENTS:

- *Wu Chi Pai Feng Wan* (White Phoenix Pills): For menstrual disorders caused by possible anemia, fatigue, amenorrhea, pain with ovulation, postpartum weakness or bleeding, low-back pain, poor appetite, and prolonged or irregular periods. Can also be used for postpartum exhaustion. Contains animal parts.
- *Tang Kwei Gin:* A Widely used liquid tonic for improving the quality of the blood. It can be used by both men and women with possible anemia or fatigue following illness, surgery, or trauma. Also good for palpitations, dizziness, poor memory, irregular menses with pale blood, amenorrhea, and postpartum weakness due to excess blood loss.
- *An Tai Wan* (For Embryo): Calms a restless fetus, premature uterine contractions, and threatened miscarriage with lower abdominal pains during pregnancy.
- *Shih San Tai Pao Wan:* Use in the first trimester of pregnancy for threatened miscarriage, fatigue, anemia, and nausea.
- *He Che Da Zao Wan* (Placenta Compound Restorative Pills): Useful for menopausal night sweats and hot flashes in women and for spermatorrhea in men when the semen is lost at night, during a dream. Both have accompanying symptoms of dizziness, tinnitus, weak and tired

legs, aching lower back, low-grade afternoon fever, fatigue, or red cheeks or hot, flushed face. Contains animal parts.

Hair

GENERAL HERBAL TREATMENTS: To restore normal hair color, dry-roast black sesame seeds and mix them with honey to make a confection. Eat several spoonfuls daily. For a condiment for grains and vegetables, dry-toast black sesame seeds and grind them with rock salt or burned sea salt (to eliminate the chlorine); proportion: 7–10 parts black sesame seeds to 1 part by volume of salt.

Headaches

GENERAL HERBAL TREATMENTS:

- For headaches caused by wind-heat syndrome, combine 9 grams each of vitex fruit, ledebouriella, and chrysanthemum flowers.
- For headaches caused by wind cold, combine 6 grams each of ligusticum and Angelica dahurica with 3 grams of asarum.
- For headaches caused by wind heat, combine 6 grams each of ligusticum, chrysanthemum flowers, gypsum, and white stiff silkworm.
- For headaches caused by wind damp, combine 6 grams each ligusticum, notopterygium, and ledebouriella.
- For headaches caused by blood stagnation, combine 6 grams of ligusticum with 9 grams each of red sage root and safflower.
- For headaches caused by blood deficiency, combine 6 grams each of ligusticum, angelica dang gui, white peony, and prepared rehmannia.
- For headaches, nausea, and vomiting caused by spleen and stomach qi weakness, combine 6 grams each of evodia and dry ginger with 9 grams each of ginseng ren shen and atractylodes bai zhu.

Heart Problems

GENERAL HERBAL TREATMENTS:

- For chest pains caused by blood stagnation of the heart meridian, combine 9 grams each of hawthorn, red sage root, and motherwort herb. Grind the mixture into a powder and take 1.5–3 grams of it 3 times daily.

- For heart palpitations, irritability, and insomnia with blood deficiency, combine 9 grams each of red sage root, zizyphus seeds, and *Polygonum multiflorum* stems.
- For coronary heart disease and angina, combine 9 grams each of hawthorn berries, motherwort, and red sage root.

Hemorrhoids

CHINESE PATENT: Fargelin Pills

CHINESE FORMULA: When hemorrhoids are caused by weakness and deficiency, use *Bu Zhong Yi Qi Tang* (Ginseng and Astragalus Combination)

Hepatitis and Jaundice

GENERAL HERBAL TREATMENTS:

- For hepatitis and jaundice, combine 9 grams each of sophora root, barberry root, dandelion root, and gardenia fruit with 6 grams of gentian root.
- For hepatitis, combine 9 grams each of philodendron, dandelion, gardenia fruit, and capillaris.
- For infectious hepatitis, take 1 teaspoon of the powder of equal parts turmeric, dandelion root, and barberry root.

Hernia and Testicular Pain

GENERAL HERBAL TREATMENTS:

- For painful and swollen testicles and hernia, combine 9 grams each of cyperus, fennel seed, and lindera root.
- For hernia and testicular pain, combine 9 grams each lindera, fennel seed, and green citrus peel.
- For hernia and testicular pain, combine 9 grams each of crushed fennel seeds and lindera root with 6 grams of evodia.

Hypertension

GENERAL HERBAL TREATMENTS:

- For hypertension with dizziness, vertigo, and blurred vision, combine

10 grams of chrysanthemum flowers, and 9 grams of cassia seeds, with 6 grams each of uncaria stems and white peony root.

- For hypertension, each morning steep 2 tablespoons of mung beans in 1 cup of boiling water and drink the liquid. At midday and evening, add another cup of boiling water each time to the strained mung beans and drink the liquid. In the evening, eat the beans.
- For hyperactive liver yang as a result of deficient liver yin with symptoms of hypertension, irritability, dizziness, vertigo, and blurred vision, combine 15 grams each of dragon bone, oyster shell, and white peony root.
- For kidney and liver yin deficiency with liver yang rising with such symptoms as hypertension, dizziness, blurred vision, and irritability, combine 15 grams each of hematite, dragon bone, oyster shell, and tortoise plastron with 9 grams each of white peony (bai shao) and achyranthes (niu xi).
- For hypertension caused by liver and kidney yin deficiency with dizziness, vertigo, and blurred vision, combine 20 grams each of crushed abalone shell, tortoise plastron, and oyster shell with 9 grams of white peony; if there are feelings of pain and distension of the head and eyes with a red face, add 6 grams of uncaria stem and 9 grams each of chrysanthemum flowers, scutellaria, and cassia seeds.
- For hyperactivity of liver yang with dizziness, distended feeling in the head, and blurred vision, combine 20 grams of crushed abalone shell with 9 grams each of prunella spike and chrysanthemum flowers.
- For liver fire rising with hypertension; red, painful, and swollen eyes; and headache, combine 9 grams each of gardenia, gentian, and crushed cassia seed.
- The most commonly used herb for hypertension in Chinese medicine is eucommia. Eucommia is available in pill form in the patents called *Fu Fang Du Zhong Pian* (Compound Cortex Eucommia Tablets) and *Jiang Ya Ping Pian* (Hypertension Repressing Tablets). Since hypertension usually is caused by kidney–adrenal deficiency, 1 pig's kidney (cleaned and sliced) is cooked with 9–15 grams of eucommia bark. This is also an excellent treatment for all kidney deficiency symptoms, including lower-back pain, weakness of the bones, and rheumatism and arthritis pains.

Immune System (to Tonify It)

General Herbal Treatments:

- For immunodeficiency and to accompany chemo and/or radiotherapy, combine 9 grams each of ligustrum berries and dendrobium with 15 grams of astragalus root; if there is digestive upset and nausea, add 9 grams each of pinellia and citrus peel.

- For immunodeficiency with symptoms of frequent colds and influenza and to prevent colds and influenza, combine 9 grams each of astragalus root, atractylodes *bai zhu,* and ledebouriella root.

CHINESE FOOD THERAPY: Astragalus congee

Impotence and Premature Ejaculation

GENERAL HERBAL TREATMENTS:

- For impotence and premature ejaculation, combine 9 grams each of eucommia bark, cornus berries, psoralea seeds, dodder seeds, and schisandra fruit.
- For impotence and/or infertility caused by kidney deficiency, take the following combination internally; 9 grams each of cnidium, cuscuta, psoralea, and schisandra.

CHINESE FORMULA: For weakness and low sexual desire, use *Huan Xiao Dan* (Lycium Combination)

Incontinence (Urinary)

GENERAL HERBAL TREATMENT: For urinary incontinence caused by deficient yang, combine 9 grams each of mantis egg case, psoralea, dragon bone, oyster shell, and cuscuta seed.

CHINESE PATENT: *Kai Kit Wan* pills

Infections and Inflammations (Boils, Carbuncles, Furuncles, and Other Infectious Conditions)

GENERAL HERBAL TREATMENTS:

- For infections, boils, and carbuncles, combine 9 grams each of honeysuckle flowers, dandelion herb and leaf, chrysanthemum flowers, and unprepared rehmannia.
- For infections, boils, and carbuncles, combine 9 grams each of dandelion, violet leaves, unprepared rehmannia, and honeysuckle flowers.
- For inflammations and infections, combine 9 grams each of forsythia

fruits, honeysuckle flowers, burdock seed, dandelion, chrysanthemum flowers, prunella, and scrophularia.
- For boils, carbuncles, and furuncles, combine 9 grams each of violet
leaves, dandelion root and leaf, and scrophularia root.

Insomnia

GENERAL HERBAL TREATMENTS:

- For insomnia caused by irritability and anxiety, combine 3 grams of
coptis and 9 grams of zizyphus seed (crushed).
- For insomnia, irritability, and palpitations caused by anxiety, combine
18 grams of lotus seed with 9 grams each of zizyphus seeds, biota
seeds, and poria hostwood (fu shen).
- For insomnia and palpitations, combine 15 grams each of dragon
bone and oyster shell with 9 grams each of zizyphus seeds and polygala root.
- For insomnia and palpitations caused by blood deficiency, combine 9
grams each of poria hostwood (fu shen), angelica dang gui, zizyphus
seeds, and biota seeds.
- For insomnia caused by deficiency of liver and heart blood, combine
12 grams of zizyphus seeds with 9 grams each of angelica dang gui,
polygala, white peony, longan berries, and polygonum stems.
- For insomnia caused by spleen qi and heart blood deficiency, combine
12 grams of crushed zizyphus seeds with codonopsis and poria hostwood (fu shen).
- For insomnia and weak memory, combine 9 grams each of polygala,
sweetflag root, and ginseng ren shen.

Lactation (to Restrain)

GENERAL HERBAL TREATMENT: To restrain lactation, decoct barley sprouts,
half of them raw and half prefried—about 30–60 grams, in 3 cups of
water. Take as needed.

Leukorrhea (Vaginal Discharge)

GENERAL HERBAL TREATMENTS:

- Take Gentiana Combination internally. To alleviate the itching, make a douche with a combination of equal parts philodendron, sophora, cnidium, and alumen.

• For trichomonas and vaginal itch, combine cnidium seeds with alumen, philodendron, and borneol and use as a douche.

• Make a strong douche of cnidium seeds.

Lower-Back Pain

GENERAL HERBAL TREATMENTS:

• For aching lower back, knees, and other joint pains, combine 9 grams each of achyranthes root, eucommia bark, loranthes, and angelica *du huo.*

• For aching soreness of the lower back (lumbago), combine 9 grams each of eucommia bark, psoralea fruit, dodder seed, and loranthes with 15 grams of walnut meats.

• For liver and kidney yang deficiency with symptoms of aching soreness of the lower back and knees and leg weakness, combine 9 grams each of teasel, eucommia bark, achyranthes, and loranthes.

• For impotence and aching soreness of the lower back, knees, and legs, combine 9 grams each of psoralea seeds, dodder seeds, eucommia bark, cistanche root, teasel root, prepared rehmannia, poria, and dioscorea with 6 grams of cornus berries.

• For aching soreness and weakness of the lower back, knee and leg weakness, or impotence, infertility, frigidity, irregular menstruation, or cold feeling in the lower back and abdomen, combine 9 grams each of morinda root, ginseng *ren shen,* cistanche, and dodder seeds.

• For deficient liver and kidneys with symptoms of aching soreness of the lower back, joint pains, knee weakness, impotence, seminal emissions, dizziness, and blurred vision, combine 9 grams each of dogwood berries, prepared rehmannia, dodder seed, psoralea, and eucommia bark.

• For lower back pain caused by kidney deficiency, use 9 grams each of cnidium, loranthes, eucommia bark, gentiana, and achyranthes.

Lung Inflammation

GENERAL HERBAL TREATMENT: For inflammation of the lungs, combine 10 grams each of houttuynia and trichosanthes fruit, 9 grams each of platycodon and mulberry bark, and 3 grams of licorice.

Mastitis

GENERAL HERBAL TREATMENTS:

- For mastitis and breast lumps, combine 9 grams each of tricho-santhes, dandelion, lonicera, and forsythia.
- For mastitis and breast cancer, combine 9 grams each of dandelion, honeysuckle flowers, forsythia fruits, and scrophularia with 4 grams of phytolacca and 3 grams of licorice.

Mind

GENERAL HERBAL TREATMENTS:

- For mental problems, combine equal parts curcuma (yu jin), sweet-flag, and gota kola
- For anger and depression with forgetfulness, combine 12 grams of albizzia bark with 9 grams each of biota, fleeceflower root, and zizy-phus seeds.
- For forgetfulness, lack of awareness, and mental weakness, combine 9 grams each of sweetflag rhizome, Gota Kola, angelica dang gui, curcuma (yu jin), ginseng ren shen, and licorice.

Morning Sickness during Pregnancy

GENERAL HERBAL TREATMENT: For morning sickness, combine 18 grams each of atractylodes bai zhu and codonopsis with 10 grams of crushed cardamon seed. Grind the mixture into a powder. Steep 1 tablespoon of it in 1 cup of boiling water, covered. Have 3 cups daily.

Motion Sickness

GENERAL HERBAL TREATMENT: For travel sickness, motion sickness, and seasickness, prepare capsules of dry ginger. Take 2 capsules with warm water beginning 20 minutes before departure and then 1 or 2 capsules every 20–30 minutes during traveling time.

Nausea and Vomiting

GENERAL HERBAL TREATMENTS:

- For vomiting and acid regurgitation caused by coldness of the stom-ach, combine 6 grams each of evodia, dry ginger, pinellia, and poria.

• For nausea and vomiting caused by cold stomach and *qi* stagnation, combine 6 grams each of galangal and dry ginger with 9 grams of pinellia.

Nervousness, Hysteria, and Insomnia

GENERAL HERBAL TREATMENTS:

• For nervousness, hysteria, insomnia, and grief, cook 5–10 jujube dates with 15 grams sprouted wheat and 9 grams of licorice.
• For nervousness, restlessness, and palpitations, combine 9 grams each of polygala and zizyphus seeds with 15 grams each of dragon bone and oyster shell.
• For mania, delusions, hysteria, and mental problems caused by invisible phlegm veiling the heart (consciousness), combine 9 grams each of polygala root, sweetflag root, and curcuma (*yu jin*).
• For nervousness, irritability, insomnia, palpitations, and anxiety, combine 9 grams each of biota seeds, zizyphus seeds, schisandra berries, and polygala.

Nonhealing Boils and Ulcers

GENERAL HERBAL TREATMENT: For nonhealing boils and ulcers that have formed pus but have failed to drain (caused by *qi* and blood deficiency), combine 9 grams each of astragalus, ginseng *ren shen*, cinnamon bark, and angelica *dang gui*.

Obesity

GENERAL HERBAL TREATMENT: The standard formulas are *Fang Feng Tong Sheng* (Ledebouriella and Platycodon Formula) with *Fang Ji Huang Qi Tang* (Stephania and Astragalus Combination), used together.
PLANETARY FORMULAS: Triphala Herbal Diet, Triphala

Pain

GENERAL HERBAL TREATMENTS:

• For pains caused by blood and *qi* stagnation, which includes most types of pains, combine equal parts of corydalis, myrrh, frankincense, angelica *dang gui*, and ligusticum (*chuan xiong*). Mix these with warm honey and roll them into a pill that contains about 6–9 grams of the powdered herbs. Take 1 pill twice daily with warm water or a little warm rice wine.

- For pains caused by *qi* and blood stagnation, treat as follows: (1) for chest pains, combine equal parts curcuma (*yu jin*), red sage root, bupleurum, bitter orange peel, and cyperus root; (2) for painful menstruation, combine equal parts curcuma (*yu jin*), bupleurum, cyperus, white peony root, and angelica *dang gui*.
- For pain caused by all types of blood stagnation, combine equal parts of the powders of myrrh, frankincense, angelica *dang gui*, ligusticum, and corydalis. Mix approximately 6 grams of these with warm honey to form a pill. Take 2 or 3 pills daily with warm water or warm rice wine.
- For acute abdominal pains and spasms, combine 9 grams each of licorice and white peony root.
- For pain and swelling caused by external injury as well as pain associated with chronic degenerative diseases, combine 12 grams of albizzia bark with 6 grams each of angelica *dang gui*, frankincense, myrrh, and corydalis.

Perspiration (Spontaneous)

GENERAL HERBAL TREATMENT: For involuntary sweating and night sweats caused by bodily weakness, combine 30 grams of Light Wheat, 9 grams each of astragalus root and ephedra root, and 15 grams of oyster shell.

Premature Ejaculation

GENERAL HERBAL TREATMENT: For seminal emissions, premature ejaculation, or clear vaginal discharge caused by kidney deficiency, combine 18 grams of lotus seeds, 10 grams of euryale seeds, and 9 grams each of dodder seeds, psoralea, and dioscorea.

Qi Deficiency (Low Energy)

GENERAL HERBAL TREATMENTS:

- For *qi* deficiency, combine equal parts ginseng *ren shen,* atractylodes bai zhu, poria, and prepared licorice in the formula Si Jun Zi Tang (Four Nobles), the representative formula for qi deficiency.

- For treating qi deficiency daily, take ginseng ren shen in commercially available honey-baked slices of the root. A few slices can be taken daily.
- For spleen and lung qi deficiency with low appetite, loose stools, and low energy, combine 9 grams each of astragalus, ginseng ren shen, and atractylodes bai zhu.
- For spleen and stomach qi deficiency with poor appetite, diarrhea, and loose stools, combine 9 grams each of dioscorea, atractylodes bai zhu, poria, and ginseng ren shen with 3 grams of prepared licorice and 5 jujube dates.
- For qi deficiency with symptoms of low appetite, combine 9 grams each of pseudostellaria, dioscorea, codonopsis, and atractylodes with sprouted millet and barley to the consistency of porridge.
- For qi deficiency with symptoms of loose stools and poor appetite, combine 5–10 Jujube Dates with 9 grams each of ginseng ren shen, atractylodes bai zhu, poria, and prepared licorice.
- For qi, blood, and yang deficiency with general exhaustion and tiredness, use Shi Quan Da Bu Tang (Ginseng and Dang Gui Ten Combination).

Qi Stagnation

GENERAL HERBAL TREATMENT:

- For liver qi stagnation with chest fullness, combine 6 grams each of bupleurum, cyperus, and green citrus.
- For qi and cold stagnation affecting the epigastric and abdominal region, possibly with symptoms of nausea, vomiting, and belching, make a powder of 1 gram of aquilaria, 6 grams of lindera, 9 grams of saussurea, and 3 grams of ginger. If there are hiccups, add 9 grams of persimmon calyx.
- For chest fullness, combine 9 grams each of cyperus, bupleurum, white peony root, and curcuma (yu jin).
- For spleen and stomach qi stagnation with symptoms of lack of appetite, borborygmus (intestinal rumbling caused by gas movement), diarrhea, and abdominal pain, make a powder of equal parts of saussurea, bitter orange peel, and citrus peel. Take 2–4 grams as

needed. If there is also *qi* deficiency, add equal parts ginseng, atractylodes, poria, and licorice root to the combination.

- For chest and costal discomfort caused by cold stagnation, combine 9 grams each of lindera, bitter orange, trichosanthes fruit, curcuma root, bupleurum, and white peony.
- For stomach and abdominal pain and stagnation, combine 9 grams each of lindera, saussurea, and citrus peel.

Revival (from Unconsciousness)

GENERAL HERBAL TREATMENT: For fainting and unconsciousness, combine equal parts musk (*she xiang*) and borneol (*bing pian*) and allow the unconscious person to smell the preparation.

Rheumatic and Arthritic Conditions

GENERAL HERBAL TREATMENTS:

- For rheumatic and arthritic pains of the shoulders and upper back, combine 9 grams each of notopterygium and ledebouriella with 6 grams of turmeric root.
- For general aches and pains, headaches, chills, and fever, combine 9 grams each of notopterygium, cimicifugu (or Western *Angelica archangelica*), black atractylodes, and pueraria root.
- For external wind-cold syndrome with fever, chills, headaches, and general achiness, combine 9 grams each of ledebouriella, schizonepeta, and notopterygium.
- For wind-heat syndrome with fever, sore throat, influenza, colds, conjunctivitis, and headaches, combine 9 grams each of ledebouriella, schizonepeta, scutellaria root, forsythia, and honeysuckle flowers with 6 grams of mint (*Herba mentha haplocalycis*).
- For rheumatic and arthritic conditions, combine 30 grams each of coix and cinnamon-twig tea cooked with rice to make a porridge. For arthralgia of all kinds and pain of the lower back, waist, legs, and feet, one of the most effective formulas combines angelica *du huo*, loranthes, large-leaf gentian, and other herbs in the formula called *Du Huo Ji Sheng Tang* (*Du Huo* Angelica and Loranthes Combination).
- Another combination for arthritic conditions is 9 grams each of angelica *du huo*, angelica *dang gui*, and loranthes with 15 grams wide-leafed

gentian. Cook this mixture in 4 cups of water down to 2 cups, take 2 cups daily.

- For arthritic pains and numbness, combine 9 grams each of clematis root, angelica *du huo*, loranthes, chaenomeles, and angelica *dang gui*.
- For rheumatic pains caused by wind dampness, combine 9 grams each of chaenomeles fruit, clematis root, stephania root, and angelica *dang gui*.
- For joint pains and spasms of the limbs, combine 9 grams each of xanthium, clematis root, cinnamon bark, atractylodes (*cang zhu*) and ligusticum. Make the mixture into a decoction and take 2 cups daily. For wind-damp obstruction (arthritic and rheumatic pains), combine 6 grams of ligusticum with 9 grams each of notopterygium, angelica *du huo*, ledebouriella, and mulberry twigs.

CHINESE PATENTS: Specific Lumbaglin, *Du Huo Ji Sheng Wan, Xiao Hu Luo Dan, Feng Shih Hsiao Tung Wan, Tian Ma Wan*

Ringworm and Scabies

GENERAL HERBAL TREATMENTS:

- Make a paste of turmeric powder, a little flour, and water and apply topically.
- For itch, ringworm, lice, and scabies, combine calamine with sulfur (*liu huang*) and *zhang nao* (camphor) and apply externally.
- For scabies, combine 1–3 grams of sulfur with calomelas (*qing fen*) and apply as a paste externally.
- For scabies and lice, combine camphor with sulfur (*liu huang*) and alumen (*ming fan*).

Skin Diseases

GENERAL HERBAL TREATMENTS:

- For rubella and itching, combine 6 grams of silkworms with 9 grams each of cicada slough, arctium seeds, and mint (*Herba mentha haplocalycis*).
- For eczema, swelling, and irritation of the nose and middle ear, combine alumen with borneol and mix with a small amount of olive or sesame oil and apply directly to the area.
- For skin diseases associated with damp heat, take *Long Dan Xie Gan Tang* (Gentiana Combination)

- For acne, take *Shi Wei Bai Du Tang* (Bupleurum and Schizonepeta Formula) or *Qing zang fang gen tang jia yi yi jen* (Ledebouriella and Coix Combination)
- For weeping eczema, genital and/or anal itch, and scabies, apply the following combination topically as a wash or powder, sophora root, stemona, alumen, borneol, and calomelas in equal parts.
- For toxic conditions with various symptoms, such as boils and swellings, combine 19 grams of houttuynia with 9 grams each of dandelion, forsythia, and lonicera and 3 grams of licorice.
- For chronic skin conditions, including eczema, psoriasis, urticaria, dermatitis, purpura, and tinea, use *Xiao Feng San* (Dang Gui and Arctium Combination).

CHINESE PATENTS: Use Margarite Acne Pills (Plum Flower brand) for acne, furuncles, skin itching, rashes, and hives; it is excellent for adolescent acne. For acute inflammations, infections of ulcerated abscesses and carbuncles with pus, and skin itching with rash and redness, use *Lien Chiao Pai Tu Pien*.

Sore Throat

GENERAL HERBAL TREATMENT: For sore throat, combine 9 grams each of scrophularia, burdock seed, platycodon root, and forsythia with 6 grams of mint.

CHINESE FOOD THERAPY: A light diet of soups (especially *mung dahl*) and diluted juices is best.

CHINESE PATENT: *Chuan Xin Lian* (Antiphlogistic Pills), one of the most reliable antibiotic, antiviral patents. It is used for acute sore throat, fevers, and swollen glands. It is useful for strep infections, tonsillitis, and viral infections with fevers. It can also be used for measles, influenza, hepatitis, boils, furuncles, mastitis, and abscesses. Topical relief can be obtained with Superior Sore Throat Powder Spray.

Summer Heat (Heat Stroke)

GENERAL HERBAL TREATMENT: For summer heat patterns with dampness, thirst that is not satisfied with drinking, vomiting, and diarrhea, combine 12 grams talcum and 6 grams of licorice.

CHINESE PATENT: *Huo Xiang Zheng Qi San* (Agastache Powder for Dispelling Turbidity and Restoring Health)

Swollen Glands

GENERAL HERBAL TREATMENTS:

- For swollen glands, combine 6 grams of silkworms with 9 grams each of fritillary and prunella.
- For swollen glands, take 1–3 grams of hornet's nest internally with frankincense, forsythia, fritillary, and prunella (1.3 grams each).

Tinnitus

GENERAL HERBAL TREATMENT: For tinnitus caused by kidney deficiency, combine 15 grams of Magnetitum and 6 grams of schisandra berries with 9 grams each of prepared rehmannia, cornus berries, and dioscorea.

CHINESE PATENTS: If tinnitus is caused by damp heat, use *Long Dan Xie Gan Wan* (Gentiana Decoction for Purging Liver Fire). If it is caused by kidney deficiency, consider *Liu Wei Di Huang Wan* (Rehmannia Six Combination) for kidney yin deficiency or *Ba Wei Di Huang Wan* (Rehmannia Eight Combination) for kidney yang deficiency.

Toothache

GENERAL HERBAL TREATMENT: Take 9 grams of angelica *du huo* steeped in warm rice wine (sake). A warm mouthful can be retained in the mouth.

Toxicity and Excess Conditions

GENERAL HERBAL TREATMENTS:

- To remove all excesses, use *Fang Feng Tong Sheng* (Ledebouriella and Platycodon Formula)
- For general toxicity, especially of the gastrointestinal tract, liver, gallbladder, and stomach, use *San Huang Xie Xin Tang* (Coptis and Rhubarb Combination).

Ulcers and Sores

GENERAL HERBAL TREATMENT: For ulcers and sores that are difficult to heal, make a powder of equal parts turmeric root, philodendron, comfrey, and coptis and apply it topically.

Urinary Stones

GENERAL HERBAL TREATMENT: For the pain of urinary stones, combine 12 grams of talcum and 4 grams of cinnamon twigs with 9 grams each of polyporus, poria, plantain seed, and alisma.

Urinary Tract Infections (Cystitis, Nephritis)

GENERAL HERBAL TREATMENTS:

• For urinary tract infections, combine 9 grams each of dianthus, plantain seeds, polyporus, and poria with 6 grams of cinnamon twigs and 20 grams of talcum.
• For urinary tract infections, combine 9 grams each of plantain seeds, alisma, and gardenia fruit with 30 grams of talcum.
• For frequent or painful urination, urinary tract infections, or mouth and tongue ulcerations, combine 6 grams of akebia, 9 grams of bamboo leaf, and 10 grams of unprepared rehmannia.

CHINESE PATENT: *Long Dan Xie Gan Wan* (Gentiana Decoction for Purging Liver Fire)

Worms and Internal Parasites

GENERAL HERBAL TREATMENT:

• For hookworm (Ancylostomatidae), combine 9 grams each of chinaberry bark and areca seed.
• For pinworms *(Enorobius vermicularis)*, combine 9 grams each of chinaberry root, stemona root, and mume plum.
• For hookworms, combine equal parts of torreya, chinaberry, and areca seed.
• For tapeworms (Cestoda), combine equal parts of torreya, pumpkin seeds, and areca seed.
• For roundworms (Nematode), combine equal parts of torreya, quisqualis, and mume plum.
• For tapeworms, take 60–120 grams of pumpkin seeds first thing in the morning on an empty stomach. After 2 hours, take 60–120 grams of Areca seeds. Another half hour later, take 15 grams of mirabilitum. This will produce a bowel movement that should discharge the tapeworms as well.

- Garlic is effective for all types of worms. It should be eaten freely for 1–3 days with rice as the only other item in the diet. It should also be taken freely with any of the above worm and parasite treatments. Take garlic once a day to prevent recurrence of any intestinal parasites.

CHINESE FORMULA: *Wu Mei San* (Mume Plum Combination)

Yang Deficiency (Low Metabolism)

GENERAL HERBAL TREATMENTS:

- For coldness, low metabolism symptoms, and deficient yang, combine 6 grams each of prepared Aconite, cinnamon bark, and dry Ginger with 3 grams of licorice. If there is accompanying dampness and fluid retention, add 9 grams of Poria.
- For stimulating metabolism, warming spleen yang, and removing cold dampness, combine 4 grams each of cinnamon bark and dry ginger with 9 grams each of atractylodes *bai zhu,* poria, and honey-prepared licorice in the formula called *Zhen Wu Tang* (Vitality Combination).
- For deficient kidney–adrenal yang with coldness, pains in the lower back, weak knees and other joint pains, diabetes, urinary weakness, and diseases associated with aging, degeneration, and weakness, combine 4 grams each of cinnamon bark, prepared aconite, and moutan peony with 9 grams each of prepared rehmannia, cornus berries, poria, and alisma in the formula called *Ba Wei Di Huang Wan* (Rehmannia Eight Combination).
- For cold mucous conditions, combine equal parts of powdered long pepper, dry ginger, and black pepper mixed with honey. Take a spoonful of the mixture as needed. A milder version for children uses 2 parts of crushed anise seeds (*Pimpinella anisum*) instead of the black pepper.
- For cold, weak digestion caused by stomach and spleen coldness, combine 6 grams each of galangal, dry ginger, atractylodes, and codonopsis.

CHINESE FOOD THERAPY: Cinnamon, ginger, and ginseng congee
CHINESE PATENT: Golden Book Tea or Sexoton Pills

Yin-Deficiency Patterns

GENERAL HERBAL TREATMENTS:

- For kidney yin deficiency with symptoms such as night sweats, nocturnal emissions, lower-back, and/or joint pains, combine 9 grams each of philodendron bark, anemarrhena, unprepared rehmannia, and dioscorea.

- For diabetes with symptoms of extreme thirst, profuse urination, and hunger, combine 9 grams each of anemarrhena, trichosanthes root, schisandra berries, ophiopogon root, and pueraria root.
- For yin deficiency symptoms of the lungs and kidneys with heat signs, such as afternoon fever, night sweats, and heat sensation in the palms, soles, and chest, combine 9 grams each of anemarrhena and philodendron.
- For yin deficiency with afternoon fever, night sweats, dizziness, blurred vision, photophobia, nocturnal emissions, and diabetes, combine 9 grams each of prepared rehmannia, lycii berries, dioscorea, cornus berries, poria, alisma, and moutan peony.
- For consumed yin from overwork, stress, excessive sex, and so on, with symptoms of dry, red tongue with a scant coat and thirst, combine 9 grams each of dendrobium, ophiopogon, American ginseng, and unprepared rehmannia.
- For deficient kidney and liver yin with symptoms of premature gray hair, dizziness, vertigo, night sweats, and blurred vision, combine 15 grams each of eclipta and black sesame seeds with 9 grams each of fleeceflower root, ligustrum, and lycii berries.
- For yin deficiency with heat, combine 9 grams each of ligustrum berries, anemarrhena, philodendron, unprepared rehmannia, poria, and alisma with 6 grams each of moutan peony and cornus berries.
- For night sweats caused by yin deficiency, combine 9 grams of biota seeds with 15 grams of oyster shell and 9 grams each of ginseng *ren shen* and schisandra berries.

CHINESE FOOD THERAPY: *su mi zhou* (ghee and honey congee)
CHINESE PATENT: *Liu Wei Di Huang Wan* (Rehmannia Six Combination)

· TWELVE ·

INTEGRATING CHINESE
HERBS AND FOODS
INTO DAILY LIFE

When I first began to study Chinese herbology, there seemed to be impenetrable language and cultural barriers. One method I used to get past those barriers was to make myself the local *may gwo ren* (American) pest by spending hours in various Chinese pharmacies observing the course of daily business. I was absolutely fascinated by the displays of strange plant, mineral, and animal parts everywhere and most of all by how these were so easily accepted by the countless numbers of Chinese who would come to their local cultural haunt to purchase their medicines. The Chinese regard their pharmacies not only as places to obtain medicine for when they are not well but also as places to purchase exotic natural health aids that can be used in countless ways, such as soups, teas, liquors, pills, baths, and ointments.

One morning, I was observing in a traditional Chinese pharmacy in Victoria, British Columbia. For about 1½ hours, literally dozens of Chinese scurried in and out asking for a large mixture of herbs they called *bo ton yok choy*. Despite the fact that I had watched very closely, I still could not figure out why they were all asking for the same combination of herbs. Since I spoke absolutely no Chinese and none of them spoke English very fluently, there was no way to ask questions. Not anticipating what I was ordering, I somehow communicated to the pharmacist that I also wanted a bag of *bo ton yok choy,* along with, to his perplexed satisfaction, a pound of each of the herbs in the formula. When he understood what I wanted, his attitude toward me suddenly improved. I had no idea what I was in for. I hoped only that I had enough money to pay the bill at the end and also that U.S. customs agents would allow me to bring these back to the United States. As it turned out, there were some thirty-six herbs in *bo ton yok choy,* and the cost did indeed stretch my meager finances to the limit. As he was wrapping each herb in a piece of folded newspaper tied with a string, I received a vague answer, accompanied by much gesticulating, to one of my burning questions: "It make the body strong—it make the lungs strong!"

I had not the vaguest notion that these very first thirty-six herbs were to be the beginning of my personal Chinese herbal pharmacy at my acupuncture and herb clinic in Santa Cruz, California. As luck would have it, they were among the most representative and commonly used herbs in Chinese herbalism. When I got home, I carefully weighed each herb in the master *bo ton yok choy* formula and used my stash to recreate the formula myself. I could tell from the little that I knew at that time that the formula was mostly a tonic. It also contained the smallest bits and pieces, however, of some rather nasty-tasting herbs, such as rhubarb, a laxative, and coptis, a bitter alterative. Their presence in the formula was very confusing, especially for a beginning Chinese herbalist with no formula training.

It was over 20 years later that I ventured to question one of my dear friends and Chinese herb suppliers, Irene Ho of the Great China Art Company: "Have you ever heard of the formula *bo ton yok choy?*" As usually happened when I attempted to speak Chinese, she was at first unable to decipher what I was asking. Perhaps I was using the wrong tone pitch that could mean the difference between an innocuous everyday word and a vulgar obscenity. Eventually, after I explained the formula and how it had been used that long-ago day in the pharmacy in Victoria, she exclaimed, "Oh! *Bo ton yok choy*—the soup of the day!" She then went on to explain to me how in her own household, when she prepared a soup or the regular morning rice porridge, called congee, she might add certain herbs according to the weather or individual needs of each family member. If, for instance, someone was having problems with too much mucus, she might add a small amount of pinellia, ginger, and citrus peel to the soup or congee; if someone was feeling particularly tired or weak, perhaps recovering from prolonged sickness, she might add a little ginseng. If the soup or congee was for someone with hypertension, then it would be prepared with green mung beans. This mixture became the "herbal formula of the day" for her family. She went on to say that traditional Chinese pharmacies often prepare such a daily mixture, based on weather and season, for their loyal clientele.

Chinese herbal medicine is a very complex subject, and mastery requires years of dedicated study. Still, perhaps, the most important use of this book for the Western layperson is to learn how to integrate Chinese herbs into their lives, as most traditional Chinese know very well how to do. The goal is to achieve the confidence to begin with a few herbs and formulas and then add to them as your needs expand. With no formal study available to me at that time, I began by simply studying those thirty-six herbs of what I took to be a popular Chinese formula that the pharmacist did not hesitate to prescribe and gave indiscriminately to everyone who walked into the pharmacy. Begin by learning the common uses of a few herbs and foods. Every herb and food has a therapeutic property. As it turns out, the distinction between Western herbs and Chinese herbs is a thin line; besides herbs of the official materia medica presented in this book, just about every common local garden weed—from dandelions to plantain—has its own Chinese name and therapeutic classification according to energy, flavors, organs and meridians affected, indications, and so forth.

In Chapter 6 (Food Therapy), I presented some of the therapeutic uses of common foods, recipes, and ways to incorporate Chinese herbs and foods in daily life. This chapter goes further to detail the use of some of the most common preparations with and without foods. Following is a list by category of use of some of the most common herbs and foods that can be prepared in various ways—as teas, as additions to soups and congees, or as alcoholic liqueurs.

USES OF COMMON CHINESE HERBS

HERB	EFFECTS	NOTES AND SUGGESTED AMOUNT FOR COMMON USE
Ginseng (ren shen)	Tonifies qi, for fatigue and tiredness; improves digestion; primarily for individuals over the age of 40	3–6 grams

HERB	EFFECTS	NOTES AND SUGGESTED AMOUNT FOR COMMON USE
Codonopsis (dang shen)	Same uses as for ginseng but about one third the potency, better suited for occasional use in all climates by people of all ages	Has a sweet flavor and warm energy; purchase by the pound so it can be used in soups and congee; dose: 6–9 grams
Astragalus (huang qi)	Tonifies qi; strengthens the immune system	Has a sweet flavor and warm energy; purchase by the pound to use in soups and congee; dose: 6–9 grams or 2–4 slices
Angelica sinensis (dang gui)	Tonifies blood; especially good for anemia, gynecological problems, and blood circulation	Somewhat bitter and sweet; dose: no more than 3 grams in congee or soup (but up to 6 grams in soup for women)
Fleeceflower (Polygonum Multiflorum; he shou wou)	Tonifies blood; regulates cholesterol and blood lipids; good for the liver and kidneys; softens the skin; restores hair color; good for bowel regularity	Comes precooked with black soybeans; slightly bitter and sweet; dose: 3–6 grams in soup or congee
Ophiopogon (mai men dong)	Yin tonic; strengthens and moistens the lungs; used for chronic lung diseases and wasting diseases	Sweet, slightly bitter, and cool; dose: up to 6 grams in soup or congee
Lycii berries (gou qi zi)	Blood and yin tonic; strengthens the liver; good for sexual energy; high in beta carotene; improves eyesight	Have a sweet flavor and a neutral energy; Chinese use them freely and refer to them as "red raisins"; use freely in soups and congee; dose: 6–20 grams
Jujube dates (da zao)	Qi tonic; good for spleen and stomach; act as sedative; counteract liver toxins; good for fatigue, loose stools, lack of appetite, restlessness, and insomnia	Have a sweet flavor and neutral energy

HERB	EFFECTS	NOTES AND SUGGESTED AMOUNT FOR COMMON USE
Walnuts (hu tao ren)	Kidney yang tonic; used for lower-back pain and urinary incontinence; also good for premature ejaculation, chronic cough, and constipation in the elderly due to Dryness	Have a sweet flavor and a warm energy; dose: 9–30 grams daily
Dioscorea (shan yao)	qi tonic for the spleen, lungs, kidneys, and stomach; used for chronic diarrhea, food Stagnation, and fatigue and for lung qi deficiency with symptoms of chronic cough and difficult breathing; good for urinary and seminal fluid incontinence and vaginal discharge, all from qi deficiency	Has a sweet flavor and neutral energy; eaten as a vegetable in both China and Japan; dose: 6–30 grams

The next group of herbs can be used for special therapeutic needs, such as improving digestion, counteracting mucus, relieving inflammation, improving circulation, warming, and stimulating metabolism.

HERBS FOR SPECIAL THERAPEUTIC NEEDS

HERB	EFFECTS AND PROPERTIES	NOTES AND SUGGESTED AMOUNT FOR COMMON USE
Herbs that warm		
Dry ginger (gan jiang)	Warms the center, benefits digestion, counteracts nausea and vomiting, warms and dries mucus; has a spicy flavor and hot energy	Dose: 3–9 grams

HERB	EFFECTS AND PROPERTIES	NOTES AND SUGGESTED AMOUNT FOR COMMON USE
Garlic (da suan)	Eliminates parasites; acts as an antibacterial and antifungal; opens the surface to treat colds; benefits digestion; treats dysentery	use freely; dose: 6–15 grams
Fennel seed (xiao hui xiang)	Regulates qi; good for digestive problems; alleviates hernia and testicular pains; has a spicy, warm energy	Dose: 3–9 grams
Cinnamon Bark (rou gui) and twigs (gui zhi)	Assist the yang of the whole body; good for coldness and blood stagnation; the twigs are used to induce perspiration and relieve circulatory problems, such as arthritis and rheumatic complaints; the bark is spicy, sweet, and hot, while the twigs are milder	Bark dose: 1–3 grams; twig dose: 3–6 grams
Black pepper (hu jiao)	Used for coldness, dampness, to increase gastric secretions, aid digestion, dry mucus, and counteract parasites; very hot and drying	Dose: 1–3 grams
Nutmeg	Used for diarrhea and as a carminative for digestion; warm and dry	Dose: 1–3 grams

HERB	EFFECTS AND PROPERTIES	NOTES AND SUGGESTED AMOUNT FOR COMMON USE
Herbs that induce sweating		
Cooling for high fever, slight chills		
Chrysanthemum flowers *(ju hua)*	Counteracts inflammation, relieves colds and fevers, calms and soothes the liver, benefits the eyes; flowers have bitter, sweet, and acrid flavors and a cool energy	Dose: 3–6 grams
Mint *(bo he)*	Most common species is Chinese *bo he,* which is somewhat different from peppermint and spearmint, but all are used to induce perspiration and aid digestion; used for the common cold, fevers, and nervous disorders; spicy flavor and cool energy	Mint should not be boiled; dose: 3–6 grams
Pueraria *(ge gen)*	Used for fevers, colds, headaches, stiff neck, hypertension, dysentery, and colitis; spicy and sweet with a cool energy	Dose: 3–9 grams
Warming for fever, slight sweat, chills		
Perilla leaf *(zi su ye)*	Used for the common cold, cough, chest congestion, abdominal bloating, nausea, and vomiting; specific for seafood poisoning; acrid flavor and warm energy	Do not boil; dose: 3–9 grams

HERB	EFFECTS AND PROPERTIES	NOTES AND SUGGESTED AMOUNT FOR COMMON USE
Scallions (cong bai)	Used for colds, influenza, and gastrointestinal upset; induces perspiration; acrid flavor and warm energy	Do not boil; Dose: 3–9 grams

Herbs that dry mucus

Pinellia (ban xia)	Used for cold phlegm, cough, dampness, nausea, and vomiting; acrid and warm energy; slightly toxic	Dose in food: 3 grams
Fresh ginger (sheng jiang)	Used for the common cold, white mucus, motion sickness, and seafood poisoning; promotes digestion; acrid and warm energy	Dose: 3–9 grams

Herbs for coughs and the lungs

Apricot seeds (xing ren)	Used for acute cough and bronchitis; also useful for dry constipation; bitter, slightly warm, and slightly toxic	Dose: 3–9 grams
Loquat leaves	Used for hot cough with yellow or blood-streaked sputum; directs the qi of the lungs and stomach downward to treat cough, hiccups, and belching; bitter and cool energy	Dose: 6–9 grams

HERB	EFFECTS AND PROPERTIES	NOTES AND SUGGESTED AMOUNT FOR COMMON USE
Cooling and detoxifying herbs		
Burdock (niu bang zi)	Seeds are used for colds, influenza, fevers, sore throats, and eruptive skin diseases; leaves can be cooked as a potherb; root is nutritive and is also diuretic and a blood purifier; can be useful for the treatment of cancer, arthritis, and rheumatic problems; seeds are bitter, spicy, and have a cool energy	Root is freely sautéed like a carrot and eaten as a vegetable; seed dose: 3–9 grams, crushed
Honeysuckle blossoms (jin yin hua)	Used for infections, fevers, common cold, influenza, and sore throat; bitter, sweet flavor and a cold energy	Dose: 3–6 grams in food
Purslane (ma chi xian)	Used for inflammations, dysentery, toxicity; slightly bitter and sweet and a cool energy	Eat freely as a steamed potherb; dose: 6–9 grams; amaranth is used similarly
Dandelion (pu gong ying)	Used for hepatitis, jaundice, conjunctivitis, urinary tract infections, mastitis, and other inflammations; also good for increasing mother's milk; bitter, sweet flavor and a cold energy	Dose: 10–30 grams

HERB	EFFECTS AND PROPERTIES	NOTES AND SUGGESTED AMOUNT FOR COMMON USE
Cassia seed (jue ming zi)	Used for conjunctivitis, hypertension, and constipation; sweet, bitter, and salty flavors and a cool energy	As a tea, the crushed roasted seeds make a great coffee substitute and can be drunk freely by those with heat, hyperlipidemia, and hypertension; dose: 6–12 grams
Prunella or self heal (xia ku cao)	Used for inflamed and swollen glands; leaves have bitter, acrid, and sweet flavors and a cold energy	Dose: 9–12 grams
Gypsum (calcium sulfate; Shi Gao)	Used for fevers, mouth sores, and toothache; acrid and sweet with a cold energy	Dose: 10 grams in congee, precooked
Herbs that stimulate appetite and relieve food stagnation		
Hawthorn berries (shan zha)	Used for heart problems, high blood pressure, and high cholesterol; stimulate appetite and relieve food congestion; sour, sweet flavors and a slightly warm energy	Dose: 9–15 grams
Sprouted barley or rice (mai ya)	Used for food stagnation, to help digest starches, and for loss of appetite; sweet flavor and a neutral energy	Dose: 9–15 grams

HERB	EFFECTS AND PROPERTIES	NOTES AND SUGGESTED AMOUNT FOR COMMON USE
Citrus peel (chen pi)	Used for digestive weakness, phlegm, food stagnation, hiccups, belching, nausea, and cough; sometimes called Chinese chewing gum because mothers typically give children a piece of tangerine peel, fresh or dried, at the first sign of a sneeze or cold; very rich in bioflavonoids and vitamin C; acrid, bitter flavors and a warm, dry energy	Dose: 3–6 grams
Diuretics		
Poria (fu ling)	Used for edema, dampness, weakness of the urinary tract, diarrhea, palpitations, vertigo, restlessness, and insomnia; sweet and bland flavors and a neutral energy	Dose: 6–9 grams
Alisma (ze xie)	Used for edema, urinary dysfunction, and diarrhea; sweet flavor and a cold energy	Dose: 6–12 grams
Coix (yi yi ren)	Used for edema, inflammation, pus, diarrhea, suppurative infections, rheumatic diseases, and cancer; sweet and bland flavors and a slightly cool energy	Dose: 15–30 grams

HERB	EFFECTS AND PROPERTIES	NOTES AND SUGGESTED AMOUNT FOR COMMON USE
Calming		
Zizyphus seeds (suan zao ren)	Used for insomnia, restlessness, nervousness, and palpitations; sweet and sour flavors and a neutral energy	Dose: 6–9 grams
Laxative		
Rhubarb (da huang)	Used for constipation; bitter flavor and a cold energy	Dose: 3–6 grams
Other food additives		
Snow herb fungus (Tremella fuciformis)	Used for problems of lung heat with thick, yellow, or green phlegm, possibly blood-streaked; sweet and bland flavor and a cooling energy	Purchased dry; presoak and add to casseroles and various dishes
Black wood ear fungus (Auricularia auricula-judae)	Good for reducing high cholesterol; often cooked with shiitake mushrooms and meat to prevent the buildup of cholesterol; sweet and bland flavors and a neutral energy	Purchased dry; presoak and add to casseroles and various dishes

HERB	EFFECTS AND PROPERTIES	NOTES AND SUGGESTED AMOUNT FOR COMMON USE
Shiitake mushrooms (black mushrooms)	Like wood ear fungus, shiitake mushroom has been found effective for lowering blood pressure and reducing cholesterol; also very good for hepatitis, diabetes, anemia, rickets, colds, influenza, gallstones, hyperacidity, stomach ulcers, and cancer; bland flavor and a neutral energy	Purchased fresh or dry; presoak and add to casseroles and various dishes
Foxnuts (Euryale ferocis; qian shi)	Used for spleen-deficiency diarrhea, clear vaginal discharge, nocturnal emission, premature ejaculation and spermatorrhea, and urinary incontinence; sweet flavor and astringent and neutral energies	Dosage: 9–15 grams. This herb is very similar to Lotus seed and they are frequently used together.
Lotus seeds (Nelumbinis nuciferae; Lian Zi)	Used for chronic diarrhea due to spleen deficiency; useful for kidney deficiency with such symptoms as premature ejaculation and vaginal discharge; also used as a heart tonic to calm the spirit in such conditions as insomnia, palpitations, and anxiety; sweet flavor and astringent and neutral energies	Commonly combined with foxnuts; should not be used by those with constipation or abdominal distension; Dose: 6–18 grams

HERB	EFFECTS AND PROPERTIES	NOTES AND SUGGESTED AMOUNT FOR COMMON USE
Lotus root	Clears hot mucus from the lungs; used for different types of bleeding from the lungs and stomach; tonifies the heart, calms the mind, regulates moods, and benefits the stomach; sweet flavor and a cooling energy	Fresh, it can be finely chopped and added to stir fried dishes. Dried, it must be soaked a long time before using it. Fresh Lotus root juice is very cooling for inflammations.
Black hair moss (fat choy)	Really a seaweed; high in iron, tonifies blood, and helps restore hair color; has a cooling energy	Used in many dishes
Water chestnuts (Eleocharis dulcis)	Used to cleanse and purify the blood; good to eat or add to foods when there are such symptoms as rashes, boils, eczema, or psoriasis; also allay hunger; sweet flavor and a cool energy	Added freely to various foods; cool, crisp texture; purchased canned or fresh, then peeled, washed, and eaten
Bamboo shoots (young shoots of Bambusa species)	Used for obesity, diabetes, fever, and phlegm; sweet flavor and slightly cold energy	Must be cooked
Green tea (Camellia sinensis)	Clears heat, lowers fire (hypertension), promotes digestion and awakens the spirits, excites the nerves, and promotes urination; has a cold energy and should not be taken by people with a cold stomach and spleen; being a diuretic, it should also be avoided by individuals with frequent urination	Freely drunk as a beverage by the Chinese

Rice Porridge (Congee)

Rice porridge—congee or jook, as it is called in Cantonese—is the traditional Chinese breakfast. It is made by prolonged cooking of 1 part rice to 8 or 9 parts water by volume. White rice is the most easily digested; it is easily prepared as congee and makes a perfect food for breakfast, convalescence, or diseases including weak digestion. Herbs cooked with rice are more smoothly absorbed, which is especially valuable for those with sensitive digestion.

Herbs are used with food in every culture. In China, the first recorded use of herbs dates back to around 2,500 years ago, and it was during the Tang and Song dynasties that Chinese physicians made extensive use of food and herb combinations and recorded specific recipes. One text, compiled during the Song, called *The Peaceful Holy Benevolent Prescriptions,* consisted of a collection of 129 prescriptions. Most of these are still commonly used, including apricot and rice congee for treating coughs, jujube seed congee for insomnia, and ginseng congee for *qi* deficiency.

As seeds, grains embody the entire yin–yang life cycle of a plant and are therefore the most energetically balanced foods. As such they are especially suitable as a staple for regular daily consumption as well as for the treatment of disease, for which they are given in a more liquid, easily digested form. One can add various other foods and herbs according to individual need. The following recipe can be reduced or expanded as needed.

BASIC RICE CONGEE

Water: 9 cups
White rice or other grain: 1 cup
Herbs: 1 ounce (28 grams)
Meat (optional): 1–2 ounces

To make various types of congees, place in a large pot the water, the white rice or other type of grain, the herbs, and meat (if desired). Cover the pot and bring the mixture to a boil, then turn down the heat to the lowest possible setting. (For this, a rice cooker, crockpot, or slow cooker is most convenient.) Allow the mixture to cook slowly and gently for 6–8 hours. For diarrhea, loose stools, nausea, vomiting, and general weakness, use sweet rice or rice that has been previously pan-toasted until it is slightly yellowish brown. In general, use brown rice to increase stamina and strength. If this is difficult to digest (it shouldn't be), white rice will do. In China, congee is eaten as the primary breakfast food. It can be served plain or with the addition of some ginger, ginger-tofu, fish, meat, or eggs and a side dish of some steamed greens. This makes the most ideal breakfast. This basic congee can be modified by adding one or more of the herbs described in the 2 tables earlier in this chapter. Following are only a few of the many possible congee recipes.

For Colds, Cough, Bronchitis, and Hypertension

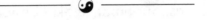

GARLIC CONGEE

Garlic: 30 grams, peeled and sliced
White rice: 1–2 cups

Boil the garlic in a pot for 1 minute and then remove it. Add 1 or 2 cups of white rice and continue to boil. After 15–20 minutes, add the cooked garlic to the rice. This can be eaten once or twice daily for breakfast or supper. Because garlic is heating, it is not recommended for patients with chronic gastritis or peptic ulcers. Garlic congee can be used for consumption, dysentery, chronic bronchitis, tuberculosis, hypertension, and arteriosclerosis.

For Colds

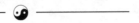

SCALLIONS AND GLUTINOUS SWEET RICE CONGEE

Scallions: 5 (or 1 small onion)
Ginger: 3–4 slices (fresh)
Glutinous white rice: 100 grams

Chop the scallions or a small onion and slice the fresh ginger and set them aside. Make rice congee. Then mash the chopped scallions and ginger to a pulp and add to the congee and simmer the mixture for 20 minutes, covered. This cures colds by inducing perspiration.

For Heat Stroke, Toxicity, Toxic Ulcers, and Hypertension

———————— ☯ ————————

MUNG BEANS AND WHITE RICE CONGEE

Mung beans (lu dou): 50 grams
White rice: 250 grams
Water: porridge consistency
Brown sugar: to taste

Cook the mung beans and white rice in water. Add brown sugar to taste.

For Infected Sores, Suppurative Skin Lesions, and Other Toxic Conditions

———————— ☯ ————————

BURDOCK ROOT CONGEE
(NIU BANG ZHOU)

Burdock root
Brown rice

Finely grate enough burdock root to get about 3 tablespoons of liquid when squeezed through a cheesecloth. Cook this with rice.

For Infections, Suppurative Skin Lesions, Sores, and Dysentery

———————— ☯ ————————

PURSLANE CONGEE *(MA CHI XIAN ZHOU)*

Purslane (fresh): 500 grams
White rice: 100 grams
Water: porridge consistency

Wash and press out the juice of the fresh Purslane *(ma chi xian)*. Add the purslane to the white rice and water and cook it. This is good for all types of dysentery, tenesmus, and abdominal distension.

For Blood Toxins and Heat Stroke

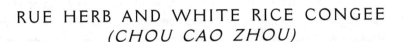

RUE HERB AND WHITE RICE CONGEE
(CHOU CAO ZHOU)

Rice congee
Rue (fresh): 50 grams

Make rice congee. Chop the fresh rue and add it to the hot congee; allow the congee to simmer for another 15–20 minutes. If using dried rue, then cook it with the rice (while making the congee).

For Cough with Phlegm

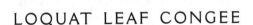

PERILLA LEAF AND APRICOT CONGEE

Apricot seed: 9 grams
Perilla leaf: 9 grams
Citrus peel: 6 grams
White rice: porridge consistency

Decoct the apricot seed *(xing ren)*, perilla leaf *(su ye*, also known as *shiso* in Japanese), and citrus peel *(chen pi)* in water. Strain the mixture and save the tea. Cook the rice in this liquid.

LOQUAT LEAF CONGEE

Loquat leaves: 15 grams
(Loquat flowers: 30 grams)
Loquat fruit (optional)
White rice: 100 grams
Water: 2¹/₂ cups

Decocting the loquat leaves in water, decocting from 1 cup down to ¹/₂ cup, then strain the leaves. To the reserved liquid add 2¹/₂ cups of water and the rice. It can be sweetened with sugar or honey to taste. Loquat fruit can be added if it is available. Loquat has a downward energy. This makes it useful for cough caused by lung heat with yellow phlegm and blood, and for vomiting caused by stomach heat, hiccups, acute gastritis, wind-heat common cold, acute bronchitis, pneumonia, and lung abscesses. It is also useful for asthma and emphysema. (For these latter 2 conditions, it is better to substitute loquat flowers for the leaves.)

For High Cholesterol and Hyperlipidemia

————————— ☯ —————————

POLYGONUM MULTIFLORUM CONGEE

Jujube dates: 5 pieces
Brown rice: 50 grams
Water: 2 cups
Polygonum multiflorum (powdered): 30 grams
Sugar: to taste

Cook the jujube dates and brown rice in the water. Add the powdered fleeceflower (*Polygonum multiflorum he shou wu*) and cook the mixture again. Before serving the congee, add sugar to taste. Eat it warm twice daily, morning and evening.

For Heart Disease

————————— ☯ —————————

GARLIC AND HAWTHORN BERRY CONGEE

Garlic: 9 grams
Hawthorn berries: 12 grams
White rice: 100 grams
Salvia miltiorrhizae (optional): 30 grams
Water

Cook the garlic, hawthorne berries, and white rice together. This is good for heart disease, chest pain, and angina pectoris. To increase the effect, add 30 grams of *Salvia miltiorrhizae (dan shen)* to the formula.

For Irregular Menstruation and Other Gynecological Problems

Chicken (female): 1 whole
Angelica dong gui: 6 grams
Brown rice: 100 grams
Water: porridge consistency

Cook the chicken (ideally a spring chicken), the Angelica *dang gui* and the rice in the water. This is useful for dysmenorrhea, stopped menstruation, post-partum recovery, and infertility caused by *qi* and blood deficiency.

For Edema, Rheumatic Diseases, and Cancer

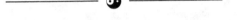

PEARL BARLEY CONGEE

Pearl barley: 50 grams
White rice: 50 grams
Water: porridge consistency

Cook the pearl barley and white rice in water until it is of porridge consistency.

For Edema and Urinary Complaints

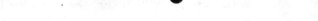

AZUKI BEAN AND BARLEY CONGEE

Azuki beans: 30 grams
Pearl barley: 30 grams
White rice: 30 grams
Citrus peel (powdered): 6 grams
Water: porridge consistency

Cook the azuki beans, pearl barley, and white rice together in the water. To this, add the powdered citrus peel *(chen pi)* after cooking. Have 2 servings daily.

For Nervousness and *Qi* Deficiency

———————— ☯ ————————

BROWN RICE AND COIX CONGEE

Brown rice: 100 grams
Coix (yi yi ren): 50 grams
Jujube dates (hong zao)
Water

Cook the brown rice, coix *(yi yi ren)*, and jujube dates *(hong zao)* in the water.

For Insomnia

———————— ☯ ————————

PORIA AND ZIZYPHUS CONGEE

Poria (fu ling): 50 grams
Zizyphus seeds (suan zao ren, finely ground): 15 grams
White rice: 100 grams
Water
Mimosa flowers (he huan hua, optional): 30 grams

Cook the poria *(fu ling)*, ground zizyphus seeds *(suan zao ren)* and the white rice together in the water. This dish is useful for insomnia, excessive dreams, and restlessness caused by heart and spleen deficiency. For emotional depression, poor memory, and restlessness, stir in 30 grams of dried mimosa flowers *(he huan hua)*.

For Yang Deficiency with Exhaustion and Cold Extremities

———————— ☯ ————————

CINNAMON, GINGER, AND GINSENG CONGEE

Cinnamon twigs (gui zhi): 6 grams
Dry ginger (gan jiang): 6 grams

Ginseng (ren shen): *3 grams*
Jujube dates (da zao): *10*
White rice: 100 grams

Decoct the cinnamon twigs *(gui zhi)*, dry ginger *(gan jiang)*, Chinese ginseng *(ren shen)*, and jujube dates *(da zao)*. After preparing the decoction, strain it and cook the white rice in the tea.

For *Qi* and Blood Deficiency

JUJUBE DATE CONGEE

White rice: 100 grams
Jujube dates (red or black): 15–30
Water: porridge consistency

The most common addition to congee is red or black jujube dates. These are very inexpensive, easily grown for that matter, and a good *qi* and blood tonic. They can be added with many other congee recipes. Cook the rice and dates in the water.

For *Qi* Deficiency

GINSENG CONGEE FOR *QI* DEFICIENCY

White rice: 100 grams
Ginseng (ren shen): *3–6 grams*
Codonopsis (dang shen): *9–15 grams*
Water
Barley malt: to taste

Add the Chinese ginseng *(ren shen)* or codonopsis *(dang shen)* to the rice. Sweeten the dish with barley malt to taste. This is ideal for individuals with *qi* deficiency and general debility. It is highly tonifying and helps prevent senility and premature aging.

To Tonify the Five Yin Organs, and Overcome Weakness; for Fevers, Cough and Blood-Streaked Sputum, Dry Constipation, and Rough, Dry Skin and Hair

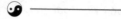

GHEE AND HONEY CONGEE *(SU MI ZHOU)*

Ghee (clarified butter): 30 grams
Honey: 15 grams
White rice congee

Mix the ghee and honey with white-rice congee.

Other Variations

There are many other congee recipes that could be included here. Many of these are taken from *The Book of Jook*, by Bob Flaws (published by Blue Poppy Press). This is a simple and wonderful book with hundreds of congee recipes. It is one of the books I have available to all my patients. Traditional Chinese cooking does not limit the use of congees only to breakfast. They can be eaten at any meal with various foods added, including some meat and other vegetables. They can also be made with different grains or other ingredients, such as wheat, which is cooling, calming, and sedating; water chestnuts, which are cooling and good for diabetes and jaundice; carrots, which are good for indigestion and chronic dysentery; spinach, which is harmonizing, lubricating for the internal organs, and sedative; pinenut, which is lubricating and relieves dry constipation; kidney, which is generally tonifying, especially to the kidneys, for all deficiency conditions with symptoms of lower-back and joint pains, impotence, premature ejaculation, and spermatorrhea; and liver, for all conditions of the liver with blood and yin deficiency.

Another Chinese name for congee is *Shui-fan*, which means "water rice." Because rice itself is diuretic, the addition of extra water increases its diuretic effects. This may mean that for those with urinary weakness and frequent urination, congee should not be eaten on a daily basis.

Chinese Casserole Cooking

Casseroles are another simple style of family cooking used by the Chinese. Like congee, casseroles do not require a lot of oil or fat. Special dishes can be easily prepared using foods and herbs therapeutically for tonifying most deficiencies. The Chinese commonly use clay pots for this type of cooking, but a covered casserole container can also be modified to prepare the most deliciously healthful lunch or dinner with the least amount of time and effort. According to Bob Flaws, this style of cooking, called *keng,* was especially dominant from the Chou (1124–249 B.C.) through the Han dynasties (206 B.C.–220 A.D.).

The tradition of vegetarianism and eating meat exist side by side in China. For the most part, certain Taoists and Buddhists follow a vegetarian diet, while most Chinese people judiciously incorporate meat into their diet. Rather than harboring strong ethical feelings about any food such as meat, traditional Chinese base their diet on using the food energy that is needed for health. Those experiencing diseases associated with deficiencies of *qi,* blood, yin, or yang should probably eat some meat on a daily basis and add appropriate herbs to their food. Casserole and soup cooking are both ideal for these types of preparations. The following recipe is one of the most popular traditional Chinese vegetarian recipes. Many variations of it can be made according to preference and the availability of different ingredients.

BUDDHA'S FEAST: VEGETARIAN CASSEROLE

Asparagus (may be omitted, or snow peas or chopped broccoli can be substituted): 1/3 pound
Chinese or green cabbage: 1/2 pound
Shiitake mushrooms (dried): 6
Cloud-ear mushrooms (a type of edible jelly fungus): 6
Daylily bud stems: 2 ounces
Water chestnuts (sliced): 1/2 can
Bamboo shoots (sliced): 1/2 can
Tofu (firm): 1/2 pound
Braised gluten (called seitan in health-food stores): 1 10-ounce can
Cellophane noodles (optional): 1/4 pound

Braising liquid:
Dry ginger: 1 teaspoon of the powder
Clarified butter (ghee): 2 tablespoons

Sesame oil: 2 teaspoons
Tamari soy sauce: 2 tablespoons
Hoisin sauce (if available): 2 tablespoons
Rice wine or sherry: 2 tablespoons
Unrefined brown sugar (Sucanat brand; optional): 1 teaspoon
Kudzu root starch (Pueraria lobata) or cornstarch (not as good
      nutritionally): 1 tablespoon
Miso paste: 1 tablespoon
Liquid in which the mushrooms were previously soaking: 1/2 cup
Water or vegetable stock (vegetable bouillon): 1/2 cup

Cut the tofu into 1-inch square cubes. Marinate it with dry ginger and tamari sauce for 15 or 20 minutes and then fry it in sesame oil or ghee. (Traditionally, tofu is considered to have a very cold energy, so in most countries where it is used, it is fried in oil with warming spices and tamari to make it more yang). Soak the dried lily buds and the cloud ear (called white or black fungus in Chinese grocery or pharmacies) along with the dried shiitake mushrooms in warm water for 1 hour. Drain and save the liquid to be added to the casserole later. When the mushrooms are soft and reconstituted, place them together with the remaining ingredients of the brazing liquid into a suitable casserole dish. Bring the mixture to a boil, then reduce the heat to medium low and simmer for 1/2 hour. Dissolve 1 tablespoon of kudzu root powder and stir it into the casserole to thicken the broth. After 1/2 hour, add the chopped remaining vegetables and simmer together for another 10 minutes. Check to see that none of the vegetables becomes overly cooked or mushy. At the same time, add the small cubes of fried tofu and chopped seitan. Sprinkle some roasted sesame oil over the casserole and serve it hot over rice or with previously cooked Chinese cellophane noodles. This recipe takes 1 hour of soaking time (which can be done overnight), 15 minutes to assemble, and 40 minutes to cook. It serves 2 people as a main course or 4–5 as part of a larger course. For nonvegetarians, add 1/2–1/3 pound of lean pork or beef. Various herbs can be added by first decocting them as a tea. This is then strained and used as part of the liquid in the preparation of this dish. Some of the herbs that can be considered include jujube dates, lotus root, astragalus, ginseng or codonopsis, and dioscorea.

BLACK MUSHROOM CHICKEN CASSEROLE

Chicken portion (a thigh or a leg): 1 small
Garlic: 1 clove

Fresh ginger: 1 thin slice
Carrot: 1
Shiitake mushrooms: 6
Cold-pressed sesame oil: enough to coat pan
Sea salt: a pinch
Tamari: 1 teaspoon
Spring onion: 1

Soak the black mushrooms in warm water for 30 minutes to 1 hour until they are reconstituted. Remove the skin and fat from the chicken. Wash and drain the chicken. Finely chop the garlic and ginger. Cut the carrot into small 1-inch segments. Thinly coat the bottom of the casserole dish with the sesame oil and heat it. When the oil is hot, stir-fry the garlic and ginger for 1 minute. Then add the chicken and the sea salt, cooking until the chicken is browned on all sides. Lower the heat and add the shiitake mushrooms and carrot and stir-fry the mixture for another 1–2 minutes. Then add the tamari and enough water (this can be a previously prepared herbal tea) until the liquid's level is halfway up the chicken and carrot. Bring the mixture to a boil, then place the casserole in an oven and bake it for 30 minutes at 350° Fahrenheit. Garnish the casserole with finely chopped spring onion. Variations:

- The water can be a strained tea that was previously made with codonopsis, *dang gui,* ginseng, or dioscorea.
- Add a whole onion or leek.
- One star anise and 1 onion can be added for a winter warming dish and for lower-back aches.
- For mucus in the lung, add a 2-inch piece of dried citrus peel *(chen pi).*
- To strengthen the lungs, add a 2-inch piece (or more) of reconstituted white snow fungus.
- For deficient liver blood, add 1 tablespoon of lycii berries *(gou qi zi)* and 3 grams of *dang gui.*
- For liver, spleen, stomach, and kidney deficiencies and symptoms of lower-back pain, add 6 dried water chestnuts (soaked overnight until soft) or walnuts, or 4 slices of dioscorea *(shan yao)* to the cooking liquid.
- For anemia, add 5 red jujube dates (with the stones removed), a little presoaked black hair moss, a 2-inch piece of presoaked black wood ear fungus, a small piece of *dang gui,* and 3 astragalus roots.
- To improve circulation, add 1 teaspoon of rice wine or sherry. This is especially good for the elderly, but it should not be added if there is hypertension. Also for circulation, one can use a tea of finely crushed *tian qi* and/or Siberian ginseng.

PIG KIDNEY, WALNUT, AND EUCOMMIA CASSEROLE

Pig kidney: 1
Eucommia ulmoidis bark (du zhong): 12 grams
Shiitake mushrooms: 6
Small onion (finely chopped): 1
Walnuts (chopped): 1 cup
Water chestnuts (sliced): 1 can
Bamboo shoots (sliced): 1 can
Peas (frozen): 1 cup
Oil (peanut or sesame): 1–2 teaspoons
Kudzu root starch or cornstarch: 1 tablespoon

Cooking liquid:
Soy sauce: 2 teaspoons
Sherry: 1 teaspoon
Fresh ginger root (finely chopped): ¹/₄ teaspoon
Unrefined brown sugar (Sucanat): ¹/₂ teaspoon
Reserved liquid from the reconstituted shiitake mushrooms and/or
  eucommia tea: ¹/₂ cup

If using dried shiitake mushrooms, soak them in warm water for approximately 30 minutes. Strain the mushrooms, saving the water they were soaked in, remove the stems, and slice the shiitakes. Cook eucommia tea in 1¹/₂ cups of water for 30 minutes. Strain and combine the eucommia tea with the shiitake soaking water. Chop the pig's kidney. Heat up a wok, and add the peanut or sesame oil. Be sure the entire pan is coated with the oil. When the wok is hot, add the chopped pig's kidney, onions, and mushrooms. Sauté the ingredients, continually mixing them until they are cooked. Place the cooking liquid in a casserole dish. Be sure to have a total of about 2 quarts liquid (add water if necessary). Bring the liquid to a boil, then reduce the heat to medium and continue cooking it, covered, for another 15 minutes. Finally, add the remainder of the ingredients and continue cooking the casserole for another 15 minutes. Add salt to taste. To thicken the mixture, dissolve kudzu root starch (or cornstarch) in a little cool water and stir it into the liquid. Continue cooking until the liquid is somewhat thickened. Serve the casserole over a bed of brown rice or noodles. Eucommia treats the liver and kidneys, relieves back pain, lowers cholesterol, and is specifically used for lowering blood pressure. This recipe is based on a famous one.

Herb Soups

At a local shoe store I frequented, there was a man of Baltic descent who was quite overweight. It was plainly hard for him to contract his bulky body to stoop down on a shoe stool to help fit our family with shoes. I thought that this man would never be able to follow any advice about health food or diet. When we went in one day, however, I was amazed to find that he had lost at least 30 pounds. I asked how he did it. He said that each day, he had only soup for lunch. Soup satisfies hunger and provides vital nutrients in an easily assimilated form without caloric bulk. Furthermore, there are various foods that can be added, such as cabbage, azuki beans, barley, and mushrooms, that actually help the body discharge excess fluid and stimulate the fat-burning process.

In Chinese medicine, herbal teas are called *tang,* which means soup. This is because the ingredients of formulas are based not on the total amount of herbs but on the dose of each, so that many ingredients can constitute a large total herb amount. Furthermore, these are usually decocted for a prolonged period (30 minutes to 1 hour)—sometimes double-decocted, which makes them quite strong and souplike.

Chinese soups provide warm, flavorful liquids that can be taken throughout the meal. In the West, we warn against drinking too much water with meals, but this really goes only for the aberration of drinking ice-cold beverages that freeze our stomach and digestion. Drinking warm water before each meal will aid digestion, as will sipping various savory soups throughout the meal. One or a number of soups are eaten between each course of a Chinese banquet.

A good, full-flavored soup is made in four stages: (1) preparation of the basic broth; (2) the addition of dried, salted, or pickled ingredients; (3) the cooking of the principal ingredients (the best soups usually have no more than 3 principal ingredients; and (4) the addition of fresh ingredients that may be aromatic and should not be subjected to prolonged cooking, such as chopped green onions, parsley, or coriander.

The Basic Broth

In nonvegetarian cooking, a basic broth is made by prolonged cooking of various meats, such as chicken, beef, lamb, or pork, or even meat bones. It can be very strengthening and is the most easily assimilable way to absorb important nutrients. The Chinese are particularly fond of a stock made of bone marrow or ox-tail soup for weakness and anemia. This broth can be kept refrigerated and reheated over the course of 5 days. With the addition of other ingredients, it will make a rich tasty broth every time.

To make a flavorful vegetarian broth, use the various peelings and normally discarded parts of vegetables, such as the tops of carrots, parsnips, celery, rutabagas, or turnips; the tough stems of shiitake mushrooms or other mushrooms; the thicker parts of the stems of the broccoli, cauliflower, and cabbage; the discarded parts of beans and peas; or water and fluids in which various dried vegetables, such as mushrooms, have been soaked. In addition, it is always a good idea to put a 4-inch piece of kombu or some other sea vegetable in the soup broth to add vital trace minerals. Other ingredients that can be added to the broth include onions, peanuts, potatoes, beans, and lentils. These are all cooked a long time in an appropriate amount of water to make stock.

Small amounts of various Chinese tonic herbs described in the tables on pages 398–400 and 400–409 can be added. Because these are more costly than vegetables, they should be cooked first for best extraction, for at least 30 minutes before the other ingredients are added. You can see that the stock can be the most nutritionally rich part of the soup. For convenience, however, there are various brands of vegetable bouillon products that can be used when there isn't time to make a good soup stock. Among these, the most healthful and nutritious is miso paste, which is discussed at length further on in this chapter (see pages 427–32). Another popular bouillon product is called marmite.

Soup Recipes

MUSHROOM SOUP

Shiitake mushrooms: 4
Regular mushrooms: 8
Basic vegetable broth or vegetable bouillon: 5 cups
Tamari soy sauce: 1 1/2 tablespoons

Yeast extract: 1 tablespoon
Butter: 2 tablespoons
Sherry: 2 tablespoons
Salt: to taste
Pepper: to taste

This soup is good for removing cholesterol and tonifying the immune system. If the shiitake mushrooms are dry, soak them in warm water for ¹/₂ hour. Cut and discard the stems and slice the tops into thin strips. Remove the stems of the fresh mushrooms and cut those tops also into thin slices. Heat the vegetable broth or water, into which has been dissolved some vegetable bouillon. Add the shiitake mushrooms, tamari soy sauce, and yeast extract. Sauté the thinly sliced fresh mushrooms in butter, turning them frequently, for approximately 3 minutes. Pour the broth into the pan with the sautéed mushrooms and continue simmering the soup for another 3 minutes. Add the sherry and seasoning to taste.

DANG GUI AND LAMB SOUP

Dang Gui (Angelica sinensis): 9–15 grams
Lamb (finely chopped): 1 pound
Walnuts (chopped): 5
Lycii berries (gou qi zi): 9 grams
Longan berries (long yan rou): 9 grams
Red jujube dates: 6
Onion (small, finely chopped): 1
Star anise seeds: 2
Fresh ginger: 2 thin slices
Rice wine or sherry: 2 tablespoons
Soy sauce: 2 teaspoons
Salt: to taste
Water: 1 quart

Dang gui has been regarded for over 2,000 years as the primary herb for most gynecological problems. It is useful for conditions related to menstrual irregularity, menopausal problems, infertility, postpartum recovery, and anemia. It is also the premier blood tonic of all Chinese herbs. Lamb is the most warming meat and is a yang tonic for the heart, spleen, and stomach. This combination is specific for blood deficiency with coldness, as it gives great strength to women and has been recommended for women to take during childbirth if they are experiencing pain. Boil the lamb in a quart of water with the scallion or onion and the ginger. Skim off any froth that gathers on the surface. Add the other ingredients, except the soy sauce and wine, and cook the mixture for another 15 minutes. Remove and discard the *dang gui* slices and ginger. Add the soy sauce, wine, and seasoning to taste and serve hot. This soup takes about ½ hour to prepare and serves 2 people.

BEEF, DIOSCOREA, AND CODONOPSIS SOUP

Beef (lean): 1 pound
Dioscorea batatas (shan yao): 15 grams
Codonopsis: 9 grams
Jujube dates (pitted): 6
Shiitake mushrooms (finely chopped): 3
Onion (finely chopped, sautéed): 1
Carrot (finely chopped): 1
Fresh Ginger: 3 slices
Parsley or chives (chopped): as garnish

This recipe is good for tonifying the spleen and stomach. First cook the codonopsis, jujube dates, and dioscorea in water. Remove the pits from the jujube dates when they are soft. Add the rest of the ingredients (the ginger should be added toward the end of cooking) and cook for 30 minutes. Serve the soup with chopped parsley or chives.

STEWED BEEF AND CARROT SOUP

Lean beef (chopped): 1 pound
Sesame oil: to coat pan
Carrots (finely chopped): 2
Onion (small, finely chopped): 1
Ginger (grated): ¼ teaspoon, or galangal root: 1 slice
Astragalus root (huang qi): 3 slices

Dioscorea root: 15 grams
Parsley (chopped): as garnish

This soup tonifies the spleen, stomach, and lungs. Make a tea of the astragalus and dioscorea. Strain and use the tea as part of the soup liquid. Sauté the chopped onion and beef in a pan with a little sesame oil until the beef is browned and the onion is transparent. Add the tea to the pan along with the chopped carrot and grated ginger or the slice of galangal root. Serve the soup with a garnish of chopped parsley.

CORDYCEPS WITH DUCK STEW

Duck: 1
Cordyceps (dong chong xia cao): 1 bundle

Cordyceps *(dong chong xia cao)* or winterworm is a dried fungus that grows on the larvae of certain caterpillars. It is very expensive and is usually harvested in the high mountains. I have heard of varieties of this fungus found in the Rocky Mountains, but there is no tradition of its use here as there is in China. Cooked with duck, it is supposed to be equivalent to the finest grade of ginseng. Cordyceps is used to build and strengthen the lungs, warm the kidneys, clear phlegm, stop bleeding, strengthen *jing* (essence) and *qi*. It can be used for chronic cough, consumption, impotence, and pain in the lower back and knees. Cordyceps is purchased tied in a bundle. Before using it, remove the string around it. Braise the duck to brown it and seal in the flavor. Stew it with an unwrapped bundle of cordyceps for at least 1 hour, or until it is well done.

The Wonders of Miso

The predecessor of miso probably originated in China as a salt-fermented food called *chiang* sometime during the Chou dynasty (722–481 B.C.). At first, the term referred to any protein-rich animal food that was preserved with salt. The substitution of soybeans for meat and fish as the basic protein of *chiang* was first described in the *Ch'imin Yaushu* (535–550 A.D.), which is the oldest agricultural encyclopedia in the world. From the book's description, it seems that fermented soybean foods had been prepared several centuries previous. The cultivation of soybeans occurred with the spread of Buddhism, which recommended vegetarianism, during the Han dynasty (206 B.C.–220 A.D.). It was also around 164 B.C. that Lord Liu An of Huai-nan invented the process of making tofu. Miso probably arrived in Japan either directly from China or from Korea around the same time as the introduction of Buddhism, sometime around the sixth century A.D. Since that time, Miso has become a characteristic staple of the Japanese diet. Today, it is made in various ways, distinguished by the local districts in Japan in which it is made. Whatever else is added, all Japanese miso varieties contain fermented soybeans. The best quality is aged and presently available throughout the United States in better natural-food stores.

Miso is one of the most perfect foods. First, because of the fermented soybeans, it is rich in easily assimilated high-quality protein. Second, it is commonly taken before or during Japanese meals because it aids the assimilation of other foods. This is because unpasteurized miso contains natural digestive enzymes, lactic acid bacteria (lactobacillus), salt-resistant yeasts, and healthful organisms found in the ingredients used to make miso. The best-quality miso is fermented over several years. This supports the breakdown of complex carbohydrates, proteins, and fats into smaller molecules in the large and small intestines. Lactobacilli present in miso are also found in other fermented foods, including salt-fermented sauerkraut and yogurt. One can only wonder why anyone would want to pay such high prices for lactobacillus products when they could have all the benefits of them with the regular consumption of miso. Remember, because enzymes and lactobacilli are live organisms, they die at temperatures over 104° Fahrenheit. This means that they are present in only unpasteurized miso. It also means that miso should never be boiled; rather, the paste should be stirred into the basic broth toward the conclusion of cooking, ideally when the temperature of the liquid is below 104°.

Contrary to what many people think, miso is actually very good for individuals who are trying to cut back on their salt intake, even though it is fermented in salt. This is because it contains only 12% salt, less than most people would ingest if they used salt alone, while imparting a rich flavor to foods. Furthermore, studies have shown that fermentation of salt with soybeans and the other ingredients changes the effect of salt on the body. It seems that the sodium chloride molecule is affected by the natural oils of the soybeans and other foods, so good-quality miso should cause no irritation or thirst. Miso is also low in fat and has absolutely no cholesterol. This makes it an ideal food for individuals who are trying to regulate their weight.

Vegetarians who exclude all animal protein and dairy can become deficient in vitamin B_{12}. The bacteria in naturally fermented miso have been found to manufacture vitamin B_{12}, making miso paste an important vegetarian food. Japanese monks, who are well known for their vitality and long life and eat no animal products, regularly consume miso. Individuals with a more alkaline blood are generally regarded as healthier. Most of the foods many consider treats, such as sugar, meat, alcohol, and coffee, weaken the body's overall health and resistance and are acid forming. In the East, miso and another fermented food, umeboshi plum, are thought of as antacids, much like Alka-Seltzer, Tums, or Milk of Magnesia in the West. Miso is similarly used to relieve acid indigestion, symptoms of hangover, and other digestive upsets. Because of this, it is used with ginger and/or garlic to prevent and/or cure colds, improve digestive metabolism, increase resistance to parasite infestations (which tend to occur in an acid environment), and neutralize blood toxins and therefore clear the skin.

Still another benefit of miso is in its ability to counteract the adverse effects of radiotherapy, antibiotics, chemotherapy, and environmental pollution. By 1972, Dr. Akizuki, his nurses, and co-workers, whose hospital was located only 1 mile from the atomic bomb blast in Hiroshima in 1945, still had experienced no side effects from radiation exposure, despite the opposite experience of others in the near vicinity. He attributed this to the fact that they regularly ate miso. Stimulated by Dr. Akizuki's claims, Japanese scientists conducted a study of miso and one of the ingredients used to make it, called natto. They found a substance they called zybicolin, which is produced by the yeasts of these products. It has the special ability to attract, absorb, and discharge such radioactive elements as strontium. Miso is also able to detoxify the harmful influences of tobacco and traffic pollution.

According to the Chinese Five Element theory and the flavor correspondences, the bean is the grain of the kidney, with salt being its corresponding flavor. The kidneys represent the deep reserves of the body and include the adrenals and hormones. Kidney tonics, such as Planetary Formula's Energetics Yin or Energetics Yang, are intended to nurture and preserve the deep energy of the body, which is represented by the various endocrine hormones. Energetics Yin has mild corticosteroid properties and nurtures the parasympathetic nervous system or yin energy, while Energetics Yang strengthens the adrenergic hormones to increase libido and stimulate warmth and motivation. It represents the sympathetic nervous system. Often when one is low, the other is as well, so that various proportions of both formulas can be taken simultaneously. In traditional Chinese medicine (TCM), it is always recommended that formulas like these be taken with a pinch of salt. Since they are in convenient pill form, I recommend they be taken with miso soup.

Miso, Brown Rice, Mushrooms, and Longevity

In areas of the world where more of the longest-living individuals are found, one of the recurring factors in that longevity is the use of whole, pure foods and fermented foods. The Chinese have always regarded the mushroom as having special properties. Mushrooms are regarded as "spirit medicine" because they are believed to nourish the *shen,* or spirit. As such, they are considered particularly important in vegetarian diets and regarded as a medicinal food that promotes longevity. Various medicinal mushrooms are used by the Chinese, but the most common is the shiitake, called the black mushroom *(Lentinula edodes).* While it was once available only by wild harvest, it has come to be the second most commonly grown mushroom in the world.* Shiitake has been used both in China and Japan for thousands of years. Recent research has substantiated the immense therapeutic properties of shiitake: antitumor, immune-regulating, antiviral, antibacterial, antiparasitic, and anticholesterol. Shiitake mushrooms have been found to be particularly valuable for treating all forms of hepatitis, including hepatitis B and C. The lentinan in shiitake mushrooms has been found to be powerfully antiviral, with the ability to increase helper T-cell and low lymphocyte counts in human immunodeficiency virus (HIV)-positive individuals.

Perhaps one of the reasons the Chinese regard mushrooms as spirit medicine is the claim found in the oldest recorded botanical monograph on another powerful Chinese medicinal mushroom, the *ling zhi* or reishi mushroom *(Ganoderma lucidum).* The Chinese claimed that it made the body lighter, which may refer to its ability to reduce cholesterol and blood lipid levels. Shiitake mushrooms have immune-potentiating properties similar to those of reishi mushrooms; however, reishi mush-

---

*Christopher Hobbs. *Medicinal Mushrooms.* (Botanica Press, Santa Cruz, CA, 1995.)

rooms are more bitter, hard, and otherwise unpalatable, except brewed as medicine or taken as powder or alcoholic extract. Therefore, they do not lend themselves to food preparations as well as do shiitake mushrooms. According to herbalist Christopher Hobbs, "eritadenine, isolated from shiitake, has been shown to lower blood levels of cholesterol and lipids. . . . Added to the diet of rats, eritadenine (0.005%) caused a 25% decrease in total cholesterol in as little as one week."* Finally, the most convenient and economical way to obtain shiitake mushrooms is to purchase them dried, by the pound, from Chinese suppliers. They can then be reconstituted with water before use.

With all of the health benefits of miso and shiitake, the combination of the two in soup makes a delicious and powerful tonic for the immune system and the core energy of the body, which resides in the kidneys. Following is a delicious recipe.

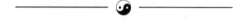

MISO-MUSHROOM SOUP

Sesame oil: 2 tablespoons
Shiitake mushrooms (thinly sliced): 6
Onion (thinly sliced): 1
Stock made from boiled and strained bonito flakes (called dashi) in 2 cups of water (if dashi is not available just use water or vegetable stock)
Dark miso paste: 3 tablespoons
Garlic clove (finely chopped): 1
Minced parsley, perilla leaves, chopped chives or leeks: about 2 tablespoons

Sauté the chopped mushrooms, onion and garlic in an iron skillet until the onions become translucent. Add the *dashi* or water and bring to a boil. Lower the heat and dissolve the miso paste into the broth, simmering another 10 minutes. Serve warm with the minced parsley, perilla, chives or leeks sprinkled on top for garnish.

The basic miso soup recipe includes a broth of various vegetables, including such sea vegetables as wakame, boiled in a broth with about

---

*Christopher Hobbs. *Medicinal Mushrooms*. (Botanica Press, Santa Cruz, CA, 1995.)

1½ tablespoons of miso stirred in for each intended serving. The best tasting miso soups usually do not contain more than 3 vegetables, excluding the basic bouillon that may be used as stock. Often, slices of braised tofu are finely cubed and added, along with a small amount of buckwheat noodles. In Japan, miso, a little brown rice, perhaps some fish or tofu, and tea is a traditional and very satisfying breakfast. Miso both has its own nutritional merits and it offers another simple way to integrate various Chinese herbs cooked in the soup as part of the diet.

Medicinal Wines

Medicinal wines and liqueurs, called *yao jiu* in China, date back well over 3,000 years. A similar tradition exists in the West: various alcoholic bitters and extracts were used in medieval monasteries, and today, there are many commercial alcoholic herb tinctures available. Herbalists understand that an extract that consists of approximately 50% alcohol (not wood or rubbing alcohol) and 50% water represents a balance of the two solvents that will best extract most herbal constituents and have medicinal value. Something near this ratio is to be found in commercially available liqueurs, such as vodka, gin, or brandy.

The Chinese, however, favor the use of a strong rice liqueur that can be purchased in Chinese grocery stores. One of the chapters of the *Yellow Emperor's Classic,* considered the single most important book on TCM, is entitled "Treatise on Fluids, Turbid Wine, and Fragrant Wine." *Fluids,* according to Bob Flaws, is a "collective term for wines." The chapter describes how medicinal wine is made using fermented rice and rice stalks. Rice, being the most balanced food, makes a good extractive for herbal wines.

In the *Tai Ping Sheng Hui Fang (Sacred and Beneficial Formulas from the Tai Ping),* compiled during the Song and Yuan Dynasties (969–1368), it is stated:

> Wine is the essence of grain. It harmonizes and nourishes the Spirit and Qi. Having a fast and strong energy, it must be used carefully. It is readily absorbed through the stomach and intestines, efficiently carrying the therapeutic energy of all medicines directly into the blood.

This view certainly agrees with the experience of herbalists down through the ages and is exemplified in the tradition of European monastic wines and liqueurs, with such popular labels as Benedictine, and the various commercial alcoholic bitters sold in liquor stores and bars. The special property of herbal wines and the various alcoholic extracts is that alcohol is able to penetrate quickly and deeply into the channels of circulation, effectively dispersing stagnant qi and blood.

Alcohol and wine are very hot in nature, and herbs steeped in wine are therefore also hotter. This makes alcohol-based herbal products especially useful when there are symptoms of stagnation and deficient yang. Medicinal wines are therefore especially good for symptoms of cold or blood and qi stagnation associated with a variety of problems, especially circulatory problems and various rheumatic type conditions. They are also preferred for long-term treatment of chronic diseases.

It is interesting that in the earlier dynasties, medicinal wines were made by fermenting the herbs and various substances with the addition of concentrated sweetening agents such as sugar, so that they would make their own alcohol. Eventually, by the time of the Qing dynasty (1644–1911), alcohol was commercially prepared and distilled. The various herbs and substances were then simply placed in the alcohol for a period of time to extract their therapeutic medicinal properties.

Alcohol-based herbal wines and tinctures are convenient to take and have a long shelf life. They are particularly good as warming tonics and for digestive and circulatory disorders. They are not appropriate for detoxification, excess heat, or yin deficiency, however. To eliminate most of the alcohol, the wine or extract can be mixed into a cup of boiling water to allow the alcohol to evaporate before ingesting the tincture.

To make wine with the herbs and various substances to be extracted in the liqueur, boil the herbs to be extracted in 1 gallon of water. Dissolve 4 pounds of sugar into the solution and allow to cool until it is around 90° to 100° Fahrenheit. Add 1 teaspoon of live wine yeast (baking yeast can also be used). Lightly cover the container and let the solution stand for 1 week or so in a warm place. You will notice the fermentation activity, but after a while, it will seem to stop. This is the time to strain off and discard the mash and lightly bottle the liqueur in narrow bottles. Next fasten a balloon, with a small needle hole punched into it, over the neck of the bottle to allow for the further escape of fermentative gases. So long as there is any further fermentation occurring, the balloon will appear somewhat inflated. Sometimes it will deflate for a time, and then when things get warm enough for fermentation to commence, it will then inflate. When it appears that all signs of fermentation are completed, the wine is done. You can then strain the liqueur through a fine cloth and return the wine to airtight capped bottles. The second and most common way to make herbal wines is to place at least 4 ounces of powdered or coarsely ground herbs into a quart of vodka, gin, or brandy. As stated before, strong rice wine is preferred in Chinese medicine. Chinese medicinal wines are recommended to be aged for a far longer period than is customarily recommended for the manufacture of Western alcoholic tinctures and extracts. Western herbalists might suggest an aging period of 2 weeks, while Chinese liqueurs are aged in several stages, usually of 3-month to 1-year intervals. The longer the mixture is aged, the stronger the flavors and energies of the resultant brew. The dose is only 1 ounce at a time to prevent inebriation.

Many valuable single herbs can be made into wines, especially with the more common method using previously distilled alcohol. Some of the single substances that are commonly used to make medicinal wines include ginseng (ren shen), deer antler (lu rong), angelica dang gui, astragalus (huang qi), Siberian ginseng (ci wu jia), rehmannia (shu di huang), eucommia (du zhong), cuscuta (tu si zi), reishi mushroom (ling zhi), poria (fu ling), calamus (shi chang pu), dioscorea (shan yao), and others too numerous to mention. One of my favorite wines, made by fermenting the herbs with the mash, is with hawthorn berries (shan zha). Other delicious medicinal wines could be similarly made with herbs such as ophiopogon (mai men dong), Jujube dates (da zao), lycii berries (gou qi zi), and mulberries (sang shen or sang zhi).

Look up the indications for the various herbs above and decide which one(s) you might like to make. As with all recipes and formulas recommended throughout the book, it is important to develop an understanding of the proper indications and contraindications for the various medicinal wines. Certainly, wines made with warm tonic ingredients should not be taken for conditions of excess, acute fevers, colds and infections, or for yin deficiency. Warm tonic wines are also generally not used in hot climates. Finally, those who are predisposed to alcohol addiction should avoid using herbs in this way. Following are a few special herbal wine formulas that I like to make.

GINSENG AND DANG GUI TEN WINE

This is one of the most commonly used tonics for general vitality. It is primarily a blood and qi tonic. It is very effective for weakness and lack of energy and can be used to promote stamina and endurance and to promote recovery after prolonged sickness. It can be used for any deficiency symptoms, chronic diseases, and all diseases except those that have signs of excess. It is not recommended during hot weather but is more suitable during the cold winter months. As with all warming tonics, it should not be used during a fever, common cold, or any acute upper-respiratory disorder.

> *Ginseng* (ren shen): *6 grams*
> *Atractylodes* (bai zhu): *6 grams*
> *Poria* (fu ling): *6 grams*
> *Licorice* (gan cao): *6 grams*
> *Prepared rehmannia* (shu di huang): *6 grams*
> *Ligusticum* (chuan xiong): *6 grams*
> *Angelica* dang gui: *6 grams*
> *White peony* (bai shao): *6 grams*
> *Cinnamon bark* (rou gui): *6 grams*
> *Astragalus* (huang qi): *6 grams*

Grind all the herbs to a powder or break them into as small pieces as possible. Place them in a wide-mouth jar, then pour in rice wine, good-quality vodka, gin, or other alcoholic beverage until there is about 1 inch of fluid above the settled herbs. Cover the bottle, store it in a dark place, and shake it once daily. Strain the wine after 2 weeks and bottle for use. Dosage: 1 ounce, once or twice daily.

JADE PILLOW ELIXIR*

This formula is especially beneficial for symptoms of nervous exhaustion, stress, and fatigue with insomnia, forgetfulness, nightmares, palpitations, and night sweats.

> *Zizyphus spinosa* (suan zao ren): *40 grams*
> *Poria* (fu ling): *10 grams*
> *Ginseng* (ren shen): *10 grams*
> *Ligusticum* (chuan xiong): *6 grams*
> *Anemarrhena* (zhi mu): *3 grams*
> *Licorice* (gan cao): *3 grams*

---

*From *Shaolin and Taoist Herbal Training Formulas*, by James Ramholz, Silk Road, with permission.

Sprouted wheat: 40 grams
Polygala: 10 grams

Grind all the ingredients as finely as possible and add them to 1 liter of vodka, brandy, or gin in a wide-mouth jar. Store the jar in a dark place for 2 weeks, strain the wine, and bottle it for use. Dosage: 1 ounce, 20 minutes before bed or 2 or 3 times daily.

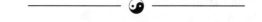

GECKO WINE *(GE JIE JIU)*

This wine is very effective for strengthening the lungs in the treatment of asthma and emphysema. In addition to tonifying the lungs, it also strengthens the kidneys, fosters the absorption of *qi* from air, and lessens wheezing. It can also be used for chronic cough, shortness of breath, and impotence. The lizards can be purchased from a Chinese pharmacy. I have used this with very reliable benefits for the chronic upper-respiratory problems described above, and I often add other valuable lung herbs, such as Astragalus *(Huang Qi)*, Ophiopogon *(Mai Men Dong)*, Platycodon *(Jie Geng)*, Apricot seed *(Xing Ren)*, Ginseng *(Ren Shen)* if there is *qi* deficiency and occasionally some Ephedra *(Ma Huang)*.

Male gecko lizard: 1
Female gecko lizard: 1

Add to 1 liter of vodka, brandy or gin in a wide mouthed jar. Store for at least 2 weeks, strain and bottle for use. Dosage: 1 ounce, 2 or 3 times daily.

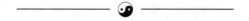

FLEXIBILITY TONIC *(SHU JIN CHIH)*

This is available as a Planetary Formula for relaxing the muscles and the tendons and therefore increasing flexibility, improving blood circulation, relieving arthritis, lower back, knee and leg pains, and numbness, and is a tonic for the Liver and Kidneys.

Angelica dang gui: *100 grams*
Achyranthes (niu xi): *120 grams*
Gambir (gou teng): *100 grams*

Angelica du huo: *120 grams*
Chaenomeles (mu gua): *120 grams*
Notopterygium (qiang huo): *80 grams*
Ligusticum (chuan xiong): *100 grams*
Lycii berries (gou qi zi): *80 grams*
Sileris (fang feng): *80 grams*
Dipsacus (xu duan): *100 grams*
Tienchi ginseng (tian qi or san qi): *100 grams*

Dosage: 1 ounce 2 or 3 times daily.

BACK EASE WINE

This wine is a formula I use to treat lower back, hip, and leg pains. It tonifies the kidneys and liver and relieves arthritic and rheumatic pains throughout the body, but especially in the lower part of the body. It is based on the well-known arthritis and back-pain formula called *Du Huo Ji Sheng Tang* (Angelica Du Huo *and Loranthes Combination*) and is available in tablet form from Planetary Formulas.

Angelica du huo (du huo): *3 parts*
Gentiana macrophyllae (qin jiao): *2 parts*
Ledebouriella (fang feng): *2 parts*
Asarum (xi xin): *1 part*
Eucommia bark (du zhong): *3 parts*
Achyranthes (niu xi): *3 parts*
Loranthes mistletoe (sang ji sheng): *4 parts*
Angelica dang gui (dang gui): *2 parts*
Ligusticum (chuan xiong): *2 parts*
Prepared rehmannia (shu di huang): *3 parts*
White peony root (bai shao): *2 parts*
Codonopsis (dang shen): *2 parts*
Poria (fu ling): *2 parts*
Cinnamon twigs (gui zhi): *2 parts*
Licorice (gan cao): *1 part*

Coarsely grind all the herbs and place them in a wide-mouth jar. Cover the herbs with vodka or brandy so that there is about 1 inch of liquid above the herb settlings. Age the wine appropriately, strain it, and bottle it for use. Dosage: 1 ounce, 2 or 3 times daily.

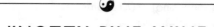

KNOTTY PINE WINE

This wine formula is one many use for athritis and rheumatic problems. It uses the knots from pine wood. These are especially high in resins, which are effective for circulation. The pine sap can also be dissolved into alcohol, which would have a similar but somewhat less regulated effect. The wine clears wind and dampness and warms the center. It is an old, effective remedy for lower-back, joint, and knee pains.

   Pine knots

Slice up the pine tree knots and cover them with vodka, gin, or brandy in a wide-mouth jar. After 7 days, strain the wine and bottle it for use. Dosage: 1–2 ounces before each meal.

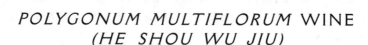

POLYGONUM MULTIFLORUM WINE (HE SHOU WU JIU)

The herb vine *Polygonum multiflorum* is becoming more common in gardens throughout the West. It is a very valuable herb, so it would be good to learn to make the following simple wine. It tonifies the kidneys and liver, nourishes the blood, raises essence, quiets the spirit, and restores normal hair color.

   Polygonum multiflorum (he shou wu): *300 grams*
   Prepared Rehmannia glutinosa (shu di huang): *300 grams (optional)*

Soak the *Polygonum multiflorum (he shou wu)* in 2 quarts of vodka, gin, or brandy, covered. After 1 month, strain the wine and bottle it for use. A particularly good herb to add to this is prepared *Rehmannia glutinosa (shu di huang)*. Dosage: 1–2 ounces before or after dinner.

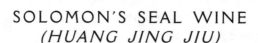

SOLOMON'S SEAL WINE (HUANG JING JIU)

Solomon's seal *(Polygonati odorati)* is used both in Western and Chinese herbalism as a tonic for the lungs and general metabolism. It can be gathered wild in the hardwood forests of southeast North America and is also available from Chinese pharmacies. It is highly regarded by the Taoists as a *qi* tonic. The Yellow Emperor, Huang Di, when asked which plant is most likely to confer immortality, replied, "the plant of the great yang," referring to Solomon's seal. Since that time, the Chinese have believed that regularly eating this herb would confer protection for the universal *jing* (essence). It is sweet and mild and warms and enters the spleen, stomach, and lung organ meridians. For anyone who suffers from serious debilitation and is recovering from illness, this herb will nourish and build the essence.

Solomon's seal (Polygonati odorati): *2 pounds*

One method used is to chop up the Solomon's seal and then soak it for a minimum of 3 months in strong rice wine (available in Chinese grocery stores) or good-quality vodka, gin, or brandy. Use enough wine to cover the herb completely. Dosage: 1 ounce, 2 or 3 times daily.

Syrups

While wines are a better medium for warm yang tonics, syrups made with a base of honey or barley malt are more nourishing and are generally better for yin or blood tonics, substances that are intended to soothe any membrane with which they come in contact, such as that of the lungs. To make a basic syrup, cook the herbs over low heat for 2 hours. Strain the herbs and keep the decoction. To the reserved herbs, add more water and repeat the same process. Repeat this one more time. Now mix all of the decoctions together and cook down to ¼ of the original amount. Stir in and dissolve approximately an equal amount of cooked honey or barley malt. Pour the syrup into an airtight dark glass container and store in a cool, dark, dry place.

OPHIOPOGON AND ASPARAGUS SYRUP

Ophiopogon root (mai men dong): *500 grams*
Asparagus root (tian men dong): *500 grams*

Cook the herbs in 15 cups of water 3 times. This syrup nourishes yin and lubricates the lungs. It is good for tuberculosis, wasting diseases, and dry cough.

DANG GUI AND MOTHERWORT SYRUP

This syrup is effective for all menstrual irregularities and symptoms associated with menopause, such as hot flashes.

>   Motherwort (yi mu cao): *500 grams*
>   Angelica dang gui: *500 grams*

Make a syrup using the herbs. Dosage: 1 tablespoon 2 or 3 times daily.

HARMONIZING HEAVEN AND EARTH SYRUP

This formula contains herbs that nourish aspects of the mind, spirit, and physical body, thus the name. It can be used as a general tonic for weakness, prostration, loss of appetite, shortness of breath, anxiety, irritability, insomnia, and nervous collapse.

>   Codonopsis (dang shen): *50 grams*
>   Astragalus (huang qi): *50 grams*
>   Lycii berries (gou qi zi): *25 grams*
>   Cistanches (rou cong rong): *25 grams*
>   Prepared Rehmannia (shu di huang): *50 grams*
>   Angelica sinensis (dang gui): *50 grams*
>   Longan berries (long yan rou): *25 grams*
>   Cimicifuga (sheng ma): *25 grams*

Make a syrup using the herbs. Dosage: 1 tablespoon twice daily.

CODONOPSIS, POLYGONUM, AND REHMANNIA SYRUP

>   Prepared rehmannia (shu di huang): *1,000 grams*
>   Codonopsis (dang shen): *500 grams*
>   Polygonum multiflorum (he shou wou): *500 grams*

Make a syrup using the herbs. Dosage: 1 tablespoonful 2 or 3 times daily. This syrup is a *qi* and blood tonic.

Natural Herb Loquat-Flavored Syrup

This formula is a popular Chinese patent syrup that is available in all Chinese pharmacies and grocery stores. It is an effective symptomatic treatment for acute and chronic cough due to weak lungs, heat, or lung dryness with sticky phlegm. It is useful in emphysema, acute bronchitis, and accompanying sinus congestion. The primary ingredient is loquat leaf (*Eriobotrya japonica*), called *pi pa ye,* and loquat fruit, called *pi pa gao.* Even the stone of the loquat has a bitter flavor and neutral energy and helps clear the throat and stop coughing. These properties are due to the presence of cyanoglycosides, which are found in several other anticough herbs, including wild cherry bark and apricot seeds (*xing ren*). Dosage: 1 tablespoon, 3 times a day; children: 1 teaspoon, 3 times a day. The syrup is sold in bottles of 5, 10, and 25 ounces (10 or 25 ounces is recommended).

Pills

Pills are easily made by mixing the herbal powder with enough honey to form it into small pellets. Some are made into larger sizes—about 1 tablespoon or more rolled into a ball.

Teas

Some non-aromatic substances, such as minerals, shells, certain roots, barks, seeds, and fruits, require decoction, while the lighter, more aromatic herbs, flowers, and some roots that contain important volatile oils need to be infused. Those that are not aromatic are generally either added last or steeped or subjected to heat for only a short period. Teas should be prepared in only a porcelain, clay, or glass pot. Good-quality stainless steel may also be used, but it is not as good because some of the properties of herbs are altered when they are brewed in metal containers.

How to Make a Decoction

Place the herb(s) in 4 cups of water. Bring the mixture to a boil, with the pot gently covered. Turn down the heat and slowly—over 30 to 45 minutes—reduce the amount of liquid down to 2 cups. Some practitioners recommend straining the first liqueur and setting it aside, then adding about half as much water to the reserved herbs and cooking the liquid down to half the amount in the same way. This could even be repeated again. Finally, strain and combine all the liqueurs together in one pot, place the pot back on the heat, and reduce the liquid down to 2 cups. The dose is usually 1 cup, two or three times daily.

How to Make an Infusion

Place the herb(s) in the selected container. Heat water in a pot until the water boils. Pour the hot water into the receptacle containing the herbs. Cover the container and allow the herbs to steep for 5 to 15 minutes or until the infusion is cool enough to drink. Strain the infusion into a cup and drink it.

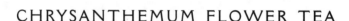

CHRYSANTHEMUM FLOWER TEA

This tea is a cooling beverage to drink during hot weather. It is calming, clears wind and heat, soothes the liver, and improves vision. It can be used for the common cold, headache, dizziness, high blood pressure, and conjunctivitis with red, inflamed eyes. This tea is as popular in China as chamomile is in the West. As a matter of fact, they both have somewhat similar uses for relieving indigestion and calming the nervous system, except that chrysanthemum flowers have more lubricating, yin-nourishing effects. The preferred species of chrysanthemum flowers to use are the full, yellow-flowered varieties.

> *Chrysanthemum flowers: 9 grams*
> *Licorice root (optional): 1 or 2 slices*

Make 2 cups of chrysanthemum flower tea by infusion. Licorice root can also be added with good effect. More water can be added for a second brewing. This tea is taken regularly, both for treatment and as a pleasant and healthful beverage. In China, I have seen carbonated sodas made of chrysanthemum flowers.

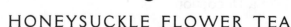

HONEYSUCKLE FLOWER TEA

One can only appreciate and wonder at the labor-intensive process of gathering enough honeysuckle blossoms to make a pound of dry weight. The blossoms are a powerful antibiotic and antiviral, commonly used for such wind-heat conditions as colds and influenza.

> *Honeysuckle flowers: 9 grams (dry weight)*
> *Licorice root (optional): 1 or 2 slices*

Prepare this tea in the same manner as chrysanthemum flower tea (see recipe above). Again, licorice can be added to enhance the properties and flavor of the brew. Honeysuckle and chrysanthemum can be combined in equal parts, with or without added licorice root, and given to patients to drink during fevers, colds, and influenza.

GLOSSARY

Terms Used in Traditional Chinese Medicine

Aromatic stomachic: Herbs that are aromatic and assist digestion by moving dampness.

Blood: Though broader in definition than this brief explanation, blood encompasses the physical blood in the body that moistens the tissues, muscles, skin, and hair and nourishes cells and organs.

Blood deficiency: A lack of blood with signs of anemia; dizziness; scanty menses or amenorrhea; emaciated body; spots in the visual field; impaired vision; numb arms or legs; dry skin, hair, or eyes; lusterless, pale face and lips; fatigue; and poor memory.

Calmative: Calms the mind and nerves; for nervous disorders.

Cold: Low metabolism.

Cold, coldness, cold signs: Lowered metabolism with such symptoms as clear to white bodily secretions, chills, body aches, poor circulation, pale complexion, lethargy, no thirst or sweating, frigidity, impotence, infertility, nighttime urination, frequent and copious urination, loose stools or diarrhea, undigested food in the stools, poor digestion, lack of appetite, aching pain in joints, slowness of speech, slow movements, low fever but severe chills, aversion to cold and craving for heat, and "hypo-" conditions, such as hypothyroidism, hypoadrenalism, and hypoglycemia.

Cooling blood: A function of herbs that clear heat out of the blood; symptoms of heat include rashes; nosebleeds; vomiting, spitting, or coughing up of blood; blood in the stool or urine; night fevers; delirium; and hemorrhage.

Damp, dampness: Excessive fluids in the body with symptoms of feelings of heaviness; sluggishness; secretions that are turbid, sluggish, sinking, viscous, copious, slimy, cloudy, or sticky; excessive leukorrhea; oozing, purulent skin eruptions; lassitude; edema; abdominal distension; chest fullness; nausea; vomiting; loss of appetite; lack of thirst; and achy, heavy, stiff, and sore joints.

Damp heat: A condition of dampness and heat with symptoms of thick, greasy, yellow secretions and phlegm; jaundice; hepatitis; dysentery; urinary difficulty or pain; furuncles; and eczema.

Deficiency: A lack of something, usually *qi*, blood, yin, yang, or essence.

Deficiency heat: Heat due to yin deficiency, resulting in emaciation and weakness with heat symptoms; deficiency heat occurs because the cooling, moistening fluids (yin) are lacking.

Deficient yang: See **Yang deficiency.**

Deficient yin: See **Yin deficiency.**

Diuretic: Eliminates excess fluids. Diuretics in Chinese medicine also enhance proper fluid metabolism by increasing absorption of fluids into the deep tissues of the body. Thus, the seemingly contradictory symptoms of edema and dry skin can be eliminated together through the use of diuretics.

Dryness: Characterized by dehydration with symptoms of extreme thirst; dry skin, hair, mouth, lips, nose, and throat; dry cough with little phlegm; and constipation.

Essence: A highly refined fluid substance that provides the basis of reproduction, development, growth, sexual power, conception, and pregnancy.

Excess: Too much of something, usually heat, cold, damp, yin, or yang.

Excess cold: A condition of too much coldness in the body; see **Cold.**

Excess heat: A condition of too much heat in the body; see **Heat.**

Excess yang: The same as excess heat, with symptoms of high fever, restlessness, red complexion, loud voice, aggressive actions, strong odors, yellow discharges, rapid pulse, and hypertension.

Excess yin: An imbalance of excessive fluids in the body, with symptoms of edema, excessive fluid retention, lethargy, a plump or swollen appearance, and overall signs of dampness; however, those with excess yin may have adequate energy.

Exterior: See **External.**

External: The location of illnesses, such as colds, influenza, fevers, skin eruptions, sore throats, and headaches, on the surface of the body.

Heat, heat signs: Hypermetabolism with symptoms of fever and concurrent little chills; restlessness; constipation; thirst; aversion to heat and craving for cold; burning digestion; infections; inflammations; dryness; red face; sweating; strong appetite; hemorrhaging; blood in the vomit, urine, stool, nose, or mucus; strong odors, sticky or thick yellow bodily excretions; irritability; scanty, dark yellow urination; and swollen, red, and painful eyes or gums and red skin eruptions; and "hyper-" conditions, such as hypertension.

Hot: Overactive metabolism.

Interior: See **Internal.**

Internal: The location of an illness, such as conditions affecting *qi,* blood, fluids, and internal organs, inside the body.

Jing: See **Essence.**

Meridians: The pathways along which *qi* circulates to supply energy and nourishment to the organs and the surface of the body.

Moves blood: See **Regulates blood.**

Nervine: Strengthens the nerves; taken for conditions of nervousness, anxiety, insomnia, emotional instability, pain, cramps, spasms, tremors, stress, muscle tension, and epilepsy.

Organs: The organs in traditional Chinese medicine are conceptualized differently than in Western medicine: organs have energetic rather than physical functions; they are dynamic, interrelated processes that occur throughout every level of the body. Yin organs include the heart, lungs, kidneys, spleen, and liver; yang organs include the small intestine, large intestine, urinary bladder, stomach, and gallbladder.

Qi: Energy, life force; *qi* circulates, protects, holds, transforms, and warms.

Qi deficiency: A lack of *qi* or energy with signs of low vitality; lethargy; weakness; shortness of breath; slow metabolism; frequent colds and influenza with slow recovery; low, soft voice; spontaneous sweating; frequent urination; and palpitations.

Regulates blood: Smooths the flow of blood in the body; symptoms for which blood regulators are taken include bleeding, hemorrhaging, excessive menstruation, localized stabbing pain, abdominal masses, ulcers, abscesses, and painful menstruation.

Regulates energy: Smooths the flow of *qi* in the body; symptoms of *qi* stagnation include dull, aching pain; abdominal distension, and pain; belching; gas; acid regurgitation; nausea; vomiting; stifling sensation in chest; pain in the sides; loss of appetite; depression; hernial pain; irregular menstruation; swollen, tender breasts; and wheezing.

Sedative: Sedates or calms the mind and spirit; conditions for which sedatives are taken include insomnia, anxiety, nervousness, irritability, fright, and hysteria.

Seven Emotions: The Seven Emotions are a major cause of illness. They are sadness, fright, fear, grief, anger, joy (overexcitability) and melancholy or pensiveness.

Shen: The overall spirit and mental faculties of a person, including enthusiasm for life, charisma, and capacity to behave appropriately, be responsive, speak coherently, think and form ideas, and live a life of joy and spiritual fulfillment.

Spirit: See *Shen.*

Stomach heat: A condition of too much heat in the stomach, with signs of bad breath, gum bleeding and swelling, mouth ulcers, frontal headaches, burning sensation in the stomach region, and extreme thirst.

TCM: Abbreviation for traditional Chinese medicine.

Tonification: Nourishing, strengthening, building, and improving the condition of either *qi,* blood, yin, or yang in the body.

Wind: Wind causes movement (or sometimes the lack of it), with symptoms of spasms, twitches, dizziness, spasms, rigidity of the muscles, deviation of the eye and mouth, stiff or rigid neck and shoulders, tremors, convulsions, vertigo, and sudden onset of colds, chills, fever, stuffy noses, and headache.

Yang: The body's capacity to generate and maintain warmth and circulation.

Yang deficiency: A condition of coldness due to lack of the heating quality of yang; symptoms include lethargy, coldness, edema, poor digestion, lower-back pain, the type of constipation caused by weak peristaltic motion, and lack of libido.

Yin: The body's substance, including blood and all other fluids in the body; these nurture and moisten the organs and tissues.

Yin deficiency: Deficiency heat that results in emaciation and weakness with heat symptoms, such as night sweats; insomnia; a burning sensation in the palms, soles, and chest; malar flush; afternoon fever; nervous exhaustion; dry throat; dry eyes; blurred vision; dizziness; and nervous tension.

Zang fu: The theory of the organs; the hollow organs *(fu)* transport and the solid organs *(zang)* store vital substances.

RECOMMENDED READING

CHINESE HERBALS

This is not intended to be an herbal bibliography. There are many valuable books on Chinese herbology; however, the following are particularly useful for beginning students of Chinese herbal medicine. A more complete bibliography can be found in the book *The Herbs of Life*.

Beinfield, Harriet, and Korngold, Efrem. *Between Heaven and Earth* (New York: Ballantine Books, 1991)

A thorough study of the Five Elements, including specific herbal formulas and cooking recipes.

Bensky, Dan, and Gamble, Andrew. *Chinese Herbal Medicine: Materia Medica* (Seattle: Eastland Press, 1986)

An extensive herbal pharmacopoeia of the traditional Chinese herbal categories and hundreds of the most commonly used Chinese herbs.

Connelly, Diane. *Traditional Acupuncture: The Law of the Five Elements* (Baltimore: Center for Traditional Acupuncture, 1979)

Presents an in-depth description of the fascinating system of Chinese Five Element theory.

Dharmananda, S. *Your Nature, Your Health* (Portland, OR: Institute for Traditional Medicine and Preventive Health Care, 1986)

Explains constitutional diagnosis based on the Five Phases, with many Chinese herbs and formulas discussed.

Fratkin, Jake. *Practical Guide to Chinese Patent Formulas* (Portland, OR: Institute for Traditional Medicine, 1986)

A listing of 200 patent formulas and their indications.

Hong-Yen, Hsu. *How to Treat Yourself with Chinese Herbs* (Los Angeles: Oriental Healing Arts Institute, 1980)

A good introductory book on the use of Chinese herbs.

Kaptchuk, Ted. *The Web That Has No Weaver* (New York: St. Martin's Press, 1983)

An excellent beginning book on traditional Chinese medicine.

Lust, John, and Tierra, Michael. *The Natural Remedy Bible* (New York: Pocket Books, 1990)

An herbal based on natural remedies for common ailments.

Ni, Maoshing. *Chinese Herbology Made Easy* (Santa Monica, CA: Seven Star Communications, 1986)

An herbal that outlines and compares specific qualities of many Chinese herbs in all the herbal categories.

Reid, Daniel. *A Handbook of Chinese Healing Herbs* (Boston: Shambhala, 1995)

A basic Chinese herbal guide to over 100 herbs and many herbal formulas.

Tang, Stephen, and Palmer, Martin. *Chinese Herbal Prescriptions* (London: Rider and Company, 1986)

A good basic book on Chinese herbs that includes several cooking recipes.

Teeguarden, Ron. *Chinese Tonic Herbs* (New York: Japan Publications, 1984)

An in-depth look at the major Chinese tonic herbs, with photographs and pre-scriptions.

Tierra, Lesley. *The Herbs of Life* (Freedom, CA: Crossing Press, 1992)

A thorough beginner's herbal on Western and Chinese herbs based on the foundations of traditional Chinese medicine. Includes specific therapies, remedies, preparations, and food energetics.

Tierra, Michael. *Planetary Herbology* (Santa Fe, NM: Lotus Press, 1988)

An extensive herbal categorizing herbs from around the world according to traditional Chinese medicine. Contains specific remedies for many ailments.

Tierra, Michael. *The Way of Herbs* (New York: Pocket Books, 1990)

A popular beginner's herbal categorizing Western herbs according to traditional Chinese medicine. Contains treatments for specific ailments.

CHINESE DIETARY BOOKS

Flaws, Bob. *The Book of Jook* (Boulder, CO: Blue Poppy Press, 1995)

An excellent book on congees, with many specific recipes.

Flaws, Bob, and Wolfe, Honora. *Prince Wen Hui's Cook* (Boulder, CO: Blue Poppy Press, 1983)

A presentation of the principles of dietary therapy using foods and some herbs, with many traditional herb-food recipes.

Jilin, Liu, and Peck, Gordon, editors. *Chinese Dietary Therapy* (New York, Churchill Livingstone, 1995)

An in-depth look at diet, foods, and their therapeutic uses, along with recipes for common ailments using herbs and foods.

Lu, Henry. *Chinese System of Food Cures* (New York: Sterling Publishing, 1986)

Explains using food and herbs for disease prevention and as disease remedies.

Lu, Henry. *Chinese Foods for Longevity* (New York: Sterling Publishing, 1990)

Includes traditional Chinese recipes for health and longevity using foods and herbs.

Ni, Maoshing, with McNease, Cathy. *Tao of Nutrition* (Santa Monica, CA: Seven Star Communications Group, 1987)

A useful book on the energetics of food, including remedies for specific diseases.

HERBAL RESOURCES

CHINESE HERBS AND PATENTS DIRECT AND BY MAIL

United States

China Herb Company
165 W. Queen Lane
Philadelphia, PA 19144
phone: (215) 843-5864, (800) 221-4372; fax: (215) 849-3338

East Earth Herbs
P.O. Box 2082
Eugene, OR 97402

Great China Herb Company
857 Washington Street
San Francisco, CA 94108
phone: (415) 982-2195

K'An Herbs
2425 Porter Street
Soquel, CA 95073
phone: (408) 438-9450

Mayway Corporation
1338 Cypress Street
Oakland, CA 94607
phone: (510) 208-3113

North South China Herbs Company
1556 Stockton Street
San Francisco, CA 94133
phone: (415) 421-4907

Nuherbs Company
3820 Penniman Avenue
Oakland, CA 94619
phone: (415) 534-4372, (800) 233-4307

Spring Wind Herb Company
2315 Fourth Street
Berkeley, CA 94710
phone: (510) 849-1820, (800) 588-4883; fax: (510) 849-4886

Tai Sang Trading Company
1018 Stockton Street
San Francisco, CA 94108
phone: (415) 981-5364

United Kingdom

East West Herbs
Langston Priory Mews
Kingham OX7 6UP
phone: 01608-658862

Neal's Yard Remedies
2 Neal's Yard
Covent Garden
London WC2H 9DP
phone: 0171-379-0705

Australia

Acupuncture Centre
173 Boundary St.
West end
QLD 4101
phone: (07) 844-2217

Chinese and Herbal Centre of Sydney
1st floor
392-394 Sussex St.
Sydney
NSW 2000
phone: (02) 261-8863

New Zealand

Chen's Traditional Chinese Herbal Medicine Ltd.
107 St. Lukes Rd
Mt. Albert
Auckland
phone: (09) 849-8239

Dragonspace
11 Mt. Eden Road
Mt. Eden
Auckland
phone: (09) 357-0753

Jamu Herbs
Shop 90
Oriental Markets
Birtomart Place
Auckland
phone: (09) 480-1709

CHINESE HERBS ON THE INTERNET

Planetherbs Online
Order Chinese herbs, formulas, extracts, and planetary formulas on the Internet.
http://supplies.planetherbs.com

CHINESE HERBAL PUBLICATIONS

North American Journal of Oriental Medicine (NAJOM)
896 West King Edward Ave.
Vancouver, B.C., Canada V5Z 2E1
phone: (604) 874-8537; fax: (604) 874-8635

The Journal of Chinese Medicine
22 Cromwell Road
Hove, Sussex BN3 #EB, England

Oriental Medicine Journal
James Ramholz
112 E. Laurel
Fort Collins, CO 80524
phone: (970) 482-5900; fax: (970) 482-4681

WESTERN HERBAL PUBLICATIONS

Australian Journal of Medical Herbalism: Quarterly publication of the National Herbalists Association of Australia (founded in 1920). Deals with all aspects of Medical Herbalism, including latest medicinal plant research findings.
National Herbalists Association of Australia, Suite 305, 3 Smail St., Broadway, NSW 2007, Australia

Canadian Journal of Herbalism: Quarterly journal of the Ontario Herbalists Association. 11 Winthrop Place, Stoney Creek, Ont L8G 3M3

HerbalGram: Quarterly journal published by the American Botanical Council and the Herb Research foundation. P.O. Box 201660, Austin, TX 78720; phone: (800) 373-7105; fax: (512) 331-1924

Medical Herbalism: A Clinical Newsletter for the Herbal Practitioner. Edited by Paul Bergner. P.O. Box 20512, Boulder, CO 80308.
Internet: http://www.medherb.com

HERBAL AND CHINESE ORGANIZATIONS AND GOVERNING BODIES

United States

American Association of Acupuncture and Oriental Medicine
(also National Commission for the Certification of Acupuncturists
c/o National Acupuncture Headquarters)
1424 16 St. NW, Suite 501
Washington DC 20036
phone: (202) 332-5794
Contact this organization for schools, certified Chinese acupuncturists and herbalists in your area.

United Kingdom

British Herbal Medicine Association
PO Box 304
Bournemouth BH7 6JZ
phone: 01202-433691

Council for Acupuncture
179 Gloucester Place
London NW1 6DX
phone: 0171-724-5330

London School of Acupuncture and Traditional Chinese Medicine
60 Bunhill Row
London EC1Y 8QD
phone: 0171-490-0513

Australia

Acupuncture Ethics and Standards Organization
PO Box 84
Merrylands
NSW 2160

Australian College of Oriental Medicine
24 Price Road
Lalorama
VIC 3766
phone: (03) 728-4073

CORRESPONDENCE COURSE

East West Herb Course
P.O. Box 712
Santa Cruz, CA 95061
phone: (800) 717-5010; fax: (408) 336-5010
Internet: http://www.planetherbs.com

Three comprehensive home-study courses in Chinese and Western herbalism are available by correspondence for beginners through professionals. Study in your own home at your own pace either the Introduction to East West Herbalism Course, the Home-Study Course in Herbal Medicine, or the comprehensive Professional Herbalist Course.

The Introduction to East West Herbalism Course is especially designed for the beginning herbal student. It encompasses seven lessons covering specific remedies for different conditions, herbal therapeutics, the use of food and herbs in health and healing, and the foundations of planetary herbal theory. Included are two books and a videotape.

The Home Study Course in Herbal Medicine is suitable for the beginning student interested in herbal medicine, those pursuing a theoretical basis in the principles of Oriental medicine and food therapy, and those who sell, grow, or manufacture herbal and health products. This course includes 12 lessons and presents the essential principles of herbs, including diet, energies, tastes, and the elements of disease and diagnosis for the application of herbs encompassing the Western, Ayurvedic, and Chinese medical systems. Herbal preparations, therapeutics, and formulary are included. This course lays the groundwork for completing the Professional Herbalist Course.

The Professional Herbalist Course is for the herbal professional or those seeking more in-depth knowledge of herbs and the practice of planetary herbology. It includes more advanced studies in the Oriental systems of diagnosis and treatment. Taking the Home-Study Course in Herbal Medicine is a suggested prerequisite. This course follows three stages. The first twelve lessons incorporate the Home-Study Course in Herbal Medicine. The next section covers an extensive and comprehensive materia medica, including herbs and medicines from around the world. The third section emphasizes clinical diagnosis of specific diseases and the maintenance of health. It then brings together all the knowledge of the previous lessons to enable you to practice as a competent herbal consultant. On completion of the Professional Herbalist Course, you will have the option of taking a final examination. Its successful completion will entitle you to a certificate in herbal studies demonstrating completion of studies with Dr. Michael Tierra, master herbalist, C.A., O.M.D.

All of these courses are an integration of Western, Chinese, and Ayurvedic herbal medicine and come with projects and lesson tests that are individually evaluated. Optional study materials are available, including audio and video cassettes.

East West Course in the U.K.
The East West Course is also offered as a full professional training and home study course in the U.K. For information, contact:
David and Sara Holland
Hartswood Marsh Green
Hartfield, E. Sussex, U.K.
TN7 4ET
phone: (011-44-1) 342-826-347; fax: (011-44-1) 342-822-312

CHINESE MEDICAL SUPPLIES (Moxibustion, Cups, Dermal Hammers, Magnets)

Oriental Medical Supplies
1950 Washington Street
Braintree, MA 02184
phone: (800) 323-1839

PLANETARY FORMULAS

Planetary Formulas are an herbal product line created by Dr. Michael Tierra over years of clinical experience. They are composed of Chinese, Western, and Ayurvedic herbs in tablet, liquid extract, or syrup form and can be used to treat a large variety of ailments and meet a great many health needs. Many are traditional

Chinese or Ayurvedic formulas, while others are single Chinese or Western herbs. These formulas may be found in most herbal retail stores under the label Planetary Formulas or they can be ordered online at http://www.supplies.planetherbs.com.

HERBAL ORGANIZATIONS

American Herbalists Guild
P.O. Box 70
Roosevelt, UT 84066
phone: (435) 722-8434

The American Herbalists Guild is a professional body of herbalists dedicated to promoting and maintaining criteria for professional practice of herbalism in North America. There is a student membership available also. The guild encompasses herbalists from all paths: Chinese, Western, naturopathic, folk, Native American, and so on. They hold annual meetings in different parts of the country and publish a beautiful quarterly herbal magazine, *The Herbalist.*

Herb Research Foundation
Rob McCale, Director
P.O. Box 2602
Longmont, CO 80501

HERBAL NURSERIES

Companion Plants
7447 N. Coolville Road
Athens, OH 457901
(614) 593-3092

Elixir Botanicals
General Delivery
Brixey, MO 65618
(417) 261-2393

Horizon Herbs
Williams, OR 97544
(541) 846-6704, Fax (541) 846-6233

Oregon Exotics
1065 Messinger Rd.
Grants Pass, OR 97527
(541) 846-7578

Richter's Nursery

One of the world's finest sources of herb plants and seeds. They ship herb seeds and plants worldwide. Visit and order from them online (www.richters.com). They are located in Ontario, Canada. Ask for a catalogue.

phone: (905) 640-6677; fax: (905) 640-6641

INTERNET HOME PAGE
http://www.planetherbs.com

This is the official web site for Dr. Michael Tierra, including the East West Herb Course, seminars, highly informative articles on herbal medicine and related topics, and an herbal forum with ongoing discussion about herbs and natural medicine. In addition, there is a secured online cybermall where you can order the East West herb courses, Planetary Formula herb products, Chinese herbs, Ayurvedic herbs, many of the herbs and formulas described in this book, books on health and healing, and specialty health and healing products.

INDEX